Economics of Healthcare - Studies and Cases

Edited by Aida Isabel Tavares

Published in London, United Kingdom

Economics of Healthcare - Studies and Cases
http://dx.doi.org/10.5772/intechopen.1001683
Edited by Aida Isabel Tavares

Contributors
Abdallah Al Farai, Adil Al Zadjali, Aida Isabel Tavares, Aiga Balode, Avinash Bhandary, Brett Baker, Cláudio Pontes Ferreira, Dominique Hamerlijnck, Ebenezer Toyin Megbowon, Ieva Bikava, Jabulile Makhalima, Janet L. Wale, Júlio Cesar Schweickardt, Katherine V. Reyes, Kawtar Zahidi, Kiera Lander, Majdouline Obtel, Maria C. G. Bautista, Maria E. C. Yap, Mohammad Al Farei, Oladipo Olalekan David, Rafael Deo F. Estanislao, Reičela Heinrihsone, Rodrigo Tobias, Saida Naji, Samson Agbo, Venus O. C. Rosales

First published in London, United Kingdom, 2026 by IntechOpen
IntechOpen is the global imprint of INTECHOPEN LIMITED, registered in England and Wales, registration number: 11086078, 167-169 Great Portland Street, London, W1W 5PF, United Kingdom

For EU product safety concerns: IN TECH d.o.o., Prolaz Marije Krucifikse Kozulić 3, 51000 Rijeka, Croatia, info@intechopen.com or visit our website at intechopen.com.

British Library Cataloguing-in-Publication Data
A catalogue record for this book is available from the British Library

Economics of Healthcare - Studies and Cases
Edited by Aida Isabel Tavares
p. cm.
Print ISBN 978-1-80632-210-7
Online ISBN 978-0-85014-890-9
eBook (PDF) ISBN 978-0-85014-892-3

Meet the editor

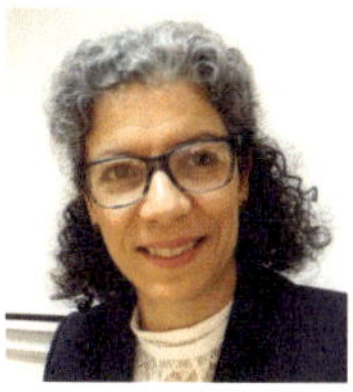

Aida Isabel Tavares holds a Ph.D. in Economic Analysis and a Ph.D. in Management - Science Applied to Decision Making. Her research areas include health economics and policy, health systems, socioeconomic determinants of health, and regulation in health markets. She has taught courses on microeconomics, public economics, and health economics. Currently, she is an Associate Professor at the Lisbon School of Economics and Management, University of Lisbon, and a researcher at the Centre of Studies and Research in Health, University of Coimbra, Portugal

Contents

Preface

In the intricate landscape of healthcare, economics serves as a vital lens through which we can analyse and comprehend the allocation of resources, the efficiency of service delivery, and the equity of health outcomes. This book, *Economics of Healthcare – Studies and Cases*, explores the complex interplay between health economics and healthcare practices, offering insights through detailed studies and real-world cases.

The design and implementation of health policies for healthcare service provision require decisions grounded in well-founded evidence. Evidence-based policymaking ensures that health interventions are effective, that resources are utilised efficiently, and that distribution is equitable. However, challenges such as limited funding, political influences, and varying stakeholder interests can hinder the development and execution of sound health policies [1–3].

Enhancing our understanding of the interactions among all components of the health system and integrating these insights with health economics and policies may pave the way for more equitable, sustainable, and resilient health systems, leading to better population health outcomes. This involves analysing factors such as the socioeconomic determinants of health, technological advancements, and the roles of various stakeholders in the health system. By adopting a comprehensive approach, policymakers can design interventions that address the root causes of health disparities and promote overall system efficiency [4, 5].

In the chapters that follow, we will explore various case studies and analyses that illustrate the application of economic principles in healthcare settings. These examples will highlight successes and challenges across different contexts, providing valuable lessons for policymakers, practitioners, and scholars interested in the economics of healthcare.

Book Content and Planning

This book is organized into two sections, each comprising different types of chapters. The first section includes original research studies, while the second section comprises perspective chapters.

The first section of the book includes three original research papers exploring the demand side of healthcare. Chapter 1, "Household Head Smoking Behavior and Household Food Insecurity in South Africa: Evidence from the National Income Dynamics Study Survey", examines how household head smoking behavior affects household food security. The analysis reveals that households with a smoking head of household experience lower food insecurity than those led by nonsmokers. Likewise, food insecurity is less prevalent in households where the head either started or continued smoking compared to those where the head remained or became a non-smoker. The demand for maternal and family planning services among beneficiaries of a cash transfer program in the Philippines is analyzed in Chapter 2, "Demand Side Predictors of the Demand and Utilization of Maternal and Family Planning Services of the Philippines' Conditional Cash Transfer Program: A Quantitative Approach". The empirical findings of this study indicate that higher program payments slightly reduce the odds of pregnancy. At the same time, factors like more children, high-mortality regions, teenage children, distance from health centers, early marriage, and low education increase them. Non-facility births are more common in remote, high-mortality areas. Antenatal visits are more frequent among those with teenage children, but decline with longer marriage duration.

Chapter 3, entitled "Who Receives the Flu Vaccine and Where? Influenza Vaccination Uptake among Europeans Aged 50+ in Bismarck-Type Health Systems", provides evidence about the motivators and barriers to flu or influenza vaccination uptake in European Bismarck-type health systems. Evidence from this analysis shows that individual characteristics influence flu vaccination decisions, though self-assessed health does not follow a linear pattern. Countries with higher health expenditure as a share of GDP have higher vaccination rates. Trust in science promotes flu vaccine uptake, while trust in government has the opposite effect, with stronger scientific trust in Western than Eastern countries. In Western countries, flu vaccination rates are inversely related to future COVID-19 vaccine coverage. The last chapter of this section, Chapter 4, "Costs of Primary Health Care in a Riverside and Rural Context of the Brazilian Amazon", estimates the costs of providing healthcare in extreme and remote areas of Brazil. The analysis focuses on the costs associated with the Basic Fluvial Health Unit used in Tefé, Amazonas State. It concludes that this approach requires significant resources but notes the need to proceed with a cost-effectiveness analysis.

The second section contains three main groups of chapters exploring different thematic areas such as healthcare funding and expenditures, the provision and supply of healthcare, and the demand side of the healthcare system.

Under the topic of healthcare funding and expenditures, Chapter 5, "Perspective Chapter: Improving Health Budgeting and Management Practices in Low Middle Income Countries (LMIC): Using 3 Country Case Studies—Nigeria, Kenya and Tanzania", argues in favor of program-based budgeting reforms to enhance spending alignment with health priorities, improve flexibility in fund usage, and increase transparency, which sustains the path toward universal health coverage. This chapter assesses the effectiveness of budgeting tools and guidelines from international organizations such as the World Bank and WHO, and concludes that they fall short in driving national progress. It also explores the advantages and limitations of budget reforms, including Public Expenditure Reviews and Medium-Term Expenditure Frameworks, highlighting the need for participatory and transparent processes. Additionally, it identifies political interference as a major obstacle to aligning health policies with resource allocation.

Chapter 6, "Perspective Chapter: Healthcare Economics in the Wake of Trauma – Navigating Costs and Care for the Injured" explores the relationship between healthcare economics and the management of traumatic injuries. It also discusses how these types of injuries may be covered by healthcare financing and policy. The work explores the continuum of post-injury care, from emergency medical treatment to long-term rehabilitation, with a focus on the economic implications at each stage. It also examines the wider effects of traumatic injuries on healthcare financing and policy, offering a comprehensive analysis of the financial impact on both individuals and the healthcare system. Then, Chapter 7, entitled “Perspective Chapter: Shifting toward Value-Based Healthcare – Lessons Learned in the Context of Breast Cancer Treatment”, evaluates the implementation of a value-based healthcare model in Latvia, widely regarded as the optimal strategy for delivering effective, efficient, high-quality, patient-centered healthcare services. This chapter examines the implementation of a value-based healthcare model that considers the optimal approach to effective, high-quality, patient-centered care. It reviews value-based healthcare theory, lessons from global applications, and challenges its adoption for breast cancer treatment in Latvia, highlighting the shift from a pay-for-service model to integrated care.

Concerning the provision of healthcare, a debate on South African healthcare policy is described in Chapter 8, “Perspective Chapter: Unravelling the Policy Paradox – A Critical Examination of Post-Apartheid South Africa’s Healthcare Development in the Context of Developmental State Goals”. The identified inequalities in health outcomes seem to be a legacy of the Apartheid regime, and the African National Congress has been unsuccessful in eliminating these traces within the healthcare system. Although South Africa’s healthcare policy appears committed to developmental goals, other policies undermine its impact by reinforcing disparities across geographic, sectoral, and racial lines. Issues such as cadre deployment and inconsistent policymaking weaken governance and hinder progress toward equitable health outcomes. The following Chapter 9 focuses on the supply of surgeries. This chapter, entitled “Perspective Chapter: Open versus Minimally Invasive Surgery Accessibility in Different Economic Level Countries”, explores disparities in the accessibility of minimally invasive surgery across countries with varying economic levels, highlighting significant differences in healthcare infrastructure, physical and human resources, and professional training. In low- and middle-income countries, limited adoption of MIS is due to challenges such as high costs, lack of specialized training, and restricted access to advanced equipment. As a result, open surgeries remain more common, particularly in public healthcare and rural areas. This chapter explores disparities in access to minimally invasive surgery, emphasizing differences in healthcare infrastructure, resources, and training, as well as global efforts to address these gaps.

Lastly, from a demand perspective and health system users, Chapter 10, “Perspective Chapter: Patient Advocacy - From a Seat at the Table to Equal Stakeholders”, suggests how patient advocacy may evolve and become more integrated into the medical product lifecycle, given the increasing intensity of innovation in healthcare products. Delays in accessing innovative, life-saving treatments remain a critical issue. This chapter explores three key pathways: i) patient involvement in the medical product lifecycle and clinical trial regulation, with a focus on the biopharmaceutical industry; ii) the role of evidence-based practice, patient-reported outcomes, and regulatory efforts to accelerate access; and iii) the evolving impact of patient advocacy, illustrated through EU public-private research funding. A different concern is described in Chapter 11, “Perspective Chapter: Sedentary Behaviors – Implications for the Future of Health”. This chapter addresses how sedentary behavior influences chronic disease risk and associated economic costs, and reviews future directions in the interaction between physical activity and health. The health risks of prolonged sedentary behavior are increasingly recognized as technology use for (tele-)work and leisure increases global screen time. Future perspectives on the relationship between physical activity and sedentary behavior are discussed. Finally, Chapter 12, "Healthcare Accessibility: Metrics, Assessment, Policies, and Barriers", examines the concept of healthcare accessibility and presents several measures, highlighting their advantages and disadvantages, in the path toward a more equitable healthcare system. A thorough assessment of these metrics highlights the potential for effectiveness and identifies areas for improvement.

In conclusion, this book endeavors to provide a comprehensive understanding of the complex relationships within healthcare systems. By examining a range of case studies and research, we aim to highlight not only the challenges healthcare systems face but also the innovative solutions and policy frameworks that can drive improvements in efficiency, equity, and access, as established in the Sustainable Development Goals [6, 7]. The diverse chapters explore critical issues from both theoretical and empirical perspectives, offering valuable insights for policymakers, practitioners, and researchers. Ultimately, the goal is to equip readers with the tools and knowledge to navigate the evolving healthcare landscape better, fostering a deeper understanding of how economic principles can help build more resilient and sustainable health systems.

Aida Isabel Tavares
ISEG, Lisbon School of Economics and Management,
CEISUC, Centre of Studies and Research in Health of the University of Coimbra,
Lisbon, Portugal

References

[1] Bullock, H.L., Lavis, J.N., Wilson, M.G. et al. Understanding the implementation of evidence-informed policies and practices from a policy perspective: a critical interpretive synthesis. *Implementation Sci* 16, 18 (2021). https://doi.org/10.1186/s13012-021-01082-7

[2] Hayman DTS, Barraclough RK, Muglia LJ, et al. Addressing the challenges of implementing evidence-based prioritisation in global health. *BMJ Glob Health*. 2023;8(6):e012450. https://doi.org/10.1136/bmjgh-2023-012450

[3] Freund, M., Zucca, A., Sanson-Fisher, R. et al. Barriers to the evaluation of evidence-based public health policy. *J Public Health Pol* 40, 114–125 (2019). https://doi.org/10.1057/s41271-018-0145-9

[4] Lavizzo-Mourey, R., Besser, R.E., & Williams, D. (2021). Understanding and Mitigating Health Inequities - Past, Current, and Future Directions. *The New England journal of medicine*, 384 18, 1681-1684. https://doi.org/10.1056/NEJMp2008628

[5] Al Meslamani, A. Z. (2024). Challenges in health economics research: insights from real-world examples. *Journal of Medical Economics*, 27(1), 215–218. https://doi.org/10.1080/13696998.2024.2310466

[6] Debie, A., Khatri, R.B. & Assefa, Y. Successes and challenges of health systems governance towards universal health coverage and global health security: a narrative review and synthesis of the literature. *Health Res Policy Sys* 20, 50 (2022)

[7] Kosiol, J., Silvester, T., Cooper, H. et al. Revolutionising health and social care: innovative solutions for a brighter tomorrow – a systematic review of the literature. *BMC Health Serv Res* 24, 809 (2024). https://doi.org/10.1186/s12913-024-11099-5

Section 1

Research Chapters

Chapter 1

Household Head Smoking Behavior and Household Food Insecurity in South Africa: Evidence from National Income Dynamics Study Survey

Ebenezer Toyin Megbowon, Oladipo Olalekan David and Jabulile Makhalima

Abstract

This study examines how the smoking behavior of household head impacts the food insecurity status of household in South Africa, with a focus on smoking behavior transition. The study used the fifth wave of the 2017 National Income Dynamics Study survey. Additionally, the smoking transition variable was computed using smoking status in waves 3 and 5 of the survey. Foster-Greer-Thorbecke food insecurity index, descriptive statistics, and logit regression techniques were deployed in the study. Surprisingly, the analysis shows that households headed by current smokers have a lower prevalence of food insecurity (compared to households whose heads are non-smokers). Similarly, household food insecurity prevalence is lesser for homes whose head initiated smoking behavior or remained a smoker compared to those whose head remained a nonsmoker or transition to nonsmoking. Nevertheless, the findings from the applied logit regression suggested that household food insecurity significantly increases when a household head is a current smoker and a consistent smoker. The finding indicates that household head smoking behavior does contribute to household food insecurity in South Africa. The need to address food insecurity at the household level is a compelling argument for tobacco smoking cessation or control in addition to health consequence concerns.

Keywords: Foster-Greer-Thorbecke index, household food insecurity, smoking behavior, smoking behavior transition, logistic regression, South Africa

1. Introduction

The importance of food for people justifies the inclusion of food security and the necessitation of the pursuit of same as a development outcome by governments of various countries and several development partners. It is known that food alongside clothing and shelter are the three basic needs of mankind [1–3]. Food plays an essential role in human sustenance and survival [4]. It is needed to build, rejuvenate, and where necessary replace worn-out body cells and tissues, to produce needed energy for warmth and physical activities and to promote the prevention of diseases, support the recovery from sickness, and aid good health in general [5, 6]. According to FAO [7], food security is the state in which everyone consistently has the means to access enough safe and nutritious food to meet their dietary requirements and preferences, ensuring a hale, hearty, and healthful life. Without a doubt, the absence of hunger and availability and at least ease of accessing nutritionally adequate, acceptable, and safe foods without theft, scavenging, use of coping strategies, or depending on crisis-related food supplies are the several dynamic reflections of a food secure situation.

Statistics from FAO et al. [8] shows that 830.2 million people (i.e., about 10.7% of the world population) experienced severe level of food insecurity between 2019 and 2021. The number of persons that were moderately as well as severely food insecure rose from about 1609.1 million people between 2014 and 2016 to about 2187.4 people between 2019 and 2021. This number also varies by region with Asia (1109.5 million) and Africa (743.5 million) accounting for the largest proportion in 2020. In South Africa, various statistical reports have provided evidence of the reality of food insecurity in the country. For instance, FAO et al. [8] reported that about 6.9% of the South African population are considered undernourished between 2019 and 2021. Likewise, the occurrence of moderate or chronic food insecurity within the entire population is 19%. Equally, with a Global Index score of 12.9 in 2022, South Africa was ranked to be having moderate hunger severity [9]. According to Statistics South Africa (Stat SA) [10], the proportion of the population who were classified as severely and moderately food insecure were estimated at 17.3% (i.e., 10.1 million South Africans) in South Africa in 2019. These international and national statistics underscore the undeniability of the reality of food insecurity in the country and justify the inclusion of food insecurity goal in the sustainable development agenda 2030. It is therefore a priority to conduct studies that identify the factors that determine household food insecurity. An important instrument to consider is one related to lifestyle risk factors.

Smoking as an unhealthy behavior or lifestyle is one of the identified direct or indirect contributors to food insecurity. Conceptually, tobacco smoking is linked with household food stock, food access, and utilization through crowding out of food expenditure, unequal spending of household income on cigarettes, and financial strain. Furthermore, the contribution of smoking to depreciated health leads to limited labor force participation, lowering of productivity at work due to ill health, and reduction of wage income, which eventually inhibits the affordability and availability of needed quality and quantity of food at the household and individual levels, [11]. WHO [12] estimated that about 1.3 billion persons are estimated to be users of tobacco products, out of which 80% live in countries that are categorized as middle- and low-income. According to Global Adult Tobacco Survey (GATS) [13], 12.7 million South African adults (i.e., 29.4% of adult population) are current users of both smoked and smokeless tobacco product. Of these statistics, 41.7% are men, while 17.9% are women. GATS [13] also reported that the median monthly expenditure on manufactured cigarettes was R263 (US$ 17.79).[1] Apparently, this smoking behavior

[1] Exchange Rate in 2021: US$ 1 = Rands 14.78

prevalence raises concern of it being a potential inhibitor of the achievement of household food security in South Africa. Therefore, given that food insecurity and smoking are prevalent in South Africa, this study's objective is to empirically investigate if and to what extent smoking behavior of household head can predict household food insecurity. The objective takes the current smoking status and smoking behavior transition patterns into consideration. The other sections of the article are organized as follows. Sections 2 and 3 provide a brief review of related previous works and methodology, respectively. Section 4 reports the outcome, discussion, and inferences regarding the analyses that were conducted. Conclusion and suggested policy directions are presented lastly in Section 5.

2. Brief literature review: empirics

Empirically, studies that have incorporated smoking behavior as an independent variable while investigating household food insecurity are very few. Moreover, available evidence on the relationships between the two issues from the literature is mixed. For example, Kang and Cho [14] demonstrated that individuals who had ever used any tobacco products, whether current or former users, had increased odds of experiencing food insecurity in comparison to those who had never used any tobacco products. Likewise, the findings from different studies [15–23] are consistent with Kang and Cho [14] in terms of association between smoking behavior and food security. Regarding health behavior transition, only Berry et al. [24] have investigated the impact of smoking transition on food security. Evidence from the modified Poisson regression utilized by the study showed that compared to those who have smoked and recently quit smoking, those who maintain smoking habit have increased risk (that is about twice as much of recent quitters) of household food insecurity.

In South Africa, a set of different research articles [25–35] have identified several demographic and socioeconomic factors (such as household head characteristics [gender, age, relationship or marital status, status in the labor market, education], number of household members, total income and income category of the household, geographical location or place of residence) that influence well-being in terms of food security. However, the potential link between health behavior and food insecurity have been unaccounted for in these studies, and it is observed as a gap in the literature in the case of South Africa. Specifically, the quantification of smoking behavior to welfare (food insecurity) impacts has been overlooked.

3. Research and methodology

3.1 Data

The study is a quantitative study that utilizes a cross-sectional research design. It uses the fifth wave of the 2017 National Income Dynamics Study (NIDS) survey, which was accessed and acquired through [36, 37] website. NIDS is a panel survey of individuals and households that reside in South Africa, conducted every 2 years from 2008 to 2017 [36, 37]. NIDS provided information on demographic and socioeconomic characteristics of individual and household including gender, level of education attained, food security, health behavior, and household size [38]. This study uses information of household heads and households from the round 5 of NIDS survey that was conducted in 2017/2018. The fifth wave of the NIDS survey was used because it is the most recent data available in South Africa that captures the key variables of interest. Furthermore, to construct a transition matrix of the targeted variable, NIDS wave 3 survey data of the targeted variable was included. The selection criteria used in this study are household heads and households in wave 5 [36, 37] whose heads were interviewed in wave 3 [36, 37] of the NIDS surveys. Consequently, a sample of 7676 households was used in this study. A detailed narrative of the dataset that was used in this article is obtainable at www.nids.uct.ac.za.

3.2 Analytical techniques

3.2.1 Foster-Greer and Thorbecke food insecurity (FGT-FI) index

FGT-FI index was used in profiling household food insecurity in this study. The FGT-FI index was adapted from Foster et al. [39], an index that is primarily used in the computation of the incidence, depth, and severity of poverty but has been extended to profile food insecurity situation in geographical areas (see [4, 40, 41]). The original FGT index is a generalized poverty index that utilizes a poverty threshold and considers the inequality among the poor (or food insecure) and allows one to vary the amount of weight on income (or expenditure) levels when analyzing poverty situation [42]. As a decomposable measure of poverty, FGT index links overall poverty with the poverty levels in population subgroups. In the context of this study, household food (in) security threshold was based on the two-thirds of the mean per capita household food expenditure (MPCHFE) [4, 40, 41]. Households whose MPCHFE is below the food security threshold were categorized as food insecure, while those whose MPCHFE is above the food security line were considered as food secure households. FGT-FI index for this study is represented by the following Eq. (1):

$$\mathrm{FGT}-\mathrm{FI}\,\alpha=\frac{\mathbf{1}}{\boldsymbol{N}}\sum_{i=1}^{q}\left(\frac{\boldsymbol{z}-\boldsymbol{y}_i}{\boldsymbol{z}}\right)^{\alpha} \tag{1}$$

where N = total households' number under consideration, z = food security line, q = number of households under the food security threshold, $\boldsymbol{y}_i$ = per capita monthly food expenditure of the *ith* household, and $\boldsymbol{z}-\boldsymbol{y}_i$ is the food expenditure shortfall of the *ith* household. The FGT-FI measure "α" take the values of 0,1,2, representing food insecurity headcount, food insecurity depth, and food insecurity severity, respectively.

3.2.2 Logit regression

The study used binary logistic regression in estimating the relationship between the variables of interest. Logit regression estimation technique was used because the dependent variable has a binary outcome. To avoid bias related to bivariate modeling, other possible determinants of household food insecurity were included as control variables in the model. Hence, the specification of binary logistic regression model for this study is stated in Eq. (2):

$$\boldsymbol{FI}_i=\varnothing_0+\varnothing_1\boldsymbol{SB}_1+\sum\varnothing_i\boldsymbol{X}_i+\boldsymbol{e}_t \tag{2}$$

Variable	Level	Measurement	Reference
Dependent Variable			
FI	Food Insecurity Status	1 if Food Insecure; 0 otherwise	
	Independent Variables		
SB	a) Current Smoking Status	1 if a current smoker; 0 otherwise	Amrullah et al. [17]
	b) Smoking Transition Pattern (S)	1 if $S_{(0,0)}$ = Not a smoker in both 2012 and 2017; 0 otherwise 1 if $S_{(0,1)}$ = Not a smoker in 2012 but a smoker in 2017; 0 otherwise 1 if $S_{(1,0)}$ = Was a smoker in 2012 but not a smoker in 2017; 0 otherwise 1 if $S_{(1,1)}$ = Was a smoker in both 2012 and 2017; 0 otherwise	[14, 24]
X_1	Gender of head	1 if male, 0 otherwise	
X_2	Age of head	Age of household head	Azwardi et al. [43]
X_3	Marital Status of Head	1 if married, 0 otherwise	
X_4	Education of Head	1 if No education, 0 Otherwise 1 if Primary, 0 Otherwise 1 if Secondary, 0 Otherwise 1 if Matric, 0 Otherwise 1 if Certificate and diploma, 0 Otherwise 1 if higher degree, 0 Otherwise	[44, 45]
X_5	Employment Status	1 if employed, 0 otherwise	[45, 46]
X_6	Household Size	Number of people in the household	[47, 48]
X_7	Health Insurance Coverage	1 if yes, 0 otherwise	[21, 49]
X_8	Household Income Quantile	1 if Quantile 1, 0 Otherwise 1 if Quantile 2, 0 Otherwise 1 if Quantile 3, 0 Otherwise 1 if Quantile 4, 0 Otherwise	[18, 21]
X_9	Population Group	1 if African, 0 Otherwise	Jonah and May [29]
X_{10}	Place of Residence	1 if Urban, 0 Otherwise	[17, 50]
X_{11}	Province	1 if WC, 0 Otherwise 1 if EC, 0 Otherwise 1 if NC, 0 Otherwise 1 if FS, 0 Otherwise 1 if KZN, 0 Otherwise 1 if NW, 0 Otherwise 1 if G, 0 Otherwise 1 if Mp, 0 Otherwise 1 if L, 0 Otherwise	

Note 1: $S_{(0,0)}$ = not a smoker in both 2012 and 2017, 0 otherwise (consistent nonsmoker); $S_{(0,1)}$ = not a smoker in 2012 but a smoker in 2017, 0 otherwise (initiate); $S_{(1,0)}$ = was a smoker in 2012 but not a smoker in 2017, 0 otherwise (quitters); $S_{(1,1)}$ = was a smoker in both 2012 and 2017, 0 otherwise (consistent smoker).
Note 2: WC, EC, NC, FS, KZN, NW, G, Mp, and L stand for Western cape, eastern cape, northern cape, Free State, KwaZulu Natal, north-west, Gauteng, Mpumalanga, and Limpopo, respectively.

Table 1.
Summary description of variables in the model.

where the dependent variable *FI* is household food insecurity status, $_0$ = the constant term, SB represents household head smoking behavior (captured by both current smoking status and smoking transition pattern "S"), $_1$ = the vector of coefficients, $\boldsymbol{X_i}$ =vector of explanatory variables, and $\boldsymbol{e_t}$ is the error term.

All the analyses in this study were conducted using STATA 15 software. **Table 1** presents the description of the variables in the model, both the dependent variable and the independent variables.

4. Results and discussion

4.1 Analysis of household food insecurity

4.1.1 FGT-FI index

As earlier mentioned, it is needed to determine the MPCHFE and the 2/3 of MPCHFE when profiling household food security. In this study, the computed MPCHFE is R498.61 (US$ 37.69) as shown in the **Table 2**. Also, the calculated 2/3 of MPCHFE, which is the food insecurity (FI) threshold used in this study, is R332.41 (US$ 25.13). The result of the FGT-FI index analysis that was used to assess the food insecurity situation in the study area is presented in **Table 2**. The food insecurity index analysis indicated that household food insecurity incidence and gap were 66.1 and 30%, respectively. The results imply that 66.1% of the households can be categorized as food insecure and that for food-insecure households to be food-secure, they will need to increase their current food spending by about 30%.

4.1.2 Distribution of food insecurity indices based on household head smoking behavior

In line with evidence from literature suggesting that socioeconomic features of the head of a household influence the well-being of households [51, 52], the disaggregation of the FGT-FI index by the smoking status of household head and household's and household head's socioeconomic and demographic characteristics are analyzed, and they are presented in **Table 3**.

It needs to be known that this profiling does not imply a cause or effect between variables of interest. **Table 3** reveals that in terms of smoking status, the reported food insecurity incidence of 58.4% is lower among households whose heads have a current

FGT Food insecurity (FGT-FI) indices	Value
FGT-FI_0 (incidence of food insecurity)	0.661
FGT-FI_1 (depth of food insecurity)	0.303
FGT-FI_2 (severity of food insecurity)	0.170
MPCHFE	R498.61 (US$ 37.69)*
Food insecurity (FI) Threshold (i.e., 2/3 of MPCHFE)	R332.41 (US$ 25.13)*

Note: "R" means Rand.
Exchange Rate in 2018: US$ 1 = Rands 13.23.
Source: Computed by Author.

Table 2.
FGT-FI index on extent of household food insecurity.

Variable	Level	Food Insecurity Indices		
		FGT-FI_0	FGT-FI_1	FGT-FI_2
SB: Current Smoking Status	No	0.676	0.311	0.173
	Yes	0.584	0.267	0.154
SB: Smoking Transition	$S_{(0,0)}$	0.677	0.311	0.173
	$S_{(0,1)}$	0.576	0.270	0.159
	$S_{(1,0)}$	0.666	0.296	0.163
	$S_{(1,1)}$	0.589	0.265	0.151

Table 3.
Decomposition of FGT-FI indices by household head smoking behavior.

smoking status than the 67.6% found among households whose heads do not smoke currently. Also, the proportion of food expenditure required to lift food insecure households whose head does not smoke currently out of food insecurity situation is higher at 31% than that of their counterpart that requires only a 22% increase in food expenditure. It is surprising to observe that households whose heads maintained a nonsmoking behavior status or transitioned out of smoking had a higher food insecurity incidence compared to those whose heads initiated a smoking behavior or remained a smoker.

4.1.3 Distribution of food insecurity indices based on households' socioeconomic and demographic characteristics

Table 4 shows that households headed by a female had a higher food insecurity incidence at 73% compared to male-headed households (53%). Also, the proportion of

Variable	Level	Food Insecurity Indices		
		FGT-FI_0	FGT-FI_1	FGT-FI_2
Gender	Female	0.730	0.344	0.195
	Male	0.533	0.228	0.124
Age of Head (Year)	22–34 years	0.522	0.224	0.120
	35–64 years	0.675	0.312	0.176
	> 64 years	0.748	0.351	0.197
Marital Status	Married	0.618	0.267	0.146
	Otherwise	0.688	0.325	0.184
Education Attainment	No Schooling	0.851	0.431	0.254
	Primary	0.802	0.391	0.226
	Secondary	0.652	0.285	0.154
	Matric	0.447	0.170	0.085
	Certificate and Diploma	0.426	0.164	0.085
	Degree	0.199	0.061	0.024
Place of Residence	Rural	0.774	0.369	0.210

Variable	Level	Food Insecurity Indices		
		FGT-FI_0	FGT-FI_1	FGT-FI_2
	Urban	0.544	0.235	0.128
Province	WC	0.473	0.185	0.098
	EC	0.705	0.323	0.181
	NC	0.589	0.272	0.157
	FS	0.607	0.266	0.142
	KZN	0.775	0.369	0.209
	NW	0.679	0.352	0.211
	Gauteng	0.492	0.204	0.109
	Mpumalanga	0.685	0.294	0.155
	Limpopo	0.722	0.345	0.198
Population Group	African	0.704	0.327	0.184
	Non-African	0.446	0.183	0.099
Health Insurance Coverage	No	0.700	0.325	0.183
	Yes	0.254	0.087	0.032
Employment Status	No	0.759	0.365	0.209
	Yes	0.254	0.221	0.117
Household Size	1–5	0.479	0.177	0.086
	6–10	0.857	0.425	0.245
	>10	0.987	0.589	0.384
Household Income Group	Quartile 1	0.742	0.363	0.211
	Quartile 2	0.721	0.340	0.192
	Quartile 3	0.705	0.328	0.185
	Quartile 4	0.520	0.212	0.111

Source: Computed by Author.

Table 4.
Decomposition of FGT-FI indices by household socioeconomic and demographic characteristics.

food expenditure required to lift female-headed food insecure households out of the food insecurity situation is higher at 34% than that of male-headed households that require only a 23% increase in food expenditure. As seen in **Table 3**, the incidence of food insecurity increased with the age of the household head. It was highest (75%) for households headed by persons of 61 years and greater. Food insecurity depth and severity were highest at 35.1 and 19.7%, respectively, among households headed by individuals greater than 60 years in age, which corresponds with [4, 53]. Contrarily, households headed by people under the age of 35 years were the least affected by food insecurity.

Table 4 further shows that the prevalence, depth, and inequality of food insecurity are higher for households residing in the Eastern Cape, KwaZulu Natal, and Limpopo provinces; rural areas; and households with a size of more than five. Likewise, in terms of food insecurity depth particularly in household socioeconomic distributions where household food insecurity incidence is prevalent, for a household to be food secure, there is a need for about 33, 43, 37, 35, and 33% raise in their monthly per capita food expenditure for households headed by a person from the African population group, with no or primary education, not employed, and without medical insurance.

4.2 Logit regression result on the impact of household head smoking behavior on household food insecurity

The estimated logit regression function's findings (i.e., estimated coefficients, standard error, and probability values) on the relationship between household head smoking behavior and household food insecurity are shown in **Table 5**. The validity of the estimation results in **Table 5** is supported by the diagnostic Pearson χ-2 goodness-of-fit test that was performed. Fit testing helps determine whether a model fits well and can be accepted or otherwise discarded. A statistically insignificant Pearson χ-2 indicates a well-fit model. In this study, the estimated goodness of fit of the models (model 1: Pearson $\chi2 = 7032.64$, $p = 0.8368$; model 2: Pearson $\chi2 = 7072.56$, $p = 0.8235$) corresponds with the desirable criteria. The validity of the goodness of fit of the models is further buttressed by the Hosmer-Lemeshow [H-L] $\chi2$ (8) results (model 1: H-L $\chi2 = 12.03$, $p = 0.1497$; model 2: H-L $\chi2 = 9.46$, $p = 0.3047$), reported in **Table 5**. Additionally, to further verify that the estimated models were unbiased and consistent, a check for possible problem of multicollinearity among the explanatory variables was performed using the variance inflation factor (VIF). The mean VIF test value of 2.26 and 2.18 obtained for models 1 and 2 is less than 10; therefore, it can be concluded that there is no multicollinearity problem. The results in **Table 5** show that household head smoking behavior, marital status, household size, and household head population group (African) increase the odds of household food insecurity. However, the odds of household food insecurity incidence are decreased by the gender and age of the head, health insurance coverage, income, and living in an urban area, Western Cape, and Gauteng provinces.

First, **Table 5** shows the odds ratio of this study's variable of interest; household head smoking behavior in terms of current status (in column 3) is statistically significant (OR = 1.161; $p < 0.01$). Similarly, the smoking behavior transition (in column 6) is statistically significant for smoking cessation (OR = 1.271; $p < 0.10$) and smoking maintenance (OR = 1.339; $p < 0.01$). These results indicate that the odds of households being food insecure are 1.16, 1.271, and 1.34 times higher when the household head is a smoker, quitted smoking, and has a consistent smoking behavior, respectively. This implies that smoking habit of household heads exerts a significant and increasing influence on the likelihood of household food insecurity. That is, having a head that smokes (especially when such head can be said to be a tobacco-smoking addict [continuous smoker]) increases the probability of a household being food insecure. This finding is consistent with several studies [14, 15, 17–19, 23] that have established an influencing effect of household head smoking behavior on household food security status. As noted earlier in this study, tobacco spending crowds out spendings on food and other necessities. Similarly, possible financial constraints are plausible reasons for the established effect of being a continuous smoker on household food insecurity probability. For the quit smoking result, it can be inferred that when stopping or trying to stop smoking, people may run into problems like nicotine withdrawal or the need for cessation assistance, which can put more financial strain on households. The expenses linked to quitting smoking, such as medication, treatment, or nicotine replacement therapy, could take money away from food purchases, which could worsen food poverty temporarily.

Variable	Level	Model 1 (Current Smoking Only)			Model 2 (Smoking Transition Pattern)		
Column 1	**Column 2**	**Column 3**	**Column 4**	**Column 5**	**Column 6**	**Column 7**	**Column 8**
		Odds Ratio	P > |z|	95% CI	Odds Ratio	P > |z|	[95% CI]
SB: Current Smoking	Yes	1.161	0.061***	0.993 – 1.356	—	—	—
	No (Reference)						
SB: Smoking Transition	$S_{(0,0)}$ (Reference)	—	—	—	—	—	—
	$S_{(0,1)}$	—	—	—	0.985	0.896	0.786–1.235
	$S_{(1,0)}$	—	—	—	1.271	0.093***	0.961 – 1.681
	$S_{(1,1)}$	—	—	—	1.339	0.002*	1.113 – 1.611
Male	Male	0.484	0.000*	0.427 – 0.549	0.472	0.000*	0.415 – 0.537
	Female (Reference)						
Age	Age	0.996	0.094***	0.992 – 1.001	0.996	0.076***	0.992 – 1.000
Marital Status	Marital Status	1.346	0.000*	1.185 – 1.530	1.351	0.000*	1.188 – 1.535
Employed	Employed	0.775	0.000*	0.686 – 0.876	0.778	0.000*	0.689 – 0.880
Health Insurance Coverage	Yes	0.456	0.000*	0.355 – 0.584	0.456	0.000*	0.356 – 0.586
Education Attainment	No Education	Ref					
	Primary	1.009	0.933	0.828–1.229	1.005	0.964	0.824–1.224
	Secondary	0.642	0.000*	0.521 – 0.790	0.644	0.000*	0.523 – 0.793
	Matric	0.384	0.000*	0.297 – 0.498	0.386	0.000*	0.298 – 0.500
	Certificate & Diploma	0.396	0.000*	0.310 – 0.505	0.398	0.000*	0.312 – 0.508
	Degree	0.195	0.000*	0.119 – 0.321	0.197	0.000*	0.119 – 0.324
Household Size	NA	9.259	0.000*	7.844 – 10.929	9.231	0.000*	7.821 – 10.896
Income Quartile	1	Ref.	—		—	—	
	2	0.775	0.001*	0.670 – 0.896	0.777	0.001*	0.672 – 0.896
	3	0.733	0.000*	0.628 – 0.855	0.732	0.000*	0.627 – 0.854
	4	0.442	0.000*	0.364 – 0.538	0.442	0.000*	0.364 – 0.538
Population Group	African	1.588	0.000*	1.294 – 1.949	1.614	0.000*	1.314 – 1.983

Variable	Level	Model 1 (Current Smoking Only)			Model 2 (Smoking Transition Pattern)		
Column 1	Column 2	Column 3	Column 4	Column 5	Column 5	Column 7	Column 8
	Non-African (Reference)						
Place of Residence	Urban	0.836	0.008*	0.732 – 0.955	0.835	0.008*	0.731 – 0.954
	Rural (Reference)						
Province	Western Cape	0.729	0.030**	0.548 – 0.971	0.718	0.023*	0.540 – 0.956
	Eastern Cape	0.897	0.375	0.706–1.140	0.891	0.348	0.701–1.133
	Northern Cape	0.991	0.952	0.7737–1.332	0.991	0.954	0.737–1.333
	Free State	0.950	0.730	0.710–1.272	0.943	0.696	0.705–1.263
	Kwa-Zulu Natal	0.848	0.128	0.686–1.049	0.850	0.133	0.688–1.051
	North-West	0.930	0.612	0.702–1.232	0.932	0.626	0.704–1.236
	Gauteng	0.716	0.009*	0.556 – 0.921	0.716	0.009*	0.556 – 0.921
	Mpumalanga	0.962	0.777	0.734–1.260	0.963	0.787	0.735–1.262
	Limpopo (Reference)	—	—		—	—	
	Constant	0.202	0.000*	0.126 – 0.325	0.201	0.000	0.125–0.323
Number of observations			7676			7676	
LR chi^2 (29)			2622.79			2631.17	
Prob > chi^2			0.0000			0.0000	
Log likelihood			−3991.9815			−3987.7919	
Pearson chi^2			7032.64			7072.56	
Prob > chi^2			0.8368			0.8235	
Hosmer-Lemeshow chi^2(8)			12.03			9.46	
Prob > chi^2			0.1497			0.3047	

Source: Computed by Author.
* = $p < 1\%$. ** = $p < 5\%$. *** = $p < 10\%$.

Table 5.
Impact of household head smoking behavior on household food insecurity: Binary logistic regression.

The results of the regression model reveal that the odds ratio for gender is less than one and statistically significant (OR = 0.484; p < 0.01). This result, which is consistent with [19, 54, 55], implies that odds of household food insecurity are predicted to be about 0.427 to 0.484 times lower for male-headed household than those headed by women, when all other variables are kept constant. A plausible reason for this result that is in favor of men is the difference in economic opportunities and assets (e.g., land and productive economic resources). Gender differences in the type of employment that is in favor of men could translate into differences in income needed to meet household expenditures. In addition, woman-led households are susceptible to food insecurity when the dependency ratio in such households is high [56].

Table 5 shows that household head's age is statistically significant (OR = 0.996; p < 0.10). According to this result, there is a decreasing likelihood of food insecurity in households as household head get older, provided that all other factors remain unchanged. The calculated odds ratio estimates specifically suggest that the probabilities of a home experiencing food insecurity are around 0.996 times lower for every unit or year that the household head's age increases. This aligns with the *a priori* statement of this study and with Azwardi et al. [43], which argued that the maturity of the household heads in terms of age affects psychological and financial stability. In a related perspective, Mthethwa and Wale [44] noted that as people grow older, they accumulate assets, experience, and strategies that could reduce their household vulnerability to food insecurity. According to Megbowon [27], the high possibility of a head in urban areas of securing a job, accumulating income over a long period time, and a robust social security program for older people in the country are plausible reasons for this finding. Also, increase in age, which is related to farming experience for rural farming household heads, leads to more output resulting in better profitability and household food security [54]. This result is however contrary to the perspective that aging of a household head leads to limited participation in economic activities and a decrease in income earning potential, thus increasing household food insecurity tendency.

The odd ratio estimated for the employment status (employed) is statistically significant (OR = 0.778; p < 0.01). This means that the odds of household having a food insecure status are predicted to be about 0.78 times lower among households having employed heads than those whose heads are unemployed. This finding is in line with the theoretical expectation of this study where it was argued that being employed is an indicator of economic empowerment, such that it can inhibit or promote access to needed food nutrients. Having an employed household head enables households to maintain higher levels of expenditure that can aid household welfare. This finding is consistent with the results of other studies [45, 46, 57], who all established that a reduced household food insecure status likelihood is linked with employed status (being employed) of the head is, the greater the chances that his or her household will be less food insecure. While unemployment increases resource and welfare deprivations, economic access to needed food for a household and availability of food would be largely guaranteed when there is a source of income, which comes when there is an economic engagement or labor market participation.

Table 5 also shows that the odds ratio of health insurance coverage is statistically significant (OR = 0.456; p < 0.01). This means that the odds of households being food insecure is 0.46 times lower when the household head is covered by medical insurance compared to those whose head is not covered by any medical insurance. This result is clearly in line with the expectations of this study, and it is also consistent with previous evidence [21, 49, 58]. Indeed, medical aid would enable individuals and households to reallocate income away from medical care, thereby leaving more funds toward food consumption. The odd ratios estimated for the education attainment categories of household head are less than one (i.e., secondary: OR = 0.644; Martic: OR = 0.386; Certificate and Diploma: OR = 0.398; Degree: OR = 0.1957) and statistically significant except for primary schooling attainment. The results imply that compared to households whose head has no education, households headed by edu cated people are less likely to experience food insecurity. It is also striking to observe that the odds of a household being food insecure reduces further as the education of the household head increases. This result is consistent with theory, *a priori* expectation, and the results found by other authors [44, 45]. This finding supports the importance of education and especially higher education in household well-being. Education provides opportunities for labor supply and employment chances and acquisition of skill and application, which could translate to better income to access household necessities and improve household well-being.

It is also shown in **Table 5** that household size's odd ratio is statistically significant (OR = 9.25; $p < 0.01$). The results indicate that the odds of household food insecurity are about 9.2 times higher when household size increases by one unit increase. This implies that an increase in households' size would further exacerbates households' food insecurity. This result is consistent with *a priori* expectation of the study and argument put forward by previous studies [47, 48, 59], that a large household is an extra burden on household resources and strain on income because of higher food consumption expenditure. According to Mota et al. [48], per capita food expenditure and availability decline as the size of the family increases, hence increasing the likelihood of food insecurity. This result is further plausible in a situation where the dependency ratio is high in a household; that is, when the number of economically active members of the household is lower than the number of non-economically active due to age, health, and unemployment.

The odds ratios of household income quartiles are less than 1 and statistically significant (i.e., quartile two: (OR = 0.775; $p < 0.01$), quartile three: (OR = 0.733; $p < 0.01$), quartile four: (OR = 0.442; $p < 0.01$)). This implies that compared to households in the quartile one income group, households in quartile two, quartile three, and quartile four are 0.775, 0.733, 0.442 less likely to experience food insecurity. However, as can be seen, the probability of being food insecure is highest for households in the quartile 4 group. This finding is related to a previous study [18]. Furthermore, in this study, the odds ratios for African are 1.588 for model 1 and 1.614 for model 2, and both are statistically significant at $p < 0.05$. It implies that households whose heads are from African population have a higher likelihood of being food insecure. The finding of this study is consistent with Jonah and May [29], where it was established that Africans had the lowest dietary diversity, and the coloreds were vulnerable when considering the Household Food Insecurity Access Scale (HFIAS) measure of food insecurity [29]. According to Jonah and May [29], the distribution of population group and food insecurity in South Africa reflects socioeconomic status where previously disadvantaged groups (Colored and Africans) have remained vulnerable. High levels of economic and social inequalities in economic opportunities, employment, purchasing power, and education access that are not in favor of Africa are plausible factors that impact the well-being including food insecurity probability of African households in the country.

The odd ratios estimated for the place of residence (urban) are statistically significant (model 1: OR = 0.835; $p < 0.01$ and model 2: OR = 0.836; $p < 0.01$). The result proposes that the odds of a household being food insecure are 0.84 times lower for urban-based households than rural area-residing households, when other variables are held constant. It can also be said that rural households and populations are more likely to be food insecure or more vulnerable to food insecurity than urban households. This finding is consistent with [19, 50, 56]. Szabo et al. [50] established that urban households are less likely to experience insufficient dietary variety and insufficient energy intake compared with rural households that are agricultural households. The result explains the advantages of residing in urban areas. In an alternative interpretation, the remoteness of rural areas, poor economic activity, poor agricultural sector performance, limited livelihood opportunities, as well as limited sources of income are plausible reasons for the negative influence of urban-based household variables on household food insecurity. These identified constraints in the rural areas limit the ability of households in the area to purchase needed food for their well-being. Bulawayo et al. [55] also argued that households in urban areas are less likely to be food insecure because they have more households' assets, and hence, more sustainable coping strategies are possible than in rural areas. Moreover, the result is unsurprising considering the higher prevalence of poverty in rural areas than in urban area in the South African context. Finally, for the provincial parameter, the odds of household food insecurity are lower for all provinces but only statistically significant at $p < 0.05$ and $p < 0.01$ for the Western Cape and Gauteng provinces, respectively. This implies that taking all other variables constant, the odds of households' food insecurity are predicted to be about 0.73 and 0.72 lower for household residing in the Western Cape and Gauteng provinces, respectively.

5. Conclusion

South Africa is one of the countries struggling with the public health challenges of food insecurity and smoking, which have been argued to be interwoven. However, while several confounders have been linked with household food insecurity, the potential relative influence of household head smoking behavior on household food insecurity has been less examined and reported globally and in South Africa. Consequently, this study provides a better understanding of the potential contribution of the smoking behavior of household heads to household food insecurity in South Africa. These findings contribute to literature understudying the dynamic relationship between smoking behavior and household food insecurity. Findings from this study indicated that while food insecurity incidence is highest for households whose head does not smoke currently or remained a nonsmoker, nevertheless, household food insecurity was found to be associated with and can be predicted by current smoking and continual smoking behavior of the household head. There are other factors that influence household food insecurity irrespective of the smoking behavior of the household head as demonstrated in this study. However, considering the interest of this study, the finding indicates that household head smoking behavior does contribute to household food insecurity in South Africa and that the case for tobacco smoking quitting or control goes beyond health outcome reasons to include the need for household food security attainment. Measures to promote quitting smoking behavior need to be promoted and intensified by the government. Therefore, given the confirmed impact of smoking behavior, concurrent (rather than isolated) interventions that can discourage smoking and smoking uptake, encourage early discontinuation of smoking addiction, and promote food security are imperative. Furthermore, intensified food insecurity reduction interventions and policies, through empowerment programs for female-headed and rural households, and toward increasing literacy and employment opportunities especially in the formal sector, are imperative. The impact of being a member of health insurance scheme on food insecurity reduction as found in this study strengthens the urgency of implementation of the national health insurance scheme in South Africa.

Conflict of interest

The authors declare no conflict of interest.

Author details

Ebenezer Toyin Megbowon[1*], Oladipo Olalekan David[2] and Jabulile Makhalima[2]

1 Department of Economics and Business Science, Walter Sisulu University, South Africa

2 Faculty of Economic and Management Sciences, School of Economic Science, North-West University, South Africa

*Address all correspondence to: megbowontoyin@gmail.com

References

[1] Maslow AH. A dynamic theory of human motivation. Psychological Review. 1958;**50**(4):370-396. DOI: 10.1037/h0054346

[2] McLeod S. Maslow's hierarchy of needs. Simply Psychology. 2007;**1**:1-18

[3] Mazzeschi R, Pisillo MR. Protection of basic needs and subsistence rights of the person. In: International Human Rights Law: Theory and Practice. Cham, Switzerland: Springer Nature; 2021. pp. 309-328

[4] Ogunniyi AI, Omotoso SO, Salman KK, Omotayo AO, Olagunju KO, Aremu AO. Socio-economic drivers of food security among rural households in Nigeria: Evidence from smallholder maize farmers. Social Indicators Research. 2021;**155**:583-599

[5] Casaer MP, Ziegler TR. Nutritional support in critical illness and recovery. The Lancet Diabetes & Endocrinology. 2015;**3**(9):734-745

[6] de Araújo FF, de Paulo FD, Neri-Numa IA, Pastore GM. Polyphenols and their applications: An approach in food chemistry and innovation potential. Food Chemistry. 2021;**338**:127535

[7] FAO. The State of Food Insecurity in the World 2001. Rome: FAO; 2002

[8] FAO, IFAD, UNICEF, WFP, and WHO. The state of food security and nutrition in the world 2022. In: Repurposing Food and Agricultural Policies to Make Healthy Diets more Affordable. Rome: FAO; 2022. DOI: 10.4060/cc0639en

[9] von Grebmer K, Bernstein J, Mukerji R, Patterson F, Wiemers M, Chéilleachair RN, et al. Global Hunger Index by Severity, Map in 2019 Global Hunger Index: The Challenge of Hunger and Climate Change. Bonn: Welthungerhilfe; and Dublin. 2019

[10] Statistics South Africa. Report-03-00-19 - Measuring Food Security in South Africa: Applying the Food Insecurity Experience Scale, 2020. Pretoria South Africs: Statistics South Africa; 2020. Available from: https://www.statssa.gov.za/publications/Report-03-00-19/Report-03-00-192020.pdf

[11] Kim-Mozeleski JE, Pandey R. The intersection of food insecurity and tobacco use: A scoping review. Health Promotion Practice. 2020;**21**:124S-138S

[12] World Health Organization. 2022. Available from: https://www.who.int/news-room/fact-sheets/detail/tobacco

[13] National Department of Health. Global Adult Tobacco Survey (GATS) Fact Sheet South Africa, 2021. Pretoria: National Department of Health; 2022. Available from: https://www.health.gov.za/wp-content/uploads/2022/05/Global-Adult-Tobacco-Survey-GATS-SA_FS-Populated__28-April-2022.pdf

[14] Kang SY, Cho HJ. Association between the use of tobacco products and food insecurity among South Korean adults. International Journal of Public Health. 2022;**67**:1604866. DOI: 10.3389/ijph.2022.1604866

[15] Ruhyana NF, Essa WY, Mardianis M. Sociodemographic factors affecting household food security in sumedang regency West Java province. AGRARIS:

Journal of Agribusiness and Rural Development Research. 2020;**6**(1):38-51

[16] Drakoulidou P, Drayton B, Shepherd L, Mihrshahi S. Sociodemographic factors associated with food insecurity: Data from the 2003–2014 New South Wales population health survey. Public Health Nutrition. 2020;**23**(11):1857-1867

[17] Amrullah ER, Ishida A, Pullaila A, Rusyiana A. Who suffers from food insecurity in Indonesia? International Journal of Social Economics. 2019;**46** (10):1186-1197

[18] Sreeramareddy CT, Ramakrishnareddy N. Association of adult tobacco use with household food access insecurity: Results from Nepal demographic and health survey, 2011. BMC Public Health. 2018;**18**(1):1-8

[19] Jumrani J, Birthal PS. Does consumption of tobacco and alcohol affect household food security? Evidence from rural India. Food Security. 2017;**9**: 255-279

[20] Gu D, Max WB, Yao T, Wang Y, Keeler C, Sung HY. Association between e-cigarette use and food insecurity among low-income adults. Tobacco Control. 2023;**32**(e2):e212-e219

[21] Asadi-Lari M, Jahromi LM, Montazeri A, Rezaee N, Mehrizi AA, Shams-Beyranvand M, et al. Socio-economic risk factors of household food insecurity and their population attributable risk: A population-based study. Medical Journal of the Islamic Republic of Iran. 2019;**33**:119

[22] Mayer M, Gueorguieva R, Ma X, White MA. Tobacco use increases risk of food insecurity: An analysis of continuous NHANES data from 1999 to 2014. Preventive Medicine. 2019;**126**: 105765

[23] Semba RD, Campbell AA, Sun K, de Pee S, Akhter N, Moench-Pfanner R, et al. Paternal smoking is associated with greater food insecurity among poor families in rural Indonesia. Asia Pacific Journal of Clinical Nutrition. 2011;**20**(4): 618-623

[24] Berry KM, Drew JA, Brady PJ, Widome R. Impact of smoking cessation on household food security. Annals of Epidemiology. 2023;**79**:49-55

[25] Musemwa L, Muchenje V, Mushunje A, Aghdasi F, Zhou L. Household food insecurity in the poorest province of South Africa: Level, causes and coping strategies. Food Security. 2015;7:647-655

[26] Ningi T, Taruvinga A, Zhou L, Ngarava S. Factors that influence household food security in Hamburg and Melani, Eastern Cape, South Africa. African Journal of Science, Technology, Innovation and Development. 2022;**14** (4):1050-1058

[27] Megbowon E. Urban household food security: An assessment of the correlates of micronutrient-sensitive dietary diversity. The Journal of Developing Areas. 2022;**56**(2):119-139

[28] David OO, Grobler W. Age progression, social interventions and food insecurity in South Africa: Logistic regression analysis. The International Journal of Social Sciences and Humanity Studies. 2020;**12**(2):289-305

[29] Jonah CM, May JD. The nexus between urbanization and food insecurity in South Africa: Does the type of dwelling matter? International Journal of Urban Sustainable Development. 2020;**12**(1):1-3

[30] Waidler J, Devereux S. Social grants, remittances, and food security: Does the

source of income matter? Food Security. 2019;**11**(3):679-702

[31] Faber M, Wenhold FA, Laurie SM. Dietary diversity and vegetable and fruit consumption of households in a resource-poor peri-urban South Africa community differ by food security status. Ecology of Food and Nutrition. 2017;**56**(1):62-80

[32] Khumalo NZ, Sibanda M. Does urban and peri-urban agriculture contribute to household food security? An assessment of the food security status of households in Tongaat, eThekwini municipality. Sustainability. 2019;**11**(4): 1082

[33] Megbowon ET, Mushunje A. Assessment of food security among households in Eastern Cape Province, South Africa: Evidence from general household survey, 2014. International Journal of Social Economics. 2018;**45**(1): 2-17

[34] Taruvinga A, Muchenje V, Mushunje A. Determinants of rural household dietary diversity: The case of Amatole and Nyandeni districts, South Africa. International Journal of Development and Sustainability. 2013;**2**(4):2233-2247

[35] De Cock N, D'Haese M, Vink N, Van Rooyen CJ, Staelens L, Schönfeldt HC, et al. Food security in rural areas of Limpopo province, South Africa. Food security. 2013;**5**:269-282

[36] Southern Africa Labour and Development Research Unit. National Income Dynamics Study 2017, Wave 5 [dataset]. Version 1.0.0 Pretoria: Department of Planning, Monitoring, and Evaluation [funding agency]. Cape Town: Southern Africa Labour and Development Research Unit [implementer], 2018. Cape Town: DataFirst [distributor], 2018. DOI: 10.25828/fw3h-v708

[37] Southern Africa Labour and Development Research Unit. National Income Dynamics StudyWave 3, 2012 [dataset]. Version 3.0.0. Pretoria: SA Presidency [funding agency]. Cape Town: Southern Africa Labour and Development Research Unit [implementer], 2016. Cape Town: DataFirst [distributor], 2016. DOI: 10.25828/7pgq-q106

[38] Brophy T, Branson N, Daniels RC, Leibbrandt M, Mlatsheni C,Woolard I. National Income Dynamics Study panel user manual. Version 1. Cape Town: Southern Africa Labour and Development Research Unit, Cape Town South Africa; 2018

[39] Foster J, Greer J, Thorbecke E. A class of decomposable poverty measures. Econometrica: Journal of the Econometric Society. 1984;**1**:761-766

[40] Omotayo AO, Aremu AO. Evaluation of factors influencing the inclusion of indigenous plants for food security among rural households in the North West Province of South Africa. Sustainability. 2020;**12**(22):9562

[41] Oluwatayo IB, Ojo AO. Effect of access to ICT on food insecurity among farming households in Nigeria. The Journal of Developing Areas. 2019;**53**(2): 155-168

[42] Odekon M, editor. The SAGE Encyclopedia of World Poverty. 2nd ed. Thousand Oaks, California: SAGE Publications, Inc.; 2015

[43] Azwardi A, Widyasthika HF, Saleh RC, Adnan N. Household food security: Evidence from South Sumatera. JEJAK: Jurnal Ekonomi dan Kebijakan. 2019; **12**(2):446-465

[44] Mthethwa S, Wale E. Household vulnerability to food insecurity in rural South Africa: Evidence from a nationally representative survey data. International Journal of Environmental Research and Public Health. 2020;**18**(4):1917

[45] Mazenda A, Molepo N, Mushayanyama T, Ngarava S. The invisible crisis: The determinants of local food insecurity in Gauteng municipalities, South Africa. British Food Journal. 2022;**124**(13):274-289

[46] Etana D, Tolossa D. Unemployment and food insecurity in urban Ethiopia. African Development Review. 2017;**29**(1):56-68

[47] Drammeh W, Hamid NA, Rohana AJ. Determinants of household food insecurity and its association with child malnutrition in Sub-Saharan Africa: A review of the literature. Current Research in Nutrition and Food Science Journal. 2019;**7**(3):610-623

[48] Mota AA, Lachore ST, Handiso YH. Assessment of food insecurity and its determinants in the rural households in Damot Gale Woreda, Wolaita zone, Southern Ethiopia. Agriculture & Food Security. 2019;**8**(1):1-1

[49] Moellman N. Healthcare and hunger: Effects of the ACA Medicaid expansions on food insecurity in America. Applied Economic Perspectives and Policy. 2020;**42**(2):168-186

[50] Szabo S, Ahmed S, Wiśniowski A, Pramanik M, Islam R, Zaman F, et al. Remittances and food security in Bangladesh: An empirical country-level analysis. Public Health Nutrition. 2022;**25**(10):2886-2896

[51] Orjiakor EC, Adediran A, Ugwu JO, Nwachukwu W. Household living conditions and food insecurity in Nigeria: A longitudinal study during COVID-19 pandemic. BMJ Open. 2023;**13**(1):e066810

[52] Hasanujzaman M, Omar MA. Household and non-household factors influencing multidimensional energy poverty in Bangladesh: Demographics, urbanization and regional differentiation via a multilevel modeling approach. Energy Research & Social Science. 2022;**92**:102803

[53] Ogundipe AA, Ogunniyi A, Olagunju K, Asaleye AJ. Poverty and income inequality in rural agrarian household of southwestern Nigeria: The gender perspective. The Open Agriculture Journal. 2019;**13**(1):51-57

[54] Awoke W, Eniyew K, Agitew G, Meseret B. Determinants of food security status of household in Central and North Gondar zone, Ethiopia. Cogent Social Sciences. 2022;**8**(1):2040138

[55] Bulawayo M, Ndulo M, Sichone J. Socioeconomic determinants of food insecurity among Zambian households: Evidence from a national household survey. Journal of Asian and African Studies. 2019;**54**(6):800-818

[56] Santos MP, Brewer JD, Lopez MA, Paz-Soldan VA, Chaparro MP. Determinants of food insecurity among households with children in villa el Salvador, Lima, Peru: The role of gender and employment, a cross-sectional study. BMC Public Health. 2022;**22**(1):717

[57] Mabuza N, Mamba SF. Food insecurity, food insecurity determinants and coping strategies in the urban space–the experience of low income households of Msunduza in Mbabane. Social Sciences & Humanities Open. 2022;**6**(1):100271

[58] Himmelstein G. Effect of the affordable care act's Medicaid expansions on food security, 2010–2016. American Journal of Public Health. 2019; **109**(9):1243-1248

[59] Ndhleve S, Dapira C, Kabiti HM, Mpongwana Z, Cishe EN, Nakin MD, et al. Household food insecurity status and determinants: The case of Botswana and South Africa. AGRARIS: Journal of Agribusiness and Rural Development Research. 2021;7(2):207-224

Chapter 2

Demand Side Predictors of the Demand and Utilization of Maternal and Family Planning Services of the Philippines' Conditional Cash Transfer Program: A Quantitative Approach

Maria C.G. Bautista, Rafael Deo F. Estanislao, Venus O.C. Rosales, Maria E.C. Yap and Katherine V. Reyes

Abstract

The study explores demand for maternal and family planning services among beneficiaries of the *Pantawid Pamilyang* Pilipino Program, a conditional cash transfer program in the Philippines. We analyzed 390 households across six provinces in the Philippines through multi-stage sampling. Three models were created: (1) pregnancy during the program, (2) facility-based delivery, and (3) non-utilization of antenatal care visits. The findings show that: (1) For every peso increase in received amounts from the program, the odds of getting pregnant decreased by 0.31%, a negative but weak association, while having more children, living in a high mortality region, having a teenage child, living far (self-perceived) from the health center, marrying at a younger age, and not completing high school also increased the odds of being pregnant. (2) Non-delivery from a health facility was likely for those who lived far from a facility and in a high mortality region, and (3) having a teenager at home increased the likelihood of seeking antenatal visits, while those who have been married longer slacked behind in terms of antenatal visits. The study points to directions for policy and research on access and use of maternal and reproductive health services, and the role of adolescent-aged children.

Keywords: demand side analyses, conditional cash transfer programs, antenatal visits, family planning, adolescent's role

1. Introduction

The *Pantawid Pamilyang* Pilipino Program, popularly known as 4Ps, is a flagship anti-poverty program that is both a social welfare and a social development intervention. As a social welfare program, it is a form of conditional cash transfer (CCT) program, providing cash grants to targeted families in extreme poverty. As a social development program, it hopes to break the cycle of intergenerational poverty by ensuring investments in education (PHP 5000 or USD 105 per year) and health (PHP 500 (USD 11) per month for a total of PHP 3000 or USD 63 per year), per household, depending on household composition. The grant is conditional to pregnant women availing themselves of antenatal care and regular health checks for women and children below 5 years old, deworming of school-aged children 6–14 years old, school enrolment of children, and attendance in family development sessions. As of 2016, the Department of Social Welfare and Development (DSWD) reported having 4,393,114 active members, of which 572,809 were from indigenous peoples (IP) households and about 219,149 households have members with disabilities. For the same period, a total of PHP 27.15 billion (USD 572 million) cash grants have been availed of, of which PHP 13.2 billion (USD 278 million) was for education and PHP 13.9 billion (USD 293 million) was for health.

The DSWD, during a 2016 Research Colloquium, showed high compliance rates for *Pantawid* families. Around 94% attendance was reported for family development sessions and 96% coverage for health visits of pregnant women and children aged 0–5. Earlier research [1] showed that *Pantawid* families had more members, roughly 6 members, compared to 4 members for non-*Pantawid* families. The family size for 23% of *Pantawid* families was at least 8 members. The *Pantawid Pamilya* 3rd Wave Impact Evaluation [2] showed that women beneficiaries did try the modern FP method at a greater rate than women who were not part of the program. The Contraceptive Prevalence Rate was reported at 52% for *Pantawid* families compared to 47% for non-*Pantawid* counterparts. The higher incidence of trial use, however, did not translate into sustained use of modern FP methods. There was a high awareness of modern family planning methods among both *Pantawid* families and non-*Pantawid* families, though *Pantawid* families are aware of more contraceptive options. Compared to an earlier national demographic and health survey (DHS)—sourced average of 84%, an impact evaluation [2] found that 76% of *Pantawid* mothers made at least four antenatal visits.

The demand for family planning and maternal health services is viewed as part of a decision-making nexus that values health intrinsically. Human capital theory posits that maximization of health is the ultimate objective of seeking health care [3]. Medical care services are inputs in the overall production of health. Consumption of medical care and other goods is determined by the amount of resources available or income, and the price and quantities of these goods. The individual maximizes welfare by choosing among a combination of goods and services that fit within the budget constraint.

Decision-making on sexual and reproductive health is influenced by education, by operating at the cognitive level of imparting information and/or through socialization that happens in these institutions. Attributing to Boongaerts, Darney et al. [4] identified the pathway through proximate determinants like age at marriage, postnatal fecundity (via breastfeeding and postnatal abstinence practices), and contraceptive use. A gender perspective would highlight the access of women to prenatal care and the extent to which their heavy domestic household and farming activities are likely to affect their health. This perspective emphasizes the social and gender roles or structures that influence women's fertility decisions and health-seeking behavior over reproductive health [5]. This study on demand for FP and MCH services by 4Ps women works around the basic demand function as influenced by a vector of individual and demographic and socio-economic aspects affecting the demand for these services by the women and their households. While not expressed among 4Ps conditions, the quality of maternal health care services forms part of the completeness of services. FP as a reproductive health issue underpins maternal care. Changes in reproductive care attitudes and practices upon participation in the 4Ps program, even if FP is not explicitly part of program conditionalities, are viewed as a consequence of life skills imparted through the family development sessions (FDS; [6]) and health center visits with a trained health worker. The information gleaned from health service encounters is expected to improve demand for reproductive health services.

This study aimed to identify demand side factors in the utilization of maternal health care and family planning services. We hypothesized that the demand side factors that may potentially be predictive for maternal health care and family planning services utilization are the following: individual characteristics of the mother and her spouse or partner such as age, education, employment, and age married, family characteristics such as years of marriage, number of children, presence of teenage child, household monthly income, locality if urban or rural, and if with high maternal mortality rate, distance from health center, transportation costs, and monthly amount received from the CCT program.

2. Methods

2.1 Study design and setting

This study was conducted in the Philippines from 2016 to 2017 and is a national multi-level mixed methods study consisting of household surveys, interviews, and focus group discussions. A regionally representative sample was obtained with a multi-stage purposive sampling design. The three major island groups, Luzon, Visayas, and Mindanao, were the first level of stratification, from which two provinces from each island group were selected: one urban and one rural. The following provinces were selected: Pampanga and Zambales for Luzon, Cebu and Western Samar for Visayas, and Compostela Valley (now Davao de Oro) and South Cotabato for Mindanao. These were selected for having one or more of the following characteristics: vulnerability to disasters, the presence of indigenous people's communities, and both high and low maternal mortality ratios. Purposive sampling was conducted for the household-level surveys, which sought *Pantawid* family members in randomly selected villages in the selected cities/municipalities. We defined a household as inclusive of those living under the same roof and sharing the same meals.

We surveyed a total of 390 households. These households received grants from the 4Ps program. Households were interviewed using an interviewer-administered survey tool covering demographic and household composition, socio-economic condition, and health service utilization, including recent experience of childbirth for those with children 5 years old and below. The main respondent was the mother grantee. The questionnaires were encoded daily and interviewers were given one opportunity to go back to the families in case some responses were unclear.

2.2 Qualitative data

Summative qualitative content analysis was conducted with the existing study variables as the initial themes. A coding and categorization tool was developed on MS Excel. Two cycles of coding were conducted to analyze the notes and transcripts, with the first using structural coding and the second using pattern coding. Analytic memos were developed throughout the coding process and then subjected to coding. Two independent coders conducted the coding and thematizing process. Coding sorts were developed and organized into themes.

2.3 Statistical analyses

Several statistical tests were used to analyze the data collected. Univariate analysis was used to describe data and to show frequencies. Bivariate analysis using the t-test and chi-square test was used to show the association between the exposure and the outcome variables. Multivariate analysis through logistic regressions was used to measure the magnitudes of the association. Only p-values of 0.05 or lower were considered significant. The STATA 12 statistics software was used for data analysis.

2.4 Dependent outcomes

Regression analyses examined several layers of women's decision-making on reproductive health care demand: (1) the factors associated with being pregnant as a 4Ps beneficiary; (2) the demand for facility-based delivery; (3) the demand for antenatal; and (4) the demand for modern contraceptive methods. The first three, the likelihood of being pregnant as a 4Ps beneficiary, facility-based deliveries, and demand for antenatal care, came out to be statistically significant and could explain 49, 8, and 11% of the variability, respectively. The discussion will therefore focus on a reduced form of the 3 demand models.

3. Results and discussion

3.1 Descriptive background of sites, women, and household respondents

The household survey covered 390 *Pantawid Pamilya* households. Maternal Mortality status of the province was determined in consultation with the DSWD Planning, Monitoring, and Evaluation Division, which identified the study provinces.

3.1.1 Locality and area characteristics

Respondents in Low MMR (**Table 1**) areas are on average a year older, have on average been married for one fewer year, and have on average one fewer household member than High MMR areas. There are fewer respondents in Low MMR areas with a child below 5 years of age than in High MMR areas, with 46.74% in Low MMR and 53.26% in High MMR. Fewer respondents in low MMR areas also have children between 6 and 18 years of age, with 45.17% in Low MMR areas and 54.83% in High MMR areas. There are far more Service workers (33 in Low MMR, 3 in High MMR)

	High MMR (n = 195)	Low MMR (n = 195)
Mean age of women respondents	35.65 ± 6.34	36.58 ± 8.04
Year married or cohabiting	14 (2 to 32)	13 (1 to 48)
Mean age when first married		
Spouse	24.70 ± 6.02	25.50 ± 6.35
Respondent	21.14 ± 4.98	22.01 ± 5.19
Household size	7 (3 to 12)	6 (2 to 11)
Children per household (18 y/o and below)	4 (1 to 9)	4 (0 to 10)
No. and % of women with children between 6 and 18 years of age	139 (53.26)	122 (46.74)
Educational attainment		
No formal education	266 (27.94)	266 (31.22)
Elementary completed	168 (17.65)	24 (2.82)
Elementary not completed	282 (29.62)	316 (37.09)
High school completed	80 (8.4)	64 (7.51)
High school not completed	123 (12.92)	147 (17.21)
Vocational completed	2 (0.21)	4 (0.47)
College completed	10 (1.05)	5 (0.59)
College not completed	21 (2.21)	26 (3.05)
Postgraduate completed	0	0
Occupation of the women respondents (n = 106)		
Technicians and associate professionals	1 (1.2)	0
Clerks	2 (2.41)	1 (1.37)
Service workers and shop and market sales owners	3 (3.61)	33 (45.21)
Farmers, forestry workers, and fishermen	4 (4.82)	2 (2.74)
Traders and related workers	0	2 (2.74)
Plant and machine operators and assemblers	0	0
Laborers and unskilled workers	12 (14.46)	28 (38.36)
Special occupations	8 (9.64)	7 (9.59)
Income of women from occupation, earnings for 2015 (mean overall and SD)		
< PHP 1000	3 (0 to 4)	4 (0 to 4)
PHP 1000–2000	60 (30.77)	62 (31.79)
PHP 2001–3000	0	0
PHP 3001–4000	0	0
> PHP 4000	3 (1.54)	6 (3.08)

Table 1.
Profile of respondents by low-high MMR status of province.

and Laborers (28 in Low MMR, 12 in High MMR) in Low MMR areas. Average income is higher in Rural areas, with an average monthly income of greater than PHP 4000 (USD 84) at 85.13% for Low MMR areas and 67.29% for High MMR areas.

In terms of the distribution of the 390 women respondents by urban-rural setting (**Table 2**), there are more respondents in urban areas who have children below 5 years of age, as well as between 6 and 18 years of age. Of the respondents in both settings, the majority were not able to reach or complete High School, with more respondents from Urban areas reaching but failing to complete High School (16.67% Urban, 12.95% Rural) but more respondents from Rural areas completing High School (4.6% Urban, 11.99% Rural). About 46.74% of women in Urban areas and 53.26% of women in Rural areas reported having children below 5 years old, while 45.17% of women in Urban areas and 54.83% of women in Rural areas reported having school-aged (6–18 years of age) children. The average household size reported is 6.

A glimpse of the provincial profile of the respondents shows the following: The richest province Cebu has the most reporting 10 years of marriage while Western Samar (a rural province) respondents reported being married longest at 16 years. Each household, including the respondent and spouse, had an average size of 6 persons. All households had on average one child below 5 years of age. On the overall, *Pantawid* respondents in the study sites, compared to the National Demographic Health Survey (NDHS) [7] results, can be considered older, married longer, have much less education, have bigger household size having on average two more children, and with less gainful employment.

	Urban (n = 215)	**Rural** (n = 175)
Mean age of women respondents	36.08 ± 6.88	36.16 ± 7.69
Year married or cohabiting	13 (1 to 35)	13 (1 to 48)
Mean age when first married		
Spouse	25.98 ± 6.28	24.39 ± 6.04
Respondent	21.97 ± 5.25	21.26 ± 4.96
Household size	6 (2 to 11)	6 (2 to 12)
Children per household (18 y/o and below)	4 (0 to 10)	4 (0 to 9)
No. and % of women with children between 6 and 18 years of age	154 (53.10)	136 (46.90)
Educational attainment		
No formal education	266 (27.2)	266 (32.2)
Elementary completed	38 (3.89)	154 (18.64)
Elementary not completed	438 (44.79)	160 (19.37)
High school completed	45 (4.6)	99 (11.99)
High school not completed	163 (16.67)	107 (12.95)
Vocational completed	6 (0.61)	0
College completed	1 (0.1)	14 (1.69)
College not completed	21 (2.15)	26 (3.15)
Postgraduate completed	0	0

Table 2.
Profile of respondents by urban-rural setting.

3.1.2 Spouse/partner's characteristics

Spouses of respondents are much older in Low MMR areas (36.5 years Low MMR, 31 years High), and were also at least a year older at marriage. Like the respondents, the majority of the spouses did not reach or complete high school, but a good number of spouses completed high school in low MMR areas (32% Low MMR, 23% High MMR). Also similar to the respondents, the largest groups of reported occupation were service workers and unskilled laborers, with almost half of spouses in both Low and High MMR areas reporting to be Laborers.

3.1.3 Family characteristics

Less than half of the households reported having 2 adult earners (41%) but 65.64% still report having an income greater than PHP 4000 (USD 84) per month. Majority report to having monthly food expenditures of less than PHP 2000 (USD 421), and nearly all (99.49%) report to having expenses for cigarettes, alcohol, and games to be less than PHP 1000 (USD 21) per month. A good number (70.77%) report having a television, while only 11.79% report to having a refrigerator. Most use either a wood or coal stove, at 87.69%. The majority source their water from faucets, with water from a spring being a distant second, at 17.95%. More than half, at 59%, have had home renovations since becoming a member of the 4Ps program. The majority, at 82.31%, report having roofs of iron sheets.

3.1.4 Health service characteristics

Health facility staff believe that poor health-seeking behavior and differences in culture inhibit utilization for some beneficiaries. This access issue is limited to those who are far from the health facility, which does not constitute the majority. Health facilities compensate by conducting outreach/missions.

Respondents living in larger villages *(barangays)* consider that travel to health facilities is costly. This is contrasted in smaller barangays when respondents consider travel costs as affordable. When household survey respondents get sick, they would prioritize going to public health centers (79.8%). It is however notable that despite this high percentage, the same set of respondents would have more regular visits to private clinics. There is also a strong preference to bring their ailing family members to private clinics and hospitals.

About 97.4% of household survey respondents are confident that they will get health care from the health facility that they visited. Only 7.3% of household survey respondents feel that health facilities are far from where they live. For those who take transportation to reach health facilities, the majority prefer tricycles.

Table 3 shows that the average grant received per month was PHP 1400 (US 29), which is roughly the same in both Low and High MMR areas. Respondents have been members of the 4Ps program on average for 4 years, but those living in High MMR areas have been members for longer, at 5 years, while the respondents in Western Samar have been members for 6 years. The single most prevalent mode of grant transfer is the On-site over the counter transaction (41.54%), which is still the method most used in High MMR areas (65%). Provinces differ, with CASH Cards being most prevalent in bigger provinces—Zambales, Cebu, and South Cotabato. A bank-backed prepaid card is a mode of grant transfer in one urbanized province. Urban settings have program members for 4 years with more than a quarter (28.37%) covered as

	Avg amounts received per household in PHP *average (min to max)*	Avg years of membership *years*	Most prevalent mode of cash transfer *% of respondents*
Overall	1400 (250 to 4000)	4	On-site over the counter transaction (41.54%)
High MMR Provinces	1400 (250 to 3600)	3	On-site over the counter transaction (65.13%)
Low MMR Provinces	1400 (500 to 4000)	5	CASH Cards (50.26%)
Urban	—	4	—
Rural	—	6	—
Pampanga	1100 (500 to 1800)	3	Landbank Prepaid card (95.38%)
Zambales	1100 (500 to 1800)	4	CASH Cards (78.46%)
Cebu	1600 (500 to 3600)	2	CASH Cards (60%)
Western Samar	2800 (1000 to 4000)	6	On-site over the counter transaction (100%)
South Cotabato	1400 (250 to 3200)	4	CASH Cards (90.77%)
Compostela Valley (Davao de Oro)	1300 (500 to 3200)	4	On-site over the counter transaction (93.85%)

Table 3.
Profile of pantawid membership.

program beneficiaries for 5 years. Those in rural settings are more dispersed, with 32.57% having been members for 6 years, and 29.14% having been a member for only a year.

4. Analytical results and discussion

4.1 Model 1: factors associated with pregnancy during 4Ps

Table 4 highlights the likelihood of being pregnant among 4Ps clientele. These factors explain 49.14% of the variability of the odds of pregnancy during the 4Ps period. The odds of getting pregnant decreased for every peso increase in amount received (OR = 0.9969, p-value<0.001), for every year increase in age when the mother first got married (OR = 0.9157, p-value<0.001), and for those who lived far from the health center (OR = 0.2246, p-value<0.02). These findings show, for instance, a negative association between the cash transfer and odds of getting pregnant, with the increase of PHP 1 (USD 0.02) received by mothers decreasing the odds of getting pregnant by 0.31%. However, with the odds ratio approaching 1 (at .99), the association of the two variables can very well be independent. The weak association may also be due to the lack of variability in the transferred cash, as shown by the narrow confidence intervals.

On the other hand, the odds of getting pregnant are increased for every increase in the number of children prior to 4Ps (OR = 2.59, p-value<0.001), for women who lived in a high MMR province (OR = 3.83, p-value<0.001), for women who had a teenager child (OR = 4.98, p-value<0.001), and for women who were unable to attain at least a high school degree (OR = 2.23, p-value<0.03). These findings show that women with

	P-Value	95% Confidence interval	Adjusted odds ratio
Amount received from *Pantawid*, per month	0.000	0.9962 to 0.9976	0.9969
No. of children before birthed child	0.000	1.8845 to 3.5762	2.5962
High MMR	0.000	1.8888 to 7.7624	3.8283
With teenage child	0.000	2.2552 to 11.0251	4.9863
Age of women when first married	0.010	0.8565 to 0.9790	0.9157
Far distance to the health center (self-perceived)	0.010	0.0726 to 0.6952	0.2247
Did not finish HS (mother)	0.020	1.1370 to 4.3766	2.2308

P-Value equals to 0.000 means p-value <0.001; R2 = 49.14%.

Table 4.
Likelihood of getting pregnant as Pantawid *members.*

teenage children have almost 5 times higher odds to get pregnant than those who do not have teenage children, reflecting perhaps the lack of vigilance in getting pregnant among relatively older but fecund women.

These results are broadly consistent with the literature. Early marriage and limited education have been shown to reduce the likelihood of pregnancy [8]. The effect of the amount received through a conditional cash transfer is less clear, as a systematic review done on CCT schemes in Latin America shows that receipt of financial incentives does not have a clear effect on fertility [9].

4.2 Model 2: demand for facility-based deliveries

A health conditionality related to maternal health is regular antenatal visits. It is surmised that once women get into the health system before deliveries, they will deliver in health facilities. **Table 5** highlights the factors affecting health facility delivery, the final model of which explains under 10 percent or just 8% of the variability in facility-based deliveries. Women in areas with high maternal mortality and living far from a health center have 3–4 times the odds of delivering outside of a health facility.

The low explanatory power of facility access may signify that variability in using health facilities for deliveries can be attributed to other factors. Literature shows how facility-based deliveries in LMICs are strongly influenced by local beliefs about what constitutes "normal" childbirth, perceptions about the quality of care they may receive, the fear of the possible costs of delivering at a facility [10], the comfort they may feel in their own home [11], and the role played by the husband in encouraging or discouraging facility-based delivery [11, 12].

	P-Value	95% Confidence interval	Adjusted odds ratio
High MMR	0.006	1.4753 to 10.1065	3.3022
Far distance to health center (self-perceived)	0.000	1.6893 to 6.4553	3.8613

P-Value <0.001; R2 = 8.05%.

Table 5.
Factors for delivery outside of health facility.

	P-Value	95% Confidence interval	Adjusted odds ratio
Years married	0.006	1.0468 to 1.3226	1.1766
With teenage child	0.018	0.0343 to 0.7267	0.1578
Far distance to health center (self-perceived)	0.148	0.6443 to 18.4265	3.4455
P-Value = 0.018; R2 = 10.89%.			

Table 6.
Factors for non-utilization of ANC.

4.3 Model 3: risk factors for non-utilization of ANC, defined as having 3 or fewer ANC visits

The likelihood of ANC non-utilization is shown in **Table 6**. The final model had an explanatory power of 10.89% and was significant at p-value<0.02.

Findings show that: (1) For every increase in years married, the odds of not availing of antenatal care increases by approximately 17.66%; (2) women with a teenage child have 0.1578 times the odds (meaning 84% less likely) of not availing of antenatal care (i.e. those with a teenage child are more likely to seek antenatal care); and (3) there was insufficient evidence to demonstrate an association between distance from the health center and absence of antenatal care. Having a teen-aged child helps with care for younger children at home, freeing the pregnant woman to have more antenatal visits.

5. Conclusion

The health conditionality, a compulsion provided by the cash grant, is anchored on a human capital perspective that a child's early years, right from conception, must be appropriately nurtured by a trained health worker or professional; and the proper care and nutrition of neonates and mothers (antenatal care) and young children (immunization and deworming) must be ensured. The standard theory posits that having more children is linked to poverty, not only in terms of direct costs of having children but also in terms of women trading off employment and income to care for children. Our study shows a significant but weak relationship between the cash transfer and the likelihood of pregnancy. Other facilitating factors that lower chances of being pregnant during *Pantawid* membership include having been married longer and being far (self-perceived) from health centers.

There may be limited understanding of their fecundity and unsystematic use of family planning, since women who already have teenage children were also more likely to get pregnant again. The challenge therefore is inculcating a greater sense of deliberation over fertility control for both couples. The low male attendance in family development sessions points to the need to bring in the husbands into the learning loop, if not through lectures, then possibly to alternative modes of delivery, through cooperatives, workplaces, and the like. The challenge of modern contraceptive uptake remains within the medical establishment to prescribe it and for health professionals to continue advising, anticipating, and being proactive with women's queries on the side effects of some methods. More work needs to be done to ensure that women deliver in health care facilities, especially in areas with already high MMR. Local government units (LGUs) have been known to send their ambulance service to pick up women about to give birth in farther areas.

There is an unanticipated significant presence in the study, the presence of a teenager or adolescent child in the family. That having an adolescent child in the family can increase chances of pregnancy and improve the likelihood of mothers seeking antenatal care may indicate the relatively long reproductive span of *Pantawid* members and that there should be no slacking in informing women that they remain fecund well into the years they may expect to be menopausing. The study affirms the need not to slack on *Pantawid*'s intended outcomes of delaying the age of marriage and completing high school as a way to break the cycle of poverty for many families. There is a need to be relentless in the pursuit of increasing awareness and utilization of family planning and maternal health care services, sustained by family development sessions as a platform for family and community transformations.

Acknowledgements

The currency conversion used was USD 1 = PHP 47.49. This is based on the official exchange rate of the World Bank for 2016, obtained from the World Bank Open Data website.

The study on which this chapter is based would not have been possible without the support of the staff and fieldworkers of the Department of Social Welfare and Development. Appreciation is also extended to the United Nations Population Fund (UNFPA) for co-funding the study and shepherding through the technical aspects of the process. These offices and their personnel are, however, not in any way responsible for the errors and omissions that may be contained in this chapter.

Author contributions

MCGB and RDFE drafted and revised this manuscript, acquired and interpreted the data, and approved the manuscript for publication. MECY and MCGB conceptualized and designed the study. MECY, RDFE, and KVR led fieldwork teams and likewise interpreted the data. VOCR conducted the statistical runs and analyzed the data.

Ethics approval

This study was approved on November 3, 2016, by the St. Frances Cabrini Medical Center and Cancer Institute – Asian Eye Institute Ethics Review Committee (ERC #2016-034).

Author details

Maria C.G. Bautista[1]*, Rafael Deo F. Estanislao[2], Venus O.C. Rosales[3], Maria E.C. Yap[4] and Katherine V. Reyes[2]

1 Graduate School of Business, Ateneo de Manila University, Philippines

2 Alliance for Improving Health Outcomes (AIHO), Philippines

3 101 Health Research, Philippines

4 ThinkWell, Philippines

*Address all correspondence to: mcbautista@ateneo.edu

References

[1] Reyes C, Tabuga A. Conditional Cash Transfer Program in the Philippines: Is it Reaching the Extremely Poor? Quezon City, Philippines: Philippine Institute of Development Studies; 2012 Available from: https://www.econstor.eu/bitstream/10419/126897/1/pidsdps1242.pdf

[2] Orbeta A, Melad K, Araos N. Reassessing the Impact of the Pantawid Pamilyang Pilipino Program: Results of the Third Wave Impact Evaluation. Quezon City, Philippines: Philippine Institute of Development Studies; 2021. Available from: https://pidswebs.pids.gov.ph/CDN/PUBLICATIONS/pidsdps2105.pdf

[3] Grossman M. The Demand for Health: A Theoretical and Empirical Investigation. New York: Columbia University Press; 1972. DOI: 10.7312/gros17900

[4] Darney BG, Weaver MR, Sosa-Rubí SG, Walker D, Serván-Mori E, Prager S, et al. The Oportunidades conditional cash transfer program: Effects on pregnancy and contraceptive use among young rural women in Mexico. International Perspectives on Sexual and Reproductive Health. 2013;**39**(04):205-214. DOI: 10.1363/3920513

[5] McCleary-Sills J, McGonagle A, Malhotra A. Women's Demand for Reproductive Control: Understanding and Addressing Gender Barriers. Washington D.C.: International Centre for Research on Women (ICRW); 2012

[6] Yap ME, Bautista MC, Reyes K, Estanislao D, Rodriguez R. Fit and dissemination of family development sessions as a learning platform for Behavioral change of *Pantawid Pamilya* Familes. Social Welfare and Development Journal. 2018:15-26

[7] National Demographic Survey. Philippine Statistics Authority: Manila, Philippines and ICF International: Maryland, USA. Vol. 2014. 2013. Available from: https://dhsprogram.com/pubs/pdf/fr294/fr294.pdf

[8] Pradhan R, Wynter K, Fisher J. Factors associated with pregnancy among adolescents in low-income and lower middle-income countries: A systematic review. Journal of Epidemiology and Community Health. 2015;**69**(9):918-924. DOI: 10.1136/jech-2014-205128

[9] Glassman A. Impact of Conditional Cash Transfers on Maternal and Newborn Health [Internet]. 2013. Available from: https://www.ncbi.nlm.nih.gov/pmc/articles/PMC4021703/

[10] Bohren MA, Hunter E, Munthe-Kaas HM, Souza JP, Vogel JP, Gülmezoglu AM. Facilitators and barriers to facility-based delivery in low- and middle-income countries: A qualitative evidence synthesis. Reproductive Health. 2014;**11**(1). DOI: 10.1186/1742-4755-11-71

[11] Orano JT. Beyond Barriers: Factors Affecting Facility-Based Childbirth among b'laan Parturients. Brussels: Longdom; 2021. Available from: https://www.longdom.org/proceedings/beyond-barriers-factors-affecting-facilitybased-childbirth-among-b39laan-parturients-59550.html

[12] Azusa S, Honda S, Dulnuan MM, Chunanon JB, Matsuyama A. Factors associated with facility-based delivery in Mayoyao, Ifugao Province, Philippines. Asia Pacific Family Medicine. 2013;**12**(1):5. DOI: 10.1186/1447-056x-12-5

Chapter 3

Who Receives the Flu Vaccine and Where? Influenza Vaccination Uptake among Europeans Aged 50+ in Bismarck-Type Health Systems

Aida Isabel Tavares

Abstract

This study investigates the individual and country-level determinants of flu-vaccine uptake in Europe, focusing on countries with Bismarck-type health system. Using logistic regression on SHARE survey data Wave 8, the analysis reveals that individual characteristics significantly influence vaccination decisions. Main results show that individual characteristics play a role in the decision to take flu vaccination. Notably, self-assessed health exhibits a non-linear, inverted U-shaped relationship with vaccine uptake. At the country level, a higher share of health expenditure in GDP is associated with greater vaccination coverage. Trust in science positively correlates with flu vaccination, while trust in national governments shows a negative association; this effect is more pronounced in western than in eastern European countries. An unexpected finding in western countries is the inverse association between flu vaccination and future COVID-19 vaccine coverage. These results contribute to understanding both micro- and macro-level factors shaping flu vaccine uptake in European Bismarck-type systems.

Keywords: flu vaccine, Bismark health systems, SHARE survey, determinant factors, +50y.o.

1. Introduction

Seasonal influenza, or common flu, is a viral respiratory disease that infects approximately 10–13% of Europeans annually [1]. The risk of infection varies across the population, with certain groups being more vulnerable, although severe complications, such as pneumonia, myocarditis, encephalitis, and death, can occur in anyone. Two primary risk groups are older people and individuals with chronic diseases. Vaccination is also recommended for other at-risk groups, such as pregnant women, children, and health care workers [2].

The underlying drivers of the yearly spread of influenza remain incompletely understood. However, minor genetic mutations are known to occur each year. Consequently, there is a need for annual influenza vaccination, with the vaccine composition updated to reflect these antigenic changes and prevent mismatches between the vaccine and circulating strains that could reduce efficacy [3]. While older adults bear the highest burden of infection and complications, they also experience the lowest vaccine effectiveness among vulnerable groups. This is largely attributed to immunosenescence, the age-related decline in immune function—which remains a significant challenge [4]. It is estimated that an average of 27,600 of respiratory deaths per winter is associated with seasonal influenza across the 28 EU countries, with over 90% occurring in individuals aged 65 and over [5]. However, there is no negative correlation between vaccination coverage and influenza mortality in this later age group [6]. Still, a lack of clear association does not imply absence of vaccine benefit.

The economic burden of influenza is substantial, arising primarily from hospitalizations and mortality. It has been estimated that up to 88% of this burden is attributable to indirect costs, and up to 75% of overall direct healthcare costs are due to hospitalizations. Additionally, among individuals aged 18 to 64, the financial burden increases with age and the presence of medical conditions. Hospital inpatient expenditures related to influenza are approximately 2.5 times higher in at-risk populations compared to those not considered at risk [7]. When focusing on older adults, 70% of hospital admissions and 77% of associated costs are attributable to individuals over 65 [5].

Across European countries, influenza vaccination is strongly recommended, but not mandatory, for older people. Most countries recommend annual vaccination starting at age 65, except for Estonia, Germany, Greece, Hungary, Netherlands, and Slovakia which use a cut-off age of 60. Austria, uniquely, recommends vaccination beginning at age 45. However, while influenza vaccination is publicly funded in all European countries, Austria, Poland, and Romania are exceptions, where vaccination is partially or fully financed through private payment [8].

The factors influencing influenza vaccination uptake, including both motivators or barriers, are well explored in the literature. The interest in this topic stems from the unique characteristics of influenza vaccines, whose effectiveness varies annually and often remains low [9]. Several systematic reviews have been published listing a set of factors, including demographic characteristics, knowledge, needs, health behaviour, beliefs, health care systems, and social support. Overall, most socioeconomic and demographic individual factors present mixed associations with vaccine uptake [10–14]. It may be useful to highlight some of the factors that influence the decision to take flu shot.

Firstly, among demographic factors, age and sex are associated with vaccination, with women and higher age being more strongly correlated with vaccination. Secondly, socioeconomic predictors include education, marital status, and professional condition. The mixed results in the literature suggest a higher likelihood of vaccination among those with higher levels of education and those who are married. Finally, health-related factors include suffering from a chronic disease, self-assessed health, and previous vaccination history. Among older adults, people with chronic diseases and poorer self-assessed health are more likely to be vaccinated. Additionally, people who have been previously vaccinated are also more prone to be vaccinated. This is related to their experience and confidence in the efficacy of the vaccines and medical science.

Concerning country characteristics, some topics are better explored than others. It is accepted that, in general, countries with higher GDP per capita tend to register higher vaccination rates [15]. Mixed effects and heterogeneity are more likely to occur when attempting to establish a relationship between public health expenditures and vaccination [16]. However, it is more likely that countries with higher public health expenditures are more willing to allocate a larger share to guarantee preventive programs for the population. Therefore, we consider the following hypotheses in our analysis:

H1: Countries with higher GDP per capita have higher rates of flu vaccination uptake.
H2: Countries with higher public health expenditure as a share of GDP have higher rates of flu vaccination uptake.

Other country characteristics potentially related to the uptake of vaccines are linked to cultural attitudes [17]. These are complex and multifaceted across countries. Among the set of cultural characteristics, we focus on trust, both in the national government and in science. There is a well-established finding that countries with higher levels of trust tend to register higher levels of vaccination rates [18–22]. Thus, we also posit the following hypotheses:

H3: Countries with higher trust in the national government have higher rates of flu vaccination uptake.
H4: Countries with higher trust in science have higher rates of flu vaccination uptake.

In this study, we introduce a new approach for assessing population attitudes toward respiratory vaccines. Instead of looking backward, we consider what happens in the future. In this case, the future refers to the COVID-19 vaccination campaign, which took place after the SHARE survey. By considering the way people accepted being vaccinated in the future, it is possible to infer insights about past experiences and the beliefs regarding vaccination. If the past experiences were positive, it is expected that the future uptake of COVID-19 vaccine would be reflect lower hesitancy rates and higher uptakes [23]. Thus, we propose another hypothesis:

H5: Countries experiencing high rates of COVID-19 vaccination, also experienced previous high rates of influenza vaccination.

Lastly, the focus of these research is on countries with Bismark-type health systems. This type of health system is characterised by the financing structure, which is based on social insurance principle, meaning a mandatory contribution paid by employers and employees based on the employee's income. The health funds are usually managed by parties independent from the government. Public financing is provided to those who are not enrolled in the employment insurance system, which may raise challenges in funding the health system during economic crisis time when unemployment raises [24]. Public resources are also used to finance public health programs, such as vaccination initiatives. This type of health systems is found mainly in central-western and eastern European countries.

The other type of health systems found in Europe is the Beveridge-type system, which is adopted by Cyprus, Denmark, Finland, Ireland, Italy, Latvia, Malta, Portugal, Spain, Sweden, and the United Kingdom.

Despite both type of health systems guarantees universal health coverage in accordance with sustainable development goal SDG 3.8, the challenges of each are different. While Beveridge-type health systems may be concerned about waiting lists and patient choice, Bismark-type health systems face more significant challenges related to higher healthcare and administrative costs [24–26]. Bismark and Beveridge health systems differ in financing and provision which shape healthcare delivery and challenges faced by each country. Consequently, it is expected that different approaches to vaccination programs will be found across these types of health systems, so the focus in this study is placed on the Birmakian-type of health systems where health care costs are a current concern. We also postulate that, despite sharing the same type of Bismarkian health system, eastern and western countries display differences concerning the country-related factors associated with individual decisions to take influenza vaccine:

> H6: The factors associated with individual decisions to take influenza vaccine differ between Eastern and Western countries.

The aim of this analysis is twofold: first, to identify the individual characteristics associated with receiving the flu-vaccine, and second, to determine which country-level characteristics may be associated with higher flu-vaccination rates. This study contributes to the literature about the motivators and barriers to influenza vaccine uptake in Europe, specifically in Bismark-type health systems, by jointly exploring micro- and macro-level explanatory factors. To achieve this aim, a logistic regression is estimated using data from Wave 8 of the SHARE survey.

2. Methods

2.1 Sample and population survey

Data utilised in our study originates from the Survey of Health, Ageing and Retirement in Europe (SHARE), Wave 8 [27, 28]. SHARE is a comprehensive international database comprising microdata on health, socio-economic status, and social and familial connections among individuals aged 50 and over who are not institutionalised. The fieldwork for Wave 8 started in October 2019 and was interrupted in March 2020 due to the outbreak of the COVID-19 pandemic. Despite this interruption, the survey continued through phone interviews, and the sample obtained remains consistent with previous waves.

Detailed information regarding methodological aspects of data collection can be found in [29]. For a comprehensive understanding of SHARE, including its description, availability, and updates, interested parties are encouraged to visit the project's official website [27]. Additional acknowledgements concerning SHARE methodology are due to Bergmann and Borsch-Suppan and Borsch-Suppan et al. [30, 31]. Our study's sample comprises 33,334 individuals from 18 European countries.

2.2 Variables

2.2.1 Outcome variable

The outcome variable is obtained from the question whether the respondent took flu vaccine. The variable is labelled 'FluVac' and takes value 1 if the respondent received an influenza vaccination in the last 12 months, and 0 otherwise.

2.2.2 Individual independent variables

Independent variables characterising individual respondent are described in **Table 1**.

From the set of individual independent variables commonly used in this type of analysis, we highlight one less common variable: Make_EndsMeet. This variable complements the income variable and captures household financial stress. While some families may find easy make ends meet, other families may struggle to pay the bills.

Variable label	Description
Demographic	
Male	Takes value 1 if respondent is male; 0 otherwise
Age	Number of years old.
Socio-economic	
Education	Number of schooling and formal education.
Income	Household annual income in constant PPP exchange rate 2019 (Germany 2015 = 1).
Make_EndsMeet	Indicator capturing household financial stress. It takes values between 1 and 4, where 1 means 'with great difficulty' and 4 means 'easily' for the household to make ends meet.
Marital status	Married. Takes value 1 if married; 0 otherwise. The reference category is including single, divorced, and widowed.
Professional situation	Employed. Takes value 1 if employed. Unemployed. Takes value 1 if unemployed. Retired. Takes value 1 if retired. Takes value 0 otherwise. The reference category is 'other' professional situation which includes permanent sick, homemaker, and others.
Health	
SAH	Self-assessed health. Categorical variable taking values from 1 to 5, where 1 means 'excellent' and 5 means 'poor'. The reference category is level 1 (excellent SAH).
Chronic	Number of self-report chronic diseases.
Inpatient	Binary variable reporting if respondent stayed over a night in hospital in the last 12 months. Take value 1 if respondent was inpatient in the previous 12 months; 0 otherwise.

Table 1.
Individual independent variables.

Regarding health-related variables, in addition to self-assessed health (SAH) and chronic diseases, we also include a report of being an inpatient in the previous 12 months, which serves as a proxy for receiving a direct recommendation from a healthcare professional. All three variables proxy not only the respondent's frailty but also their potential contact with healthcare providers, which may influence influenza vaccine uptake.

2.2.3 Country independent variables

The country-level independent variables include the trust in government and trust in science, as well as the share of total public health expenditures, financed through both taxes and mandatory contributions, as a percentage of GDP. This indicator serves as a proxy for the priority a country assigns to the health sector.

Another variable, Eastern_Eur, distinguishes between eastern (including former soviet countries) and western countries. Not only are the historical and geopolitical contexts of these countries different, but a significant economic difference, namely GDP and GDP per capita, may help explain disparities in health outcomes and health

Variable label	Description and source
Country	Country dummy variable.
Eastern_Eur	Dummy variable takes value 1 if country is Eastern Europe: Bulgaria, Croatia, Czechia, Estonia, Hungary, Latvia, Lithuania, Poland, Romania, Slovakia, Slovenia. Otherwise takes value 0 for countries Austria, Belgium, France, Germany, Greece, Netherlands, and Switzerland.
Trust_Gov	Indicator of trust in national government measuring the share of people who trust the national government in 2020. Source: OWD
Trust_Science	Indicator of trust in science measuring the share of people who trust science in 2020. Source: OWD.
OneDoseCovid_Vac	Share of country population who have taken at least one dose of COVID vaccine in 2021. Source: OWD. Except for Bulgaria, Hungary, Romania, and Slovakia in 2023. Source: ECDC.
THE/GDP	Public finance indicator measuring the total health expenditures as a share of GDP in 2018. Source: Eurostat database.

Table 2.
Country characteristic variables.

care provision. Eastern countries are mainly characterised by a lower level of these economic variables.

Finally, we include a variable, labelled OneDoseCovid_Vac, to capture potential experience with vaccination and beliefs in the effectiveness of vaccination. This variable acts as a proxy for intertemporal attitudes toward respiratory vaccines (**Table 2**).

2.3 Quantitative approach

Following a descriptive statistical analysis, the quantitative method employed to examine the factors associated with flu vaccination uptake is logistic regression. The estimation results are presented as odd ratios. Additionally, several goodness-of-fit measures are computed, including *linktest*, Pearson statistic, area under the ROC (receiver operating characteristic) curve, sensitivity, specificity, accuracy, and the information criteria AIC and BIC.

Logistic regression estimation is estimated using three different model specifications, based on the country-level variables included. The first specification includes country dummy variables; second includes only the total public health expenditures as a percentage of GDP; and the third specification includes a dummy variable for eastern countries, trust variables, and the national COVID-19 vaccination rate (at least one dose). Additionally, separate logistic regressions are estimated for eastern and western countries, with results presented in the Appendix. All estimations and computations are performed in STATA.14.

3. Results

We begin this section by presenting some descriptive statistics. The average flu or influenza vaccination uptake among respondents aged over 50 in the 18 European countries is about 30%. This figure is highly heterogenous across countries as shown,

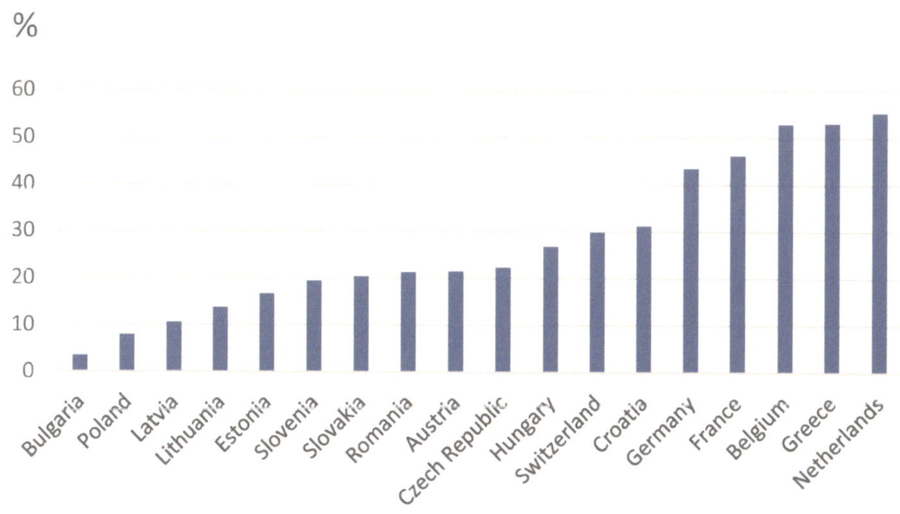

Figure 1.
Percentage of people taking flu vaccine.

in **Figure 1**. It is evident that eastern European countries tend to exhibit significantly lower vaccination rates compared to their western counterparts. The country with the lowest reported uptake is Bulgaria, where 3.47% respondents indicated they have received a flu vaccine, while the Netherlands has the highest uptake, with 55.4% of people reporting vaccination. Austria, although a Western country, records the lowest vaccination rate; notably, it is also the only Western country where influenza vaccination is not publicly funded.

In **Table 3**, the descriptive statistics for the individual-level independent variables are presented.

Most respondents are female, the mean age is nearly 71 years, and the average number of years of education is about 11. Most respondents are married and retired. Regarding health indicators, the majority report a self-assessed health status below 'fair' and suffer from an average of two chronic conditions. Additionally, a small percentage of 16.7% of respondents reported spending at least one night in the hospital in the past 12 months.

Concerning the country characteristics, for which data are presented in Appendix (**Table A1**), we report the pairwise correlations between variables in **Table 4**. Among these correlations, it is worth noting the very high correlation (around 88%) between the share of THE_GDP and the eastern countries variable. This correlation is expected, as eastern European countries tend to have lower levels of both GDP and THE compared to Western European countries. This extremely high correlation prevents the joint inclusion of the THE_GDP and Eastern_ countries variable in the logistic regression due to multicollinearity. Another noteworthy correlation is between Trust in Science and the percentage of people receiving at least one dose of the COVID-19 vaccine in 2021. The correlation, being below 50%, indicates a weak association, which allows for speculative interpretations of potential inconsistencies in public behaviour.

We now present the results of the logistic regression explaining the factors associated flu vaccination uptake.

The results are reported in **Table 5**, which displays three model specifications: the first includes country fixed effects, the second incorporates the percentage of THE in

Variable	Obs	Mean	Std. dev.
Demographic			
Male	33,334	0.419	0.493
Age (years)	33,334	70.553	9.277
Socio-economic			
Education (years)	33,334	11.277	3.960
Income (euros/year)	33,334	22589.06	34570.14
Make_EndsMeet (1 & 2)	32,966	0.405	1.003
Married	33,334	0.659	0.474
Employed	33,334	0.174	0.379
Unemployed	33,334	0.019	0.135
Retired	33,334	0.706	0.456
Health			
SAH (self-assessed health)			
1	33,334	0.045	0.208
2	33,334	0.149	0.356
3	33,334	0.395	0.489
4	33,334	0.297	0.457
5	33,334	0.113	0.317
Chronic (number of diseases)	33,334	1.962	1.639
Inpatient	33,334	0.167	0.373

Note: Obs means observations; Std. dev means standard deviation.

Table 3.
Descriptive statistics for individual independent variables.

	Eastern	FLUvac	Trust_ Gov	Trust_ Science	OneDose Covid_vac
Trust_Gov	−0.6097	0.1209			
	(0.000)	(0.000)			
Trust_Science	−0.2101	0.0849	0.5048		
	(0.000)	(0.000)	(0.000)		
OneDoseCovid_vac	−0.7194	0.2320	0.5327	0.4831	
	(0.000)	(0.000)	(0.000)	(0.000)	
THE_GDP	−0.8804	0.2374	0.7510	0.4918	0.6825
	(0.000)	(0.000)	(0.000)	(0.000)	(0.000)

Note: in parenthesis p-values.

Table 4.
Pairwise correlations across country variables.

Variable	Specification 1		Specification 2		Specification 3	
	OR	P > |z|	OR	P > |z|	OR	P > |z|
Demographic						
Male	0.968	0.255	1.027	0.322	0.983	0.543
Age	1.045	0.000	1.046	0.000	1.046	0.000
Socio-economic						
Education	1.027	0.000	1.030	0.000	1.033	0.000
Income	1.000	0.080	1.000	0.010	1.000	0.053
Make_ends_meet	1.152	0.000	0.950	0.001	1.069	0.000
Alone/single/widow (REF)						
Married	1.282	0.000	1.409	0.000	1.364	0.000
Other labor status (REF)						
Employed	0.892	0.058	0.652	0.000	0.835	0.002
Unemployed	0.564	0.000	0.393	0.000	0.539	0.000
Retired	1.049	0.332	0.704	0.000	0.929	0.121
Health						
SAH 1 – excellent (REF)						
2 – very good	1.419	0.000	1.304	0.000	1.303	0.000
3 – good	1.657	0.000	1.398	0.000	1.522	0.000
4 – fair	1.818	0.000	1.375	0.000	1.622	0.000
5 – poor	1.309	0.002	0.949	0.518	1.181	0.046
Chronic	1.159	0.000	1.149	0.000	1.138	0.000
Inpatient	1.278	0.000	1.122	0.001	1.192	0.000
Country						
Germany	2.923	0.000				
Netherlands	5.398	0.000				
France	3.562	0.000				
Greece	6.695	0.000				
Switzerland	1.860	0.000				
Belgium	4.673	0.000				
Czech Republic	0.981	0.819				
Poland	0.355	0.000				
Hungary	1.721	0.000				
Slovenia	0.986	0.872				
Estonia	0.766	0.002				
Croatia	2.268	0.000				
Lithuania	0.683	0.000				
Bulgaria	0.191	0.000				
Latvia	0.583	0.000				

Variable	Specification 1		Specification 2		Specification 3	
	OR	P > |z|	OR	P > |z|	OR	P > |z|
Romania	1.587	0.000				
Slovakia	1.755	0.000				
Country characteristics						
THE_GDP			1.297	0.000		
EasternEur					0.183	0.000
Trust_Gov					0.982	0.000
Trust_Science					1.023	0.000
OneDoseCovid_Vac					0.998	0.425
_cons	0.002	0.000	0.001	0.000	0.004	0.000
Number of obs	32,855		32,855		32,855	
Wald chi2(32)	4526.590		3053.370		3981.550	
Prob > chi2	0.000		0.000		0.000	
Pseudo R2	0.155		0.090		0.124	
Pearson chi2 (Prob>chi2)	33605.990	(0.001)	32965.82	(0.267)	33295.80	(0.028)
Area under ROC curve	0.761		0.704		0.735	
AIC	34053.90		36613.88		35283.65	
BIC	34331.09		36756.67		35451.65	
Sensitivity	0.406		0.235		0.346	
Specificity	0.904		0.928		0.908	
Correctly classified	0.754		0.719		0.739	

Note: OR means odd-ratio; p-value of 0.000 means p-value < 0.001; REF means reference category.

Table 5.
Logistic regression estimation results.

GDP as a country-level characteristics, and the third includes a set of country-specific factors potentially influencing vaccine uptake.

Findings concerning individual characteristics show that "sex," "income," or financial strain ("make ends meet") are not significant and exhibit little association with flu vaccination uptake. On the other hand, "education" and being "married" positively influence the decision to take the vaccine.

A more concerning finding is that individuals who are labour active, whether "employed" or "unemployed," are less likely to get vaccinated, likely because these people tend to be younger. Lastly, health-related individual factors indicate that "self-assessed health" (SAH) is significant and promotes vaccination, although there is no linear relationship between the level of SAH and the likelihood of vaccination. As expected, people suffering from "chronic" diseases or those who have been hospitalised ("inpatient") are also more likely to take a flu vaccine.

Findings concerning country characteristics reveal that countries with higher percentage of total health expenditure as a share of GDP are nearly 30% (OR = 1.297, p-value < 0.001) more likely to have a higher flu vaccination rate, thus confirming hypothesis H2. Eastern countries exhibit a substantial reduction of 81.7% (OR = 0.183, p-value < 0.001) in the odds of flu vaccination compared with western countries. The effects of trust in government and science are more nuanced. While countries with higher levels of trust in science show a 2% increase in the odds of flu vaccination (confirming hypothesis H4), countries with higher levels of trust in the national government have a nearly 2% decrease in the odds of flu vaccination (OR = 0.982, p-value < 0.001), contrary to the expectations outlined in hypothesis H3. The potential cultural effect of vaccination, measured by the uptake of COVID-19 vaccine, was not supported by the data, as no empirical evidence confirms this relationship (hypothesis H5 is not confirmed).

Concerning the model's goodness of fit, specification 1 appears to provide the best fit data, with a higher area under ROC curve, lower AIC and BIC values, better accuracy in correctly classified cases.

Additionally, two separate logistic regressions for Eastern and Western countries were estimated. The results are presented in the Appendix, **Table A2**.

Evidence comparing these two groups of countries reveals several notable differences (H6 is confirmed). While western countries display the inverse U-shaped relationship between self-assessed health, with 'fair' health status having a peak odds, and flu vaccination, eastern countries exhibit a flatter and more stable relationship. Trust in science is a stronger predictor in western countries (OR = 1.38, p-value < 0.001) compared to eastern countries (OR = 1.039, p-value < 0.001). Lastly, there is no evidence of a relationship between flu vaccination and the COVID-19 vaccination uptake in eastern countries, while a deterrent effect of current flu vaccination on future COVID-19 vaccination is observed in western countries, suggesting other factors may be influencing these patterns and warranting further investigation.

A summary of the results found for country characteristics is presented in **Table 6**.

Hypothesis concerning country characteristics	Testing variable	Estimated correlation sign	Reference
H1: Countries with higher GDP per capita have higher rates of flu vaccination uptake.	Countries and/or THE_GDP	Positive	[15, 16]
H2: Countries with higher public health expenditure as a share of GDP have higher rates of flu vaccination uptake.	THE_GDP	Positive	[15, 16]
H3: Countries with higher trust in the national government have higher rates of flu vaccination uptake.	Trust_Gov	Negative	[17–22]
H4: Countries with higher trust in science have higher rates of flu vaccination uptake	Trust_ Science	Positive	[17–22]
H5: Countries experiencing high rates of COVID-19 vaccination, also experienced previous high rates of influenza vaccination.	OneDoseCovid_Vac	Non-significative	[23]
H6: The factors associated with individual decisions to take influenza vaccine differ between eastern and western countries.	Eastern_Eur Additional to group comparison.	Negative	[24–26]

Table 6.
Summary results for country characteristics.

4. Discussion

The analysis presented here had a dual purpose: firstly, to identify the individual characteristics linked to the decision to take flu vaccine, and secondly, to ascertain which national characteristics may predispose populations to higher flu vaccination acceptance. This research adds to the existing literature on micro- and macro-factors associated to flu vaccination in Europe, particularly in Bismarck-type health systems.

The key findings of this research are grouped into individual and country characteristics. First group of findings relates to individual factors associated with taking flu vaccine [10–14]. Labor-active individuals, either employed or unemployed, are less likely to get vaccinated. On the one hand, these people tend to be younger; on the other hand, employed individuals may not find the time to have the flu shot and unemployed people may consider it unimportant since it does not cause labour costs due to absenteeism. However, this result tends to disappear when the analysis accounts for Eastern and Western countries separately, with no evidence found for employed individuals in Western countries.

Self-assessed health does not display a linear relationship with the likelihood of flu vaccine uptake, a finding not consistently reported in other studies [4, 10, 12]. Instead, there is an inverted U-shape relationship, with the peak occurring at the "fair" level of self-assessed health status. However, when analysing eastern and western countries separately, some differences become apparent. In eastern countries, more education increases the odds of vaccination by about 4%, while in western countries the effect is reduced to 1.7%. While the inverted U-shape holds for self-assessed health in western countries, is more stable to happen in eastern countries, with the peak occurring at median health levels.

The second group of key finding concerns the country-independent variables. Countries with higher priority on health, as indicated by the share of health expenditures in the GDP, tend to have a higher likelihood of flu vaccination uptake, with nearly 30% higher odds. However, when the analysis is conducted separately for eastern and western countries, we find no evidence of this relationship in eastern countries and even a negative association between health expenditures and the odds of taking the flu vaccine. This result does not correspond with previous literature and may be worth of future research.

On the other hand, in eastern countries, people are nearly 82% less likely to get vaccinated compared to western countries, as expected from previous studies. These differences may be explained by several reasons such as historical determinants, poor communication in the health and science toward people, lack of health education, difficult access, and low trust in the government or in general [32, 33].

Trust in science plays a role in flu vaccination uptake, whereas the opposite is true for trust in the national government, which seems to have a negative effect across all countries [18–22]. Nevertheless, trust in science is stronger in Western countries than in Eastern countries, most likely due to differences in education levels among older people.

Finally, past experience and beliefs do not seem to be reflected in future vaccination 70 decisions, except in Western countries. In these countries evidence shows that the odds of taking 71 flu vaccine in the present are inversely related to COVID-19 vaccine coverage. This result is unexpected and raises questions about intertemporal behavioural consistency and how other factors may influence past experiences. Despite this surprising finding, new evidence suggests an inverse correlation between flu vaccination and COVID-19 vaccination [34]. According to this study, the likelihood of the elderly getting vaccinated against COVID-19 is much higher than that of receiving the flu vaccine.

These findings contribute to the discussion in the literature on the factors associated with the flu vaccination uptake, which has specific characteristics compared to other vaccines that are typically administered only once in a lifetime. This study highlights the heterogeneity across Bismark countries in terms of flu vaccination, which becomes more pronounced when comparing eastern and western countries.

Other findings from this analysis align with existing literature, which shows that individual characteristics vary by country, groups of countries, timing, demographic groups, surveys, and so on [10–14]. Our study found no evidence linking flu vaccination uptake with sex or retirement status. Common factors associated with flu vaccination uptake include older age, higher education levels, and being married.

From a policy design perspective, some measures focused on education and health literacy may be suggested. Primary care doctors and community pharmacists could provide basic scientific information to reduce vaccination misconceptions. Additionally, countries where higher health spending does not translate into higher vaccine uptake may need to reorient investments toward community-based outreach, transparent communication campaigns, and mechanisms that rebuild institutional trust; the behavioural nudges approach may also be considered in seasonal vaccination to increment spillover effects between different vaccines.

5. Limitations

The analysis presented here, based on a logistic regression, does not account for all potential factors that may influence the individual decision to take flu vaccines such as the consultations with primary care and specialists, past vaccination experience, peer effects, and others. Additionally, it does not consider the potential role of private insurance, which may influence vaccination decisions to prevent future healthcare costs. Finally, this analysis does not allow to make causal inference. Cross-sectional logistic regression establishes associations or correlations, not causality, except perhaps in the case of intertemporal variables.

Another limitation worth mentioning is related to the sample. SHARE Wave 8 took place in a very turbulent time [29–31]. It started by collecting data in a face-to-face computer-assisted personal interview (CAPI). Since then, a specific survey was carried out via computer-assisted telephone interviews (CATI). So, the sources of data are both CAPI and CATI which may imply that in some sensitive variables the answers by respondents may not be completely comparable. The pandemic has also caused some dropouts, reducing the sample in some countries, even though the sample sizes allow for consistent analysis [29–31]. Moreover, as countries were hit differently across time, that means that the data collection was different across countries, which implies a cautious comparison [29–31]. Nevertheless, this study focuses only on a single wave of SHARE, and it does not perform a longitudinal analysis. Also, its focus is mainly on the country level rather than on the individual level.

6. Conclusion

The Bismark-type health system in European encompass a heterogeneous group of countries that can broadly be classified into eastern and western countries. Despite structural similarities, notable differences in vaccination-related factors justify the need for context-specific analysis.

The findings support policies focused on improving education, a consistent determinant of vaccination uptake. While trust in science plays a relatively minor role, this underscores the need for better science communication strategies to enhance public trust. Finally, further investigation into the inverted U-shape relationship between self-assessed health and flu vaccination could help design interventions that address vaccine hesitancy by targeting underlying beliefs, expectations, and perceived health risks.

Acknowledgements

The author AIT acknowledges that CEISUC/CiBB is funded by national funds through FCT – Foundation for Science and Technology, I.P., under the Multiannual Financing of R&D Units.

Conflict of interest

The authors declare no conflict of interest.

Declaration of generative AI and AI-assisted technologies in the writing process

During the preparation of this work, the author used ChatGPT in order to improve the readability and language of the manuscript.

A. Appendix

	Trust the national government	Trust in science	At least one COVID vaccine dose	THE/GDP
	2020	2020	2021	2018
Austria	73.4	89.5	75.03	10.35
Belgium	54.9	93.4	76.70	10.86
Bulgaria	40.4	81.9	30.50[a]	7.33
Croatia	42.0	89.5	56.06	6.73
Czechia	45.8	94.8	65.03	6.83
Estonia	56.0	91.8	63.50	6.69
France	56.3	94.1	78.50	11.21
Germany	82.0	96.7	75.27	11.48
Greece	40.7	83.0	71.92	8.12
Hungary	48.6	93.6	65.30[a]	6.58
Latvia	39.6	85.1	71.01	6.19

	Trust the national government	Trust in science	At least one COVID vaccine dose	THE/GDP
	2020	2020	2021	2018
Lithuania	55.1	83.6	69.74	6.53
Netherlands	78.5	90.3	70.68	10.20
Poland	33.6	87.2	54.38	6.31
Romania	24.3	79.5	42.50[a]	5.52
Slovakia	53.5	92.3	52.00[a]	6.67
Slovenia	48.1	88.9	58.99	8.28
Switzerland	93.3	89.3	68.26	10.77

[a]*2023, ECDC.*
Source: Our-World-in-Data (ourworldindata.org/) and ECDC (https://www.ecdc.europa.eu/en); THE/GDP - Eurostat (https://ec.europa.eu/eurostat/data/database).

Table A1.
Data on country characteristics.

	Eastern countries		Western countries	
	OR	P > z	OR	P > z
Male	0.932	0.097	0.986	0.712
Age	1.029	0.000	1.055	0.000
Education	1.041	0.000	1.017	0.000
Income	1.000	0.011	1.000	0.079
SAH				
2	1.586	0.006	1.238	0.010
3	1.523	0.009	1.478	0.000
4	1.538	0.009	1.693	0.000
5	1.200	0.296	1.354	0.005
Married	1.401	0.000	1.221	0.000
Employed	1.062	0.578	0.759	0.000
Unemployed	0.427	0.001	0.680	0.023
Retired	1.079	0.442	1.069	0.262
Make_EndMeet	1.146	0.000	1.111	0.000
Chronic	1.121	0.000	1.159	0.000
Inpatient	1.305	0.000	1.220	0.000
THE_GDP	0.945	0.119	0.648	0.000
Trust_Gov	0.994	0.080	0.939	0.000
Trust_Science	1.039	0.000	1.384	0.000
OneDoseCovid_Vac	0.997	0.314	0.727	0.000
_cons	0.000	0.000	0.069	0.012
Number of obs	17,416		15,439	

	Eastern countries		Western countries	
	OR	P > z	OR	P > z
Wald chi2(19)	579.86		1831.31	
Prob > chi2	0.00		0.00	
Pseudo R2	0.04		0.11	
Area under ROC curve	0.6369		0.7230	

Table A2.
Logistic regression for group of countries.

Author details

Aida Isabel Tavares[1,2]

1 ISEG, UL – Lisbon School of Economics and Management, University of Lisbon, Lisbon, Portugal

2 CEISUC – Centre for Health Studies and Research, University of Coimbra, Coimbra, Portugal

*Address all correspondence to: aitavar@gmail.com; atavares@iseg.ulisboa.pt

References

[1] European Centre for Disease Prevention and Control (ECDC). 2023. Available from: https://www.ecdc.europa.eu/en/seasonal-influenza

[2] European Centre for Disease Prevention and Control (ECDC). 2023. Available from: https://www.ecdc.europa.eu/en/seasonal-influenza/prevention-and-control/vaccines/risk-groups

[3] Kim H, Webster RG, Webby RJ. Influenza virus: Dealing with a drifting and shifting pathogen. Viral Immunology. 2018;**31**:174-183

[4] Bartoszko JJ, Loeb M. The burden of influenza in older adults: Meeting the challenge. Aging Clinical and Experimental Research. 2019;**33**:711-717

[5] Lemaitre M, Fayssoil F, Carrat F, et al. Estimating the burden of influenza-related and associated hospitalizations and deaths in France: An eight-season data study, 2010–2018. Influenza and Other Respiratory Viruses. 2021;**16**:717-725

[6] Paget J, Danielle Iuliano A, Taylor RJ, et al. Estimates of mortality associated with seasonal influenza for the European Union from the GLaMOR project. Vaccine. 2022;**40**(9):1361-1369

[7] de Courville C, Cadarette SM, Wissinger EL, Alvarez FP. The economic burden of influenza among adults aged 18 to 64: A systematic literature review. Influenza and Other Respiratory Viruses. 2022;**16**:376-385

[8] European Centre for Disease Prevention and Control (ECDC). 2023. Available from: https://vaccine-schedule.ecdc.europa.eu/Scheduler/ByDisease?SelectedDiseaseId=15&SelectedCountryIdByDisease=-1

[9] Osterholm MT, Kelley NS, Sommer A, Belongia EA. Efficacy and effectiveness of influenza vaccines: A systematic review and meta-analysis. The Lancet Infectious Diseases. 2012;**12**:36-44. DOI: 10.1016/S1473-3099(11)70295-X

[10] Bish A, Yardley L, Nicoll A, Michie S. Factors associated with uptake of vaccination against pandemic influenza: A systematic review. Vaccine. 2011;**29**(38):6472-6484

[11] Yeung MP, Lam FL, Coker RJ. Factors associated with the uptake of seasonal influenza vaccination in adults: A systematic review. Journal of Public Health. 2016;**38**(4):746-753

[12] Kohlhammer Y, Schnoor M, Schwartz M, et al. Determinants of influenza and pneumococcal vaccination in elderly people: A systematic review. Public Health. 2007;**121**(10):742-751

[13] Schmid P, Rauber D, Betsch C, et al. Barriers of influenza vaccination intention and behavior – A systematic review of influenza vaccine hesitancy, 2005 – 2016. PLoS One. 2017;**12**(1):e0170550. DOI: 10.1371/journal.pone.0170550

[14] Viswanath K, Bekalu M, Dhawan D, et al. Individual and social determinants of COVID-19 vaccine uptake. BMC Public Health. 2021;**21**:818. DOI: 10.1186/s12889-021-10862-1

[15] Moradpour J, Shajarizadeh A, Carter J, et al. The impact of national income and vaccine hesitancy on country-level COVID-19 vaccine uptake.

PLoS One. 2023;**18**(11):e0293184. DOI: 10.1371/journal.pone.0293184

[16] Ethgen O, Rémy V, Wargo K. Vaccination budget in Europe: An update. Human Vaccines & Immunotherapeutics. 2018;**14**(12): 2911-2915. DOI: 10.1080/ 21645515.2018.1504528

[17] Leonhardt JM, Pezzuti T. Vaccination acceptance across cultures: The roles of collectivism, empathy, and homophily. Journal of International Marketing. 2022;**30**(2):13-27. DOI: 10.1177/1069031X211073179

[18] Viskupi F, Wiltse DL, Meyer BA. Trust in physicians and trust in government predict COVID-19 vaccine uptake. Social Science Quarterly. 2022; **103**(3):509-520. DOI: 10.1111/ssqu. 13147

[19] Jennings W, Valgarosson V, McKay L, et al. Trust and vaccine hesitancy during the COVID-19 pandemic: A cross-national analysis. Vaccine X. 2023;**14**:100299. DOI: 10.1016/j.jvacx.2023.100299

[20] Thornton J. Covid-19: Trust in government and other people linked with lower infection rate and higher vaccination uptake. BMJ. 2022;**376**:o292. DOI: 10.1136/bmj.o292

[21] Bajos N, Spire A, Silberzan L, et al. When lack of Trust in the Government and in scientists reinforces social inequalities in vaccination against COVID-19. Frontiers in Public Health. 2022;**10**:908152. DOI: 10.3389/ fpubh.2022.908152

[22] Sturgis P, Brunton-Smith I, Jackson J. Trust in science, social consensus and vaccine confidence. Nature Human Behaviour. 2021;**5**: 1528-1534. DOI: 10.1038/s41562-021-01115-7

[23] Kumar D, Chandra R, Mathur M, et al. Vaccine hesitancy: Understanding better to address better. Israel Journal Health Policy Research. 2016;**5**:2. DOI: 10.1186/s13584-016-0062-y

[24] Liaropoulos L, Goranitis I. Health care financing and the sustainability of health systems. International Journal for Equity in Health. 2015;**14**:80. DOI: 10.1186/s12939-015-0208-5

[25] Or Z, Cases C, Lisac M, Vrangbaek K, Winblad U, Bevan G. Are health problems systemic? Politics of access and choice under Beveridge and Bismarck systems. Health Economics, Policy and Law. 2010;**5**:269-293

[26] van der Zee J, Kroneman MW. Bismarck or Beveridge: A beauty contest between dinosaurs. BMC Health Services Research. 2007;7:94. DOI: 10.1186/ 1472-6963-7-94

[27] SHARE. 2023. Available from: https://share-eric.eu/data/data-documentation/waves-overview/ wave-8

[28] Börsch-Supan A. Survey of Health, Ageing and Retirement in Europe (SHARE) Wave 8. Release Version: 8.0.0. SHARE-ERIC. Data set; 2022. Available from: https://share-eric.eu/ data/data-documentation/waves-overview/wave-8. DOI: 10.6103/SHARE. w8.800

[29] Scherpenzeel A, Axt K, Bergmann M, et al. Collecting survey data among the 50+ population during the COVID-19 outbreak: The survey of health, ageing and retirement in Europe (SHARE). Survey Research Methods. 2020;**14**(2):217-221

[30] Bergmann M, Börsch-Supan A, editors. SHARE Wave 8 Methodology: Collecting Cross-National Survey Data in

Times of COVID-19. Munich: MEA, Max Planck Institute for Social Law and Social Policy; 2021. Available from: https://share-eric.eu/data/data-documentation/waves-overview/wave-8

[31] Börsch-Supan A, Brandt M, Hunkler C, Kneip T, Korbmacher J, Malter F, et al. Data resource profile: The survey of health, ageing and retirement in Europe (SHARE). International Journal of Epidemiology. 2013. Available from: https://share-eric.eu/data/data-documentation/waves-overview/wave-8. DOI: 10.1093/ije/dyt088

[32] ILC. 2023. Shifting the Narrative: Improving vaccine uptake in Central & Eastern Europe'. Available from: https://ilcuk.org.uk/vaccine-confidence-in-ce-europe/

[33] Fan G, Song H, Yip S, Zhang T, He D. Impact of low vaccine coverage on the resurgence of COVID-19 in Central and Eastern Europe. One Health (Amsterdam, Netherlands). 2022;**14**: 100402. DOI: 10.1016/j.onehlt.2022.100402

[34] Tang S, Ji L, Bishwajit G, Guo S. Uptake of COVID-19 and influenza vaccines in relation to preexisting chronic conditions in the European countries. BMC Geriatrics. 2024;**24**(1): 56. DOI: 10.1186/s12877-023-04623-5

Chapter 4

Costs of Primary Health Care in a Riverside and Rural Context of the Brazilian Amazon

Cláudio Pontes Ferreira, Júlio Cesar Schweickardt and Rodrigo Tobias

Abstract

Access to healthcare is a particular challenge in extreme and remote contexts. In Brazil, primary care has led to remarkable improvements in healthcare access in peri-urban and rural contexts such as Basic Fluvial Health Unit. This chapter's objective is to demonstrate the costs of a Basic Fluvial Health Unit in the municipality of Tefé in Amazonas State, Brazil. This experience reports the health costs for the Legal Amazon region. We use primary data collected directly from the municipal management, thus obtaining a real value per displacement in service, maintenance, logistics, HR and health supplies. In nine trips made in 10 months, with a total cost of R$ 761,705.87 (U$190,426.47), human resources represented 64.62% of the total costs analysed, followed by inputs for health actions (17.72%), and fuel (12.11%). It was demonstrated that the allocated resources represent a significant amount for the development of actions to promote the health of riverside populations by the Basic Fluvial Health Unit in Tefé, observing the seasonality of the rivers and rainfall arranged in the fluid territory of the Brazilian Amazon region.

Keywords: cost analysis, primary health care, access to health services, fluid territory, health promotion

1. Introduction

The Basic River Health Units (UBSF) were created in 2013 as a strategy to take healthcare into the Amazon territory to isolated populations in the Legal Amazon [1–4]. Epidemiological data show that the absence of a health service within the territory greatly increases morbidity rates. Because the main access is by river, the riverside populations find it very difficult to reach health services, as, on average, they have to travel 60.4 kilometres, taking an average of 4.2 hours to reach the urban area of the municipality [5, 6].

Studies in riverine areas show high rates of hypertension, with around 26% of the adult population living in these areas, increasing across the age range, with a predominance of males [7]. This new health technology model was designed to meet the needs of riverine populations, which were previously met by boats without adequate structures in so-called health campaigns. This strategy aimed to combat the inequality

IntechOpen

that exists in this immense territory, cut off by rivers, lakes, and streams, to meet a specific and unique demand. At the same time as it filled this care gap, it brought to the debate the costs of the Amazon and the need to understand these values of doing health in the Amazonian context [8–10].

There is a great need for economic studies that incorporate the Amazonian factor and quantify the costs of healthcare in the northern region [11, 12]. We need more research because we know that a lot of health programme funding disregards the Amazon factor, since fixed and variable costs change according to the "coming and going of the waters" because even fixed costs, such as the health team, for example, can change during the period when the river is flowing, this is the "liquid territory" of the riverside populations [13–16].

In the Amazon region, primary care has made significant progress. The creation of specific Primary Care teams for the region, such as the Riverine Family Health Teams (ESFRIb) and the River Family Health Team (ESFF), has played a fundamental role in expanding health services in hard-to-reach areas and strengthening links between health professionals and local communities. Between 2011 and 2017, there was a 68-fold increase in the number of riverine health teams set up, resulting in 205. As for the UBSF, there were 4 in 2013, rising to 8 more in 2018, as 7 of the 12 units were accredited, observing the federal financial inducement [17].

Specifically in Amazonas, there is an urgent need for an applied study of the Amazonian factor in the day-to-day running of health services and the tools of health economics that can help in this analysis [11]. Studies on economic evaluations and analyses can provide an important tool for management, helping with decision-making.

We therefore have the challenge of measuring the costs in the Amazon. These additional values generated, for example, by difficulties in travelling, transport, communication, logistics and access routes to riverside areas, are hardly ever demonstrated. This is why studies into these impacts are so important [18]. Only with scientific evidence can we discuss whether the amounts passed on by the Ministry of Health meet these specific needs.

Understanding the costs of this new care model is the problem that generated the research question. To this end, cost analysis tools can help improve planning processes and are important for analysing and establishing priorities for future programmes or actions planned for the northern region [19].

Understanding the costs of the innovative care model is the problem that generated the research question. Based on questioning the costs involved in the maintenance and operation of the health unit to produce healthcare in riverside areas of a municipality of great social vulnerability, this study aims to analyse the costs of a River UBS in the municipality of Tefé, Amazonas.

2. Methods

This is a descriptive, quantitative case study on economic evaluation through cost analysis, with the aim of analysing the costs of a basic health unit in the municipality of Tefé-AM between June 2018 and March 2019, according to **Figure 1**.

In order to carry out the proposed work, it was decided to carry out the survey directly at Tefé City Hall, with the support of the Municipal Health Department, where the data was collected before each trip.

The municipality has 89 communities. The UBSF will serve 30 communities, with 432 registered families and a population of 2051 people to be served. The others are

DOI: http://dx.doi.org/10.5772/intechopen.1004776

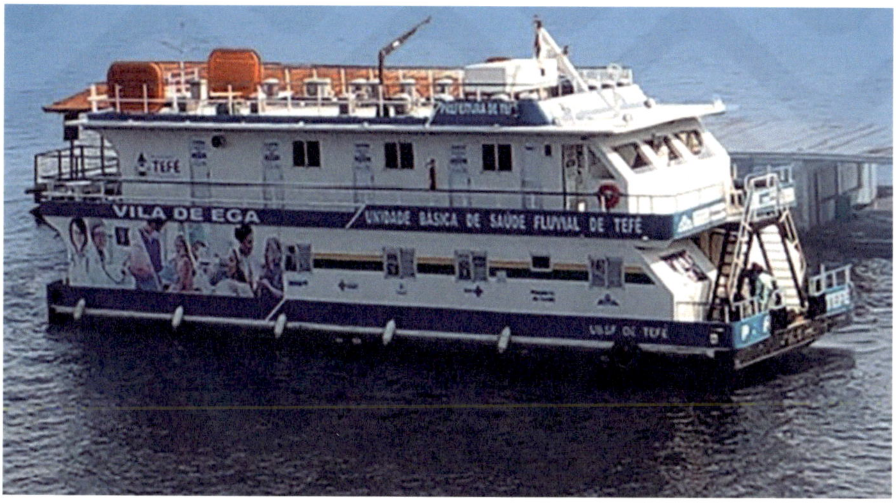

Figure 1.
Vila de Ega Tefé-AM River Health Unit, 2020. Source: Tefé City Hall.

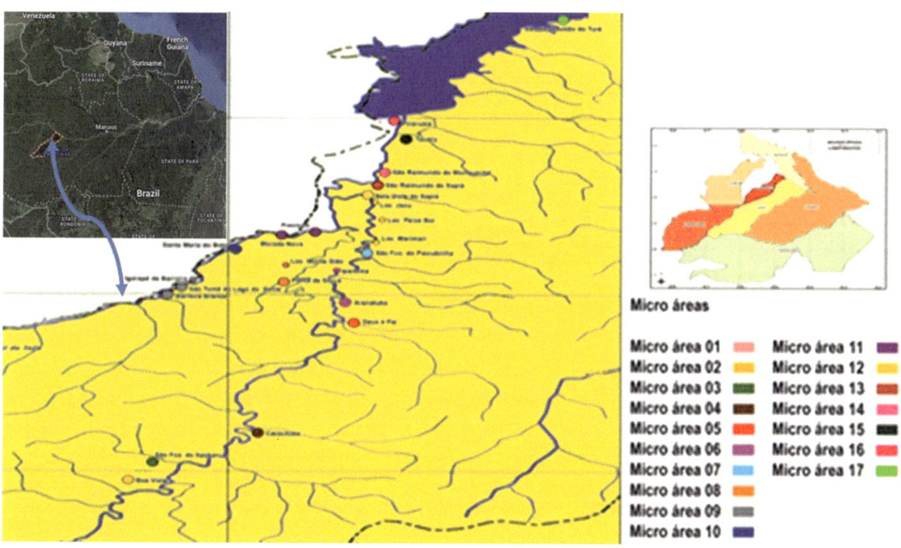

Figure 2.
Area of UBS Fluvial Vila de Ega operation, Tefé-AM, 2020. Source: Municipal Secretariat of Tefé-AM.

covered by the riverine family health strategy—eSFR. This population is covered by team 15—eSFFSB—Fluvial Family Health Team with Oral Health, which serves the riverside population on the Solimões River, Lago do Jutica, and Lago do Catuá, as **Figure 2** shown below [20].

The recurring cost of the basic unit was stratified by journeys, thus obtaining a real cost per journey on duty, i.e. an estimate for each journey to provide care: UBSF structure, UBSF equipment, fuel, cooking gas, foodstuffs, hygiene and cleaning materials, boat maintenance, office supplies, human resources, and health products. The cost considered for the salaries of the professionals who work at the UBSF was gross. For the other costing items, information was collected directly from Tefé City

Hall using a spreadsheet [21]. The results were presented in Brazilian currency (Real: R$) corresponding to U$ 0.25.

The study project is part of the research project of the Laboratory of History, Public Policies and Health in the Amazon - LAHPSA entitled "Access of the riverside population to the Urgency and Emergency Network in the State of Amazonas" and approved by the Research Ethics Committee—CEP of the Federal University of Amazonas, under CAAE: 99460918.3.0000.5020.

3. Results

The UBSF in Tefé made nine (9) trips during the period studied, from June 2018 to March 2019, covering ten (10) areas served: three trips to area 10, two to area 11, one to area 14, one to area 19 and three to area 21.

The UBSFs work 20 days a month in a defined area, including travelling by river to the communities and providing direct care to the riverside population. On other days, the boat can be moored in the harbor, at the municipality's headquarters, so that the River Family Health Teams (eSFF) can carry out planning and continuing education activities with other professionals. In this scenario, the longest trip that the UBSF made lasted 18 days, and the shortest trip lasted 8 days.

The total cost of these trips, as shown in **Table 1**, was R$761,705.87 (U$190.426.47), representing a monthly average of R$84,633.99.

Macro area	Location	Travel date	Travel cost	FNS transfer
Area 21	Tefé River	23/06/2018 to 04/07/2018	R$ 103,920.79 (U$25,980.20)	R$ 0.00
Area 11	Vila do Caiambé/Lake Caiambé	07/08/2018 to 15/08/2018	R$ 75,058.80 (U$18,764.70)	R$ 90,000 (U$22,500)
Area 10	Solimões River, Jutica Lake, Catuá	23/08/2018 to 07/09/2018	R$ 61,929.38 (U$15,482.34)	R$ 90,000.00 (U$22,500.00)
Area 21	Tefé River	14/09/2018 to 02/10/2018	R$ 87,392.78 (U$21,848.20)	R$ 90,000 (U$22,500)
Area 10	Solimões River, Jutica Lake, Catuá	22/11/2018 to 02/12/2018	R$ 72,757.53 (U$18,189.38)	R$ 111,390 (U$27,847.50)
Area 11	Vila do Caiambé/Lake Caiambé	13/12/2018 to 22/12/2018	R$ 78,281.27 (U$19,570.31)	R$ 146,558 (U$36,659)
Area 14 and Area 19	Tarará Island, Tefé and Bacuri Coast, Curupira	08/01/2019 to 19/01/2019	R$ 116,790.38 (U$29,197.60)	R$ 146,558 (U$36,659)
Area 21	Tefé River	09/02/2019 to 21/02/2019	R$ 99,227.04 (U$24,806.76)	R$ 146,558 (U$36,659)
Area 10	Solimões River, Jutica Lake, Catuá	02/03/2018 to 12/03/2019	R$ 66,347.90 (U$16,586.98)	R$ 149,390 (U$37,347.50)
Total			R$ 761,705.87 (U$190,426.47)	R$ 970,454.00 (U$242,613.50)

Source: From the research.

Table 1.
UBSF travel schedule, associated costs and federal funding transfers (FNS) for Tefé-AM, in 2018 and 2019.

Federal funding for UBSF is conditional on accreditation and the implementation of strategies and programmes. The monthly funding incentive is R$90,000.00 (U$22,500.00) in the oral health modality. However, according to GM/MS Accreditation Ordinance No. 2145, of 17 July 2018, the municipality was accredited with an expanded team, plus logistical and support points, which, after accreditation and implementation, amounted to a monthly transfer of R$149,390.00 (U$37,347.50).

Considering the expenditure per trip, which totalled R$761,705.87 (U$190,426.47), and the total transferred by the Ministry of Health for costs, which totalled R$970,454.00 (U$242,613.50), in this specific case there was a surplus of R$208,748.13 (U$52,187.03).

During the period analysed, there was no record of counterpart funding from municipal or state sources earmarked for the recurring cost of the health unit's actions.

Stratifying the journeys, the cost arising from area 21 represented R$290,540.61 (U$72,635.15 corresponding 38.14%), followed by area 10 with R$201,034.81 (U$50,258.70 corresponding 26.39%), area 11 with R$153,340.07 (U$38,335.20 corresponding 20.13%) and areas 14 and 19 together with R$116,790.38 (U$29,197.60 corresponding 15.33%).

An analysis of the total costs shows that human resources account for 64.62%, totalling R$ 492,209.25 (U$123,052.31), followed by the consumption of medicines with 17.72% and fuel with 12.11%, according to **Table 2**.

4. Discussion

It is clear that the River BHU is an innovative project, as it has corrected years of inequality due to the lack of care in distant and remote communities in the Amazon, since there was no institutionalised care model suitable for this type of care; it has expanded access, offering these riverside communities various basic health services, such as medical and nursing consultations, emergency care, immunisation, prenatal care; the river units have equipment and technologies that facilitate the diagnosis and treatment of the users they serve. This new arrangement has established a territory where the population will be linked to a basic health unit and registered in national information systems.

Thus, we have the challenge of measuring the costs in the Amazon. These additional amounts generated, for example, by difficulties in travelling, transport, communication, logistics and access routes to riverside areas, are hardly ever demonstrated [9]. Only with scientific evidence can we discuss whether the amounts passed on by the Ministry of Health meet these specific needs. To this end, cost analysis tools can help improve planning processes and are important for analysing and setting priorities [10].

The main finding relates to the cost specified in the survey. The total cost of UBSF trips generated a total of R$761,705.87 (U$123,052.31) during the period analysed, with an average monthly cost of R$84,633.99 (U$21,158.50). The highest costs were related to human resources (64.62%), inputs for health actions (17.72%), fuel (12.11%) and the rest (5.54%).

These findings directly contribute to demonstrating that the basic amounts passed on by the Ministry of Health only cover the costs of travelling, considering the value of R$ 80,000 (U$20,000) without oral health and 90,000 (U$22,500) with oral health. In this report, the municipality accredited the unit with logistical points and an extended team.

Cost component	Type of resource	Nature of Cost	Expenses	%
Human resources	Costing	Fixed	R$ 492,209.25 (U$123,052.31)	64.62
Supplies (medicines and surgical chemicals)	Costing	Variable	R$ 135,000 (U$33,750)	17.72
Fuel	Costing	Variable	R$ 92,272.24 (U$23,068.06)	12.11
Foodstuffs	Costing	Variable	R$ 30,599.22 (U$7649.80)	4.02
Office and IT supplies	Costing	Variable	R$ 6257.79 (U$1561.95)	0.82
Maintenance of the UBSF	Costing	Fixed	R$ 2558.97 (U$639.74)	0.34
Hygiene and cleaning materials	Costing	Variable	R$ 1816.40 (U$454.10)	0.24
Cooking gas	Costing	Variable	R$ 992.00 (U$248.00)	0.13
Total			R$ 761,705.87 (U$190.426.47)	100.00

Source: From the research.

Table 2.
Breakdown of measured costs, by type and nature, at the UBSF, Tefé-AM, 2020.

The discussion begins by comparing the cost of a traditional family health strategy with a fluvial one. The research findings show an average gross cost of R$123,052.31 (U$30,763.08) thousand for the fluvial family health team, which is much higher than the national average for traditional family health teams, which was R$18,000 (U$4500) without charges and approximately R$24,400 (U$6100) with labour charges for the ESF, according to an IPEA survey in 2013. This same study showed that of the five Brazilian regions analysed, the Midwest had the highest average, at R$25,600 (U$6400) per ESF [22].

In another comparison, the average monthly expenditure identified in this study is much higher than the average expenditure of a Family Health Programme unit in a municipality in Bahia, which was R$17,302 (U$4325.50)/unit/month in 2005. At that time, funding from the federal government was R$2834 (U$708.50)/unit/month, showing that there was underfunding on the part of the federal government [23].

Regarding inputs, such as medicines, dental, laboratory and chemical-surgical materials for the development of actions, these accounted for 17.72% of the total value. An average of R$33,750.00 (U$8437.50) per trip in this period, for an estimated population of 2051 inhabitants, which comprises the area in which the River Unit operates. Compared to another study carried out in a town in Rio Grande do Norte, a UBS with two family health teams spent R$23,833.00 (U$5958.25) on medicines and hospital medical supplies for a population of 9780 people [24].

Still on the subject of the cost of medicines, as can be seen in **Table 2**, the cost of medicines in the nine trips made by the UBSF totalled R$135,000 (U$33,750). A study carried out in 2007, in the city of Fortaleza, in the IV Regional Executive Secretariat, showed that the basic units with the three highest expenses for medicines totalled the first with R$135,283.36 (U$33,820.84), followed by R$129,813.82 (U$32,453.46) and the third with R$129,258.59 (U$32,314.65) [25]. In this scenario, there was a great deal of pent-up demand caused by the lack of health services in the riverside area of the city of Tefé.

Nevertheless, this study made it possible to see, as shown in **Table 1**, that the three trips to area 21 had the highest costs, corresponding to R$290,540.61 (U$72,635.15) (two hundred and ninety thousand, five hundred and forty reais and sixty-one cents). On the other hand, the least expensive trips were those made to areas 14 and 19, equalling R$116,790.38 (U$29,197.60) (one hundred and sixteen thousand, seven hundred and ninety reais and thirty-eight cents). Therefore, the study shows that there are differences in the costs of trips made to the same area in different months, as seen in **Table 1**, which can be attributed to the seasonality of the rivers, travelling time, climatic conditions and the endemic diseases associated with them and treated by the health team.

Following the analysis in **Table 2**, we have the costs of feeding the UBSF team during all the trips made, totalling R$30,599.22 (U$7649.81) thousand, or 4.02% of the total. Considering a study of the costs of the Family Health Programme in a municipality in Paraíba (2005–2006), taking into account the 19 existing Family Health Programme teams, we have a figure of R$40,800.00 (U$10,200) and R$69,600.00 (U$17,400) thousand for 2005 and 2006 respectively, and in percentage terms, we have 2.2% and 3.7% of the total. Therefore, when comparing these figures, we see that one of the Amazonian costs corresponds to the food of one team on board, which is equivalent to almost 19 ESFs in a northeastern region in 2005 [26].

The Ministry of Health is the main funding agent for the UBSF/eSFF. In the specific case of the Vila de Ega basic River Unit, the costs of travelling compared to the funds transferred by the National Health Fund to cover the cost of the actions were sufficient during the period studied to meet the needs of the care activities, generating a balance of R$208,748.13 (U$52,187.03) thousand, which, due to the seasonality of the rivers, must be spent on future travel.

Some limitations of the study and the results are worth mentioning, such as the absence of computerised control by the municipality, such as purchases, stocks, and warehouses, making management more precise, and information on spending by cost centre. To minimise these limitations, a single person was appointed to collect the cost information, using a standard form to collect the data.

It is also worth highlighting the fact that the research is a single case study and does not allow comparisons with other river units but only with traditional basic units. In this study, only fixed and variable costs were measured, and further economic evaluation studies are needed to present a costing method.

As a result, the study concluded that the costs of the UBS Fluvial during the seasonal period of river floods and the beginning of droughts, as well as that federal transfers, represent a significant amount of resources that support Amazonian municipalities in carrying out basic riverine care. However, it should be borne in mind that the seasonal regime of the rivers can determine the variation in variable costs, since the more days spent travelling, as happens during the dry season, the more the UBSF's costs can gradually increase. This means an increase in the amount of food, given the five meals a day for the multi-professional health and support teams on board, and the number of travelling days, given that the journey has to follow the main riverbed and without "holes" or shortcuts, and the amount of fuel and maintenance visits to the boat. It is worth pointing out that the other resources invested come from the municipality, since there is no state policy for basic care with financial support.

Although the results of the research pointed to evidence in the field of cost accounting and health economics, it is suggested that we move forward with new studies that estimate the cost-effectiveness and cost-efficiency of the model of river-based basic health units, seeking this coexistence of understanding the net territory in order to estimate the Amazonian cost of the national basic care policy and other public policies that will require displacement and multi-professional teams in order to promote the citizenship of riverside dwellers.

Acknowledgements

The authors would like to thank the Municipal Secretary of Tefé in Amazonas State, in the name of the Manager Maria Adriana Moreira, for the partnership in the development of the research. To the Amazonas Research Support Fund (FAPEAM), LAHPSA/ILMD/FIOCRUZ AM and Michele Rocha El Kadri for their considerations about the study.

Conflict of interest

There is no conflict of interest between the authors of the manuscript.

Appendices and nomenclature

CNS	National Health Council
eSFF	River Family Health Teams
eSFR	Riverside Family Health Teams
FAPEAM	Amazonas Research Support Foundation
FNS	National Health Fund
LAHPSA	Laboratory of History, Public Policies and Health in the Amazon
MS	Ministry of Health
UBSF	Basic River Health Unit
UFAM	Federal University of Amazonas

Author details

Cláudio Pontes Ferreira, Júlio Cesar Schweickardt and Rodrigo Tobias*
Laboratory of History, Public Policies and Health, Leônidas and Maria Deane Institute (ILMD/Fiocruz Amazonas), Manaus, Amazonas, Brazil

*Address all correspondence to: tobiasrodrigo@gmail.com

References

[1] Brazil. Ordinance no 2.436 of 21 September 2017. 2017. Available from: https://bvsms.saude.gov.br/bvs/saudelegis/gm/2017/prt2436_22_09_2017.html [Accessed: February 23, 2023]

[2] de Lima RT, Fernandes TG, da Balieiro AA, dos Costa F, de Schramm JM, Schweickardt JC, et al. Primary Care in Brazil and the More Doctors Programme: An analysis of production indicators. Ciência & Saúde Coletiva. 2016;**21**:2685-2696. DOI: 10.1590/1413-81232015219.15412016

[3] Schweickardt JC, Ferla AA, de Lima RT, Kadri M. História Das Políticas de Saúde No Amazonas: Da Zona Franca Ao SUS, 1967-1990, 01 ed

[4] da Reis MH, Portugal JK, Mariño JM, da Barros W, de Dantas JS, Souza TT, et al. O impacto do adventento de uma Unidade Básica de Saúde Fluvial na assistência aos povos ribeirinhos do Amazonas. Revista Eletrônica Acervo Saúde. 2020;**53**:e3631

[5] Guimarães AF, Barbosa VLM, Silva MP, Portugal JK, Reis MH, Gama AS, et al. Acesso a Serviços de Saúde Por Ribeirinhos de Um Município No Interior Do Estado Do Amazonas, Brasil. Revista Pan-Amazônica de Saúde. 2020;**11**:e202000178. DOI: 10.5123/s2176-6223202000178

[6] Garnelo L, Lima JG, Rocha ESC, Herkrath FJ. Access to and coverage of primary health care for rural and urban populations in the northern region of Brazil. Saúde Em Debate. 2018;**42**:81-99. DOI: 10.1590/0103-11042018S106

[7] Oliveira B et al. Prevalence of arterial hypertension in riverside communities of the Madeira River, Western Brazilian Amazon. Cadernos de Saúde Pública. 2013;**29**:1617-1630. DOI: 10.1590/0102-311X00146212

[8] de Lima RT, Fernandes TG, Martins Júnior PJA, Portela CS, et al. Saúde em vista: uma análise da Atenção Primária à Saúde em áreas ribeirinhas e rurais amazônicas. Ciência & Saúde Coletiva. 2021;**26**:2053-2064. DOI: 10.1590/1413-81232021266.02672021

[9] Kadri MRE, Santos BS, et al. Unidade Básica de Saúde Fluvial: um novo modelo da Atenção Básica para a Amazônia, Brasil. Interface – Comunicação, Saúde, Educação. 2019;**23**:e180613. DOI: 10.1590/Interface.180613

[10] Silva R et al. Dental caries in a riverside population in the State of Rondônia, Amazon region, Brazil, 2005/2006. Cadernos de Saúde Pública. 2008;**24**:2347-2353. DOI: 10.1590/S0102-311X2008001000015

[11] Silva EN, Silva MT, Pereira MG. Health economic evaluation studies: Definition and applicability to health systems and services. Epidemiologia e Serviços de Saúde. 2016;**25**:205-207. DOI: 10.5123/S1679-49742016000100023

[12] Sancho LG, Dain S. Evaluation in health and economic evaluation in health: Introduction to the debate on their points of intersection. Ciência & Saúde Coletiva. 2012;**17**:765-774. DOI: 10.1590/S1413-81232012000300024

[13] Ugá MAD. Instrumentos de avaliação econômica dos serviços de saúde: alcance e limitações. 1995. Available from: http://www.ipea.gov.br

[14] Lourenço Ó, Silva V. Economic evaluation of health programmes

- essentials on concepts, methodology, difficulties and opportunities. Revista Portuguesa de Medicina Geral e Familiar. 2008;**24**(6):729-752. DOI: 10.32385/rpmgf.v24i6.10572

[15] Schweickardt, Lima RT, Simões AL, Freitas CM, de Alves V. In-formes da atenção básica: aprendizados de intensidade por círculos em rede (Prospecting Techno-Assistance Models in Primary Health Care) - Volume 1. JÚLIO CÉSAR. Available from: https://editora.redeunida.org.br/project/in-formes-da-atencao-basica-aprendizados-de-intensidade-por-circulos-em-rede-prospeccao-de-modelos-tecnoassistenciais-na-atencao-basica-em-saude-volume-1-2/ [Accessed: February 23, 2023]

[16] Kadri MR, Wilson DR, Schweickardt JC, Linn JG, Farias LNG, Moreira A, et al. The Igarau fluvial Mobile clinic: Lessons learned while implementing an innovative primary care approach in rural Amazonia, Brazil. International Journal of Nursery Midwifery. 2017;**9**(4):41-45. DOI: 10.5897/IJNM2017.0256

[17] Schweickardt JC, Lima RT de et al. Educação permanente em gestão regionalizada da saúde: Saberes e fazeres no território do Amazonas. Editora Rede Unida. Available from: https://editora.redeunida.org.br/project/educacao- permanente-em-gestao-regionalizada-da-saude-saberes-e-fazeres-no-territorio-do- amazonas/ [Accessed: February 23, 2023]

[18] Deslandes SF. Concepções em pesquisa social: articulações com o campo da avaliação em serviços de saúde. Cadernos de Saúde Pública. 1997;**13**:103-107. DOI: 10.1590/S0102-311X1997000100020

[19] de Castro ALB, Machado CV. A política de atenção primária à saúde no Brasil: notas sobre a regulação e o financiamento federal. Cadernos de Saúde Pública. 2010;**26**:693-705. DOI: 10.1590/S0102-311X2010000400012

[20] Tefé Municipal Health Plan: 2018 to 2021

[21] Santos SM et al. Estimation of direct costs of the municipal dengue control programme of Goiânia-GO. Epidemiologia e Serviços de Saúde. 2015;**24**:661-670. DOI: 10.5123/S1679-49742015000400008

[22] da Vieira R, Servo LM. Estimates of human resources costs in primary care: Family Health Teams (ESF) and Oral Health Teams (ESB). 2013. Available from: http://www.ipea.gov.br

[23] Rosa MRR, Coelho TCB. What do the costs of the family health programme in a municipality in Bahia say? Ciência & Saúde Coletiva. 2011;**16**:1863-1873. DOI: 10.1590/S1413-81232011000300021

[24] da Carvalho D, Soares FC, Dantas MG, Oliveira RM. Analysing the efficiency of public spending in basic health units in the municipality of Parnamirim/RN. Anais do Congresso Brasileiro de Custos-ABC. 2017

[25] Chaves ES. Expenditure on medicines dispensed in Primary Health Care in Fortaleza, CE, and influential co-factors in 2007 [Dissertation]. Fortaleza: Federal University of Ceará; 2009. 159 p

[26] de Barbosa E, de Rêgo T, Rezende I. O custo do Programa de Saúde a Família: um estudo de caso no Município de Sapé/PB. Anais do Congresso Brasileiro de Custos-ABC. 2008

Section 2

Perspective Chapters

Chapter 5

Perspective Chapter: Improving Health Budgeting and Management Practices in Low Middle Income Countries (LMIC): Using 3 Country Case Studies—Nigeria, Kenya and Tanzania

Samson Agbo

Abstract

This chapter examines the budgeting and management issues in health sectors of Nigeria, Kenya, and Tanzania, relating to their goal of achieving universal health coverage (UHC) by 2030. Highlighting the World Health Organization's 2010 report, it points out financial inefficiencies accounting for 30–40% of health spending, which obstruct progress towards the Sustainable Development Goal (SDG) target 3.8. It identifies key obstacles including poor planning, corruption, inadequate skills, weak governance, and lack of social accountability. The text evaluates the effectiveness of budgeting tools and guidance provided by international organizations like the World Bank and WHO, finding them insufficient for national advancement. It discusses the benefits and limitations of budget reforms, such as Public Expenditure Reviews (PERs) and Medium-Term Expenditure Frameworks (MTEF), emphasizing the importance of participatory and transparent practices. It notes political interference as a significant barrier to aligning health policies with resource allocation. Concluding, the chapter advocates for program-based budgeting reforms to enhance health spending alignment with sector priorities, flexibility in fund usage, and transparency. It suggests capacity building, improved community engagement, open government collaboration, and evidence-based practices as ways to advance towards UHC. These reforms are seen as critical for fostering transparent, high-quality budget management in the health sector.

Keywords: budget, management, MTEF, programme-based budgeting, operational, efficiency, inclusion, transparency, accountability, LMIC

1. Introduction

1.1 Overview of health budgeting and management in LMICs

This chapter provides a comprehensive overview of the challenges and dynamics surrounding health systems in Low- and Middle-Income Countries (LMICs). It begins by highlighting the persistent challenges faced by LMICs in the realm of health systems, including limited financial resources, inefficient healthcare systems, and disparities in access for vulnerable families. The author identifies crucial actions to address these issues, such as improving budget allocation for health by adequate planning, implementing cost-effective interventions, and exploring innovative financing mechanisms like health insurance. Furthermore, the importance of enhancing governance, transparency, reducing corruption, fostering inclusion, and fostering international collaborations is emphasized as vital components contributing to more sustainable health financing and management in LMICs [1].

Budgets are seen as both political and technical tools. When used optimally, they have the potential to reflect a government's policy priorities, allow for the efficient use of public resources and ensure transparency and accountability in the use of those resources. Public budgeting is the process by which governments prepare and approve strategic allocations of public resources. From the perspective of Public Finance Management (PFM), robust public budgeting serves several important functions: it sets expenditure ceilings, promotes fiscal discipline and financial accountability, and enhances efficiency in public spending [2, 3].

Budget formulation is an important part of the budgeting process. The way budgets are presented, formulated, and structured has an underrated influence on actual budget implementation. If multiple budget classifications can be used to present budgets, the dominant classification selected ends up shaping budget appropriations. The choice of budget classification is therefore crucial for actual spending as it largely defines how money is received and spent by different budget holders, as well as how public money is controlled and accounted for (e.g., by consumption of inputs versus by achieved service outputs). Because programme budgets force the allocation and appropriation of public resources by policy goals and outputs, they have been one of the most promising PFM mechanisms to help link public resources to priorities and needs for a sector. It is a major reform to foster public sector performance, tested in nearly all countries across the world. In many LMICs, budgets have long been formulated and spent by inputs, a common occurrence that often creates inflexible budget structures which are too rigid to adapt to service delivery needs [4].

The programme-budgeting approach offers an opportunity to introduce flexibility and greater orientation towards services. Despite the potential benefits of the reform, health sector stakeholders have often lacked a solid understanding of the approach, its key merits, and its requirements for success. When reforms are introduced, there is often a desire to define a common framework across sectors. However, there is often limited guidance given to sector stakeholders on how they can engage in the reform, which means the reforms are often poorly understood, only partially implemented, and not tailored to the sector's needs [5–7].

The chapter analyses the evolving landscape in LMICs, where stakeholders, including donors, UN partners, policymakers, politicians, and program managers, are increasingly seeking fit-for-purpose and evidence-based frameworks. This shift reflects a growing demand for efficient identification of priority health interventions and value-for-money healthcare delivery options.

The acknowledgement that public spending must align with the proclamations in human rights instruments underscores the importance of tangible government commitment to realizing these rights through the budget. This insight adds depth to the discussion, highlighting the interplay between policy declarations and concrete financial actions [8].

The purpose of a budget is articulated clearly in the chapter, emphasizing its role in planning, organizing, tracking, and improving the financial situation of a government. The division of resources for government functions is noted as a crucial aspect, linking the budgetary process directly to the practical implementation of government responsibilities.

Overall, this chapter explores the complexities of health systems in LMICs. It effectively combines a concise analysis of challenges with actionable solutions, emphasizing the interconnectedness of financial, governance, and transparency aspects in health budgeting. The inclusion of the human rights perspective adds a compelling layer to the narrative, emphasizing the need for concrete financial commitments to realize these rights. The chapter sets a strong foundation for the subsequent exploration of specific case studies and frameworks in the broader context of health budgeting and management in LMICs [8, 9].

1.2 Importance of efficient resource allocation and management for health outcomes

This chapter critically examines the significance of efficient resource allocation and management in the context of health outcomes, with a specific focus on Low- and Middle-Income Countries (LMICs). The author reviewed four generic arguments of public investment in health, which include rights-based, economic, social, and political perspectives, although not the central theme of the contribution. [10–12].

The narrative then delves into the challenges faced by LMICs such as Nigeria, Kenya, and Tanzania in health budget preparation and management over the past two decades. The common issues identified include inadequate funding, inefficient allocation, and suboptimal financial management systems. The World Health Organization (WHO) and World Bank (WB) have provided best practices guidance and tools in 2022 to address these challenges, emphasizing transparent budgeting processes, stakeholder engagement, and performance-based budgeting [12].

Looking at the diverse political-economic landscapes of the mentioned countries, the findings illustrate how Nigeria contends with corruption and underfunded infrastructure, Kenya struggles with urban-rural health disparities, and Tanzania faces limitations due to scarce resources. These nuances highlight the need for country tailored health systems strategies in LMICs. The chapter underscores the budget as a paramount instrument for governments to invest in better health, addressing poverty and social determinants. It elucidates the cyclical and functional stages of the budget process, emphasizing formulation, enactment, execution, and evaluation/audit. The argument is that the budget process is a critical negotiation between present benefits and future investments, making it pivotal for improved population health and well-being. A notable aspect explored is the interplay between a sound budget system, good governance, and democratization. Thus, the emphasis on transparency as a key feature of budget-making, empowering citizens to challenge proposals. The role of the legislature in representing the people is discussed, highlighting challenges in many African countries such as lack of evidence and weak governance committee systems [11].

The discussion extends to post-implementation aspects, including internal budget auditing for accountability. However, in the review one notes considerable delays in the publication of such audit reports, a significant concern.

The weak link between policy planning and budget planning in African countries is identified as a serious limitation, affecting the proper reflection of strategic priorities in expenditure frameworks. The capacity of budget implementing agencies is deemed crucial, and the chapter discusses efforts by LMICs, with the support of WHO and World Bank, to address capacity limitations through budget reforms [9, 11].

The concluding section outlines the scope and methods of the chapter, which reviews health budgeting from an efficiency and equity lens based on WHO (2022) guidance and framework on "how to make budgets work for health". It promises a comprehensive analysis of case studies from Kenya, Nigeria, and Tanzania, aiming to provide strategic solutions to the challenges faced by these countries in health resource preparation, allocation, and management [12].

In summary, this chapter combines theoretical underpinnings with practical insights, providing a comprehensive overview of the challenges and potential solutions related to health budgeting in LMICs. The mix method approach, including key informant interviews and qualitative questionnaires, added depth to the analysis. The chapter holds promise for offering valuable insights applicable globally to strengthen health systems and improve healthcare outcomes in LMICs.

1.3 Objectives

Summing up, the objectives of this chapter are as follows:

1. Analyzing health budgeting processes and management challenges in Kenya, Nigeria, and Tanzania.

2. Identifying successful strategies and best practices.

3. Proposing recommendations for improved health budgeting and its management.

2. Health budgeting landscape in Kenya

2.1 Overview of health budgeting in Kenya

2.1.1 Political structure

Kenya operates as a unitary state with a devolved system of governance, consisting of 47 counties. Health services are devolved, and each county is responsible for planning and implementing its health budget.

2.1.2 Budget allocation structure

Counties have the authority to allocate budgets for health services based on their local needs and priorities. The national government supports counties through conditional grants and funding mechanisms.

2.1.3 Policy landscape

Kenya has a National Health Sector Strategic Plan outlining policies and strategies for the health sector. Devolution has led to increased autonomy for counties in decision-making regarding health service delivery and budgeting.

2.1.4 Political significance

Health is a key agenda in political discussions and campaigns, reflecting its significance in addressing public concerns.

2.1.5 Challenges in healthcare

Challenges persist, including disparities in resource distribution among counties, workforce shortages, and the need for improved infrastructure.

2.1.6 Health budgeting process

Counties engage in a budgeting process that involves planning, allocation, and execution of resources for health services. The national government provides financial support through conditional grants and oversight to ensure alignment with national health policies.

This review provides an in-depth understanding of the budget process in Kenya, emphasizing its significance in government planning and decision-making. The budget cycle commences in August of the current year and concludes in December of the following year, aligning with the fiscal year, which runs from July 1st to June 30th.

The structure of a financial quarter in Kenya, comprises 3 months, facilitating a clear timeline for budget-related activities. Public participation is emphasized throughout the budget process at both the national and county levels. Key legislations and regulations, including the Constitution, Public Finance Management Act, Public Finance Management Regulations, and County Governments Act, guide the budget planning process, ensuring alignment with public needs and government policy.

A notable aspect of the budget process in Kenya is its continuous and overlapping nature. The chapter highlights the intricate timeline spanning formulation and approval (10 months), implementation (12 months), and audit and evaluation (6 months). However, it acknowledges that adherence to deadlines is not always consistent across government levels and agencies, as shown in **Figure 1** [13].

The importance of vigilance is key regarding any deviations from the defined timelines, particularly during general election years, which may impact the budget process. Advertisements for budget hearings or forums are usually published in newspapers, government websites, and social media, providing avenues for public awareness and participation.

In summary, the stages of the budget process in Kenya for both the national and county governments follow these key stages: which includes integrated development planning, financial and economic policy determination, budget estimation, approval, enactment, implementation, and ongoing evaluation and reporting. Public participation is underscored as a crucial element, with the responsibility placed on the Cabinet Secretary for Finance to ensure its inclusion in the budget process. This review provides a comprehensive guide to the intricacies of the budgeting process in Kenya,

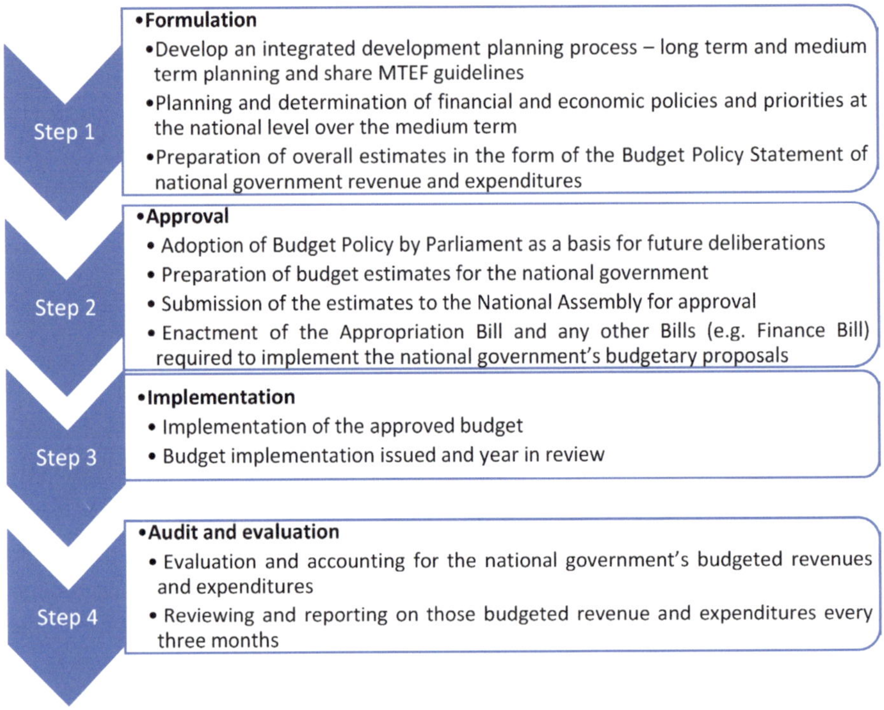

Figure 1.
Stages of budget process in Kenya. Source: Kenya Parliamentary Act (2012) updated Public 2020. Available from: https://countytoolkit.devolution.go.ke/sites/default/files/resources/ibp_kenya_budget_calendar_2015.pdf; https://vivaafricallp.com/wpcontent/uploads/Budget%20Making%20Process%20in%20Kenya.pdf.

with valuable insights into the stages, timelines, and legislative frameworks that shape the nation's fiscal landscape, as shown in **Figure 1** [14].

2.2 Status, trend, and issues with healthcare expenditure in Kenya

The 2021/2022 Public Expenditure Review (PER) on healthcare in Kenya reflects positive trends and achievements in the country's health system and financing. Over the past decade, Kenya has improved access to quality care, resulting in better health outcomes. However, demographic, and epidemiological transitions pose challenges that require adapting service delivery models.

Kenya is undergoing a health financing shift, with the government playing a more significant role as contributions from donors and corporations decrease. Despite substantial increases in health spending, there's a need for efficient planning and management to achieve universal health coverage (UHC). Total public spending on health doubled from KSh 96 billion in FY2014/15 to KSh 228 billion in FY2019/20, surpassing 2% of GDP [15].

The national government's role in health financing has increased, especially during the COVID-19 pandemic and UHC initiatives. Clarity in defining roles between national and county governments is crucial. Public financial management (PFM) capacity has improved, but unspent resources persist, affecting UHC goals. Systemic weaknesses, including delayed fund releases, contribute to suboptimal budget execution [15, 16].

Changes in Ministry of Health (MoH) expenditure reflect a shift towards UHC, with increased spending on health policy and social protection programs. Health spending is skewed towards secondary and tertiary care, emphasizing the need to prioritize primary health care for equity and efficiency.

Devolution has altered funds flow, giving more control to county governments but creating challenges in PFM and health financing. The PER identifies opportunities to increase value for money in the health sector, emphasizing the importance of efficiency due to limited fiscal space. A comparison of spending, service coverage, and outcomes reveals suboptimal returns, with inefficiencies in devolved functions, management, governance, and transparency [13, 14].

Noteworthy inefficiencies include high rates of absenteeism among health workers and challenges in diagnosing and treating common conditions. Potential savings from absenteeism alone are estimated at $58 million in FY 2019/20, representing around 5% of total health expenditure. The PER emphasizes the need for improvements in HRH and the allocation and use of medical equipment [14, 15].

2.2.1 Challenges in health funding and budget execution

- *Inadequate funding*: One of the persistent challenges in Kenya's healthcare system has been insufficient funding. The healthcare sector often faces budgetary constraints, leading to challenges in providing quality services, maintaining infrastructure, and retaining skilled healthcare professionals.

- *Unequal distribution of resources*: There has been a notable disparity in healthcare resource distribution between urban and rural areas. Urban centers tend to receive more attention and resources, leaving rural areas with limited access to essential healthcare services.

- *Dependency on donor funding*: Kenya's healthcare system has, at times, relied heavily on donor funding. While external assistance is essential, over-dependence on it can result in vulnerability to fluctuations in donor priorities and potential gaps in sustained funding.

- *Challenges in implementation of devolution*: Kenya implemented a devolved system of government, and healthcare services were devolved to the county level. However, challenges related to the equitable distribution of resources, varying capacities among counties, and management issues have emerged.

- *High out-of-pocket spending*: A significant proportion of healthcare financing in Kenya comes from out-of-pocket spending by individuals. This can be a barrier to healthcare access, especially for low-income populations, and may lead to financial hardships for households.

- *Corruption and mismanagement*: Issues related to corruption and mismanagement within the healthcare system can divert funds away from their intended purposes, impacting the overall efficiency and effectiveness of healthcare delivery.

- *Health insurance coverage gaps*: While efforts have been made to increase health insurance coverage in Kenya, there are still gaps in reaching the entire population. Many individuals, especially in informal sectors, may lack access to health insurance, limiting their ability to afford necessary medical services.

- *Emerging health challenges*: The emergence of new health challenges, such as the COVID-19 pandemic, has strained healthcare resources. Responding to such crises requires additional funding and resources, potentially exacerbating existing financial constraints.

- *Misalignment of budget timing*: Some consultative activities expected to take place between these key dates are not mentioned in the revised Act 2020. For example, the meetings by the Executive to discuss and approve certain documents. This limits full participation of the public, key stakeholders, and transparency in the process [13].

2.2.2 Status of healthcare budgeting, engaging key stakeholders and their roles

- *Government funding*: The Kenyan government allocates a portion of its budget to the health sector, covering various aspects such as infrastructure development, personnel salaries, and medical supplies.

- *Budget cycle*: The budgeting process in Kenya is cyclical and annual, involving formulation, enactment, execution, and evaluation/audit stages. It serves as a crucial instrument for government investment in better health and addresses poverty and social determinants of health.

- *Public participation*: The budget process allows for public participation at different stages, fostering transparency and inclusivity. This engagement ensures that the healthcare budget aligns with public needs and government policies.

- *Legislation and regulations*: The budget planning process in Kenya is guided by legislation and regulations, including the Constitution, Public Finance Management Act, Public Finance Management Regulations, and County Governments Act.

- *Oversight by parliament and county assemblies*: Budget oversight is conducted by the Parliament at the national level and County Assemblies at the county level. These bodies play a crucial role in scrutinizing and approving budgetary allocations for the health sector.

- *Continuous budget process*: The budget process is continuous and overlaps, with the formulation and approval stage lasting from August 30 of the current year to June 30 of the coming year, the implementation stage from July 1 of the coming year to June 30 of the year after, and the audit and evaluation stage from July 1 of the year after to December 30 of the same year [14, 16].

2.2.2.1 Key stakeholders and their roles

- *Ministries of health and finance*: These government bodies are central in the budgeting process. The Ministry of Health identifies health priorities and needs, while the Ministry of Finance plays a role in budget formulation, allocation, and financial planning.

- *Parliament and county assemblies*: These legislative bodies provide oversight during the budget process. They review, debate, and approve budgetary allocations for the health sector, ensuring accountability and transparency.

- *Public participation*: Citizens participate in the budget process through public hearings and forums. This involvement ensures that the budget reflects the needs and priorities of the population.

- *County governments*: At the county level, county governments are actively involved in budgeting for health services. They identify local health priorities, allocate resources, and oversee the implementation of healthcare programs.

- *Healthcare implementing agencies*: These include health facilities, departments, and agencies responsible for executing healthcare programs. They play a crucial role in translating budgetary allocations into actual health outcomes.

- *Auditors*: Independent auditors conduct internal budget auditing to ensure funds are used as stipulated and due processes are followed. Their role is crucial in maintaining accountability and transparency in the utilization of healthcare funds.

- *Private sector and NGOs*: These entities may also be stakeholders, particularly in public-private partnerships and donor-funded programs. They contribute resources, expertise, and support to complement government efforts in healthcare delivery.

2.2.3 Insufficient budget allocation, poor financial management and accountability

Poor financial management and accountability, especially with devolution at the county level, in Kenya, has significantly impacted health outputs and outcomes in various ways. Some of the key consequences are:

- *Inadequate resource allocation*: Poor financial management may result in inadequate allocation of resources to the health sector at the county level. This can lead to insufficient funding for critical areas such as healthcare infrastructure, personnel, and essential medical supplies.

- *Limited access to quality healthcare*: Inefficient financial management can hinder the establishment and maintenance of healthcare facilities, leading to limited access to quality healthcare services for residents. This is particularly detrimental in rural areas where healthcare infrastructure may be lacking or poorly maintained.

- *Delayed or incomplete health projects*: Lack of accountability may contribute to delays or incomplete implementation of health projects. Funds may be mismanaged or misappropriated, leading to incomplete construction of hospitals, clinics, or other essential healthcare facilities.

- *Shortage of healthcare personnel*: Poor financial management can result in delayed or irregular payment of salaries for healthcare workers. This can lead to demotivation, low morale, and even migration of qualified healthcare professionals, resulting in a shortage of skilled personnel.

- *Decreased quality of health services*: Inadequate funding and financial mismanagement can compromise the quality of health services provided at the county level. Insufficient resources may lead to poorly maintained equipment, inadequate training for healthcare staff, and a lack of essential medicines.

- *Increase in preventable diseases*: Limited resources and poor financial management may result in inadequate preventive measures and health education programs. This could contribute to the spread of preventable diseases and negatively impact public health outcomes.

- *Lack of emergency response capacity*: Ineffective financial management may hinder the county's ability to respond to health emergencies promptly. This includes the procurement of emergency medical supplies, establishing emergency response teams, and conducting necessary training.

- *Underinvestment in public health initiatives*: Poor financial management may lead to a lack of investment in public health initiatives, such as vaccination campaigns, disease surveillance, and health promotion programs. This can increase the vulnerability of the population to infectious diseases.

- *Underutilization of health information systems*: Inefficient financial management practices may lead to the underutilization of health information systems and data. This can hinder evidence-based decision-making, strategic planning, and monitoring of health outcomes.

- *Erosion of public trust*: Poor financial management and accountability practices erode public trust in the healthcare system. When citizens perceive mismanagement of funds or corruption, it can lead to decreased confidence in the health services provided, discouraging utilization and adherence to health recommendations [15].

2.2.4 Health service coverage

2.2.4.1 Overview of health service coverage

Health service coverage in Kenya has seen significant improvements over the years, partly due to initiatives aimed at achieving Universal Health Coverage (UHC), one of the key pillars of the country's Big Four Agenda. However, despite these advancements, the country still faces numerous challenges in ensuring comprehensive health service coverage for all its citizens.

2.3 Case studies: findings from the Kenya review

- *National health insurance fund (NHIF) expansion*: Kenya has made strides in expanding coverage through the NHIF, which aims to provide affordable health insurance to all Kenyans. This includes both inpatient and outpatient services, maternity care, and dialysis, among others.

- *Community health services*: The government has also focused on strengthening community health services to provide primary care at the grassroots level, which is critical for early detection and management of diseases.

- *Infrastructure and equipment*: Significant investments have been made in upgrading health facilities and equipping them with modern medical equipment, aimed at improving service delivery across the country.

- *Human resources for health*: Efforts to increase the number and capacity of healthcare workers have been ongoing, including training and deploying more personnel to underserved areas.

2.3.1 Challenges

- *Financial constraints*: Despite NHIF, many Kenyans still face financial barriers to accessing healthcare services due to high out-of-pocket expenses, limited NHIF coverage for certain treatments, and the exclusion of some vulnerable populations.

- *Geographical inequities*: Access to health services remains uneven, with rural and marginalized areas suffering from a lack of facilities, healthcare workers, and essential medicines compared to urban centers.

- *Quality of care*: There are concerns about the quality of healthcare services, with reports of shortages of essential drugs, inadequate healthcare infrastructure, and occasional lapses in the standard of care.

- *Disease burden*: Kenya continues to battle both communicable diseases, such as HIV/AIDS, tuberculosis, and malaria, and an increasing prevalence of non-communicable diseases (NCDs), including diabetes and hypertension, which strain the healthcare system.

- *Health system strengthening*: Challenges remain in strengthening health system pillars, including health information systems, supply chain management, governance, and financing mechanisms, to support effective and efficient service delivery.

- *COVID-19 pandemic*: The recent COVID-19 pandemic has further exposed and exacerbated existing weaknesses in the health system, including the capacity to respond to health emergencies [13–15].

2.3.2 Successful initiatives and programs in Kenya

There are available documents, legislation and operational guide tools like the PFM, Health Acts, and other budget guidance notes across governments. The adopted processes include the conduct of PERs and PETS, including PFM reviews. The national government budget implementation reports are available on the National Treasury's website. Although, the county governments budget implementation reports are on their websites as well, but some counties are notorious for not uploading these quarterly reports on time and regularly.

2.3.3 Lessons learned and their applicability to other LMICs

Healthcare budgeting in Kenya involves multiple stakeholders, including government bodies, legislators, the public, and implementing agencies. Collaboration and engagement among these stakeholders are essential for effective and transparent budgeting, ultimately leading to improved healthcare outcomes.

In conclusion, while Kenya has made commendable progress in expanding health service coverage, significant challenges remain in achieving universal health coverage. Addressing these challenges requires a multi-faceted approach that includes increasing investment in health, strengthening health system governance, enhancing the quality of care, and ensuring equitable access to health services across the country.

2.3.4 Policy recommendations

To address these challenges, it is essential for county governments in Kenya to prioritize transparent financial management, strengthen accountability mechanisms, and ensure that allocated resources are efficiently utilized for the improvement of health outputs and outcomes.

This includes robust oversight, regular audits, and the implementation of audit reports and policies that promote fiscal responsibility and integrity in the healthcare sector.

3. Health budgeting challenges in Nigeria

3.1 Overview of health budgeting in Nigeria

- *Political structure*: Nigeria is a federation comprised of 36 States, 774 Local Government Areas (LGAs), and a Federal Capital Territory (FCT). Health responsibilities are distributed across the federal, state, and local governments, with each tier accountable for primary, secondary, and tertiary healthcare delivery.

- *Budget allocation structure*: Each tier of government manages its health budget allocation and implementation, emphasizing decentralization. The State and local governments often share responsibilities for priority projects through a joint account, as outlined in the 2014 Health Act [17].

- *Policy landscape:* Health is on the concurrent list, indicating shared responsibilities among the three tiers of government. The Health Act of 2014 and the Basic Health Care Provision Fund (BHCPF) provide additional health financing options for States and LGAs.

- *Political significance:* Health holds a prominent position in political party manifestos, and a robust health agenda is a key tool in political campaigns. A three-phased scenario exists, and health is part of several political manifestos.

- *Challenges in healthcare:* Nigeria faces challenges in achieving comprehensive healthcare service coverage and effective budgeting, impacting the accessibility and quality of healthcare for its population.

- *Health budgeting process:* The process involves formulation, approval, implementation, and evaluation of budgetary allocations to the health sector. Joint accounts managed by the State play a role in budget execution and resource distribution [17, 18].

3.1.1 Healthcare services coverage in Nigeria

- *Limited access*: A significant portion of the Nigerian population faces challenges in accessing primary healthcare services, particularly in rural and underserved areas. Infrastructure deficiencies, inadequate healthcare facilities, and workforce shortages contribute to this limitation. Less than 10 per cent of these facilities are operational.

- *Out-of-pocket expenses*: Most of the healthcare financing comes from out-of-pocket expenses, leading to financial barriers that limit access to essential health services. This is especially problematic for low-income individuals who may have to forego necessary medical care due to cost.

- *Inequitable distribution*: There is an inequitable distribution of healthcare resources between urban and rural areas, leading to disparities in service availability and quality. Urban centers tend to have better access to healthcare facilities and skilled personnel.

- *Health insurance challenges*: Health insurance coverage remains low, with a significant portion of the population lacking insurance. This contributes to the financial burden on individuals and hampers efforts to achieve universal health coverage.

3.2 Lessons from Nigeria

In assessing Nigeria's healthcare financing and examination of key budgeting challenges, it is important to note the following:

- *Government funding*: The funding remains inadequate, less than the 2001 AU countries agreed 15 per cent of their annual budget allocated to the health sector (also known as the Abuja Declaration) [19]. The Nigerian government allocates funds in the national budget for healthcare, covering various aspects such as infrastructure development, personnel salaries, and procurement of medical supplies shown in **Figure 2** [18, 21, 22]. The healthcare sector often receives insufficient budgetary allocations, leading to challenges in maintaining and improving healthcare infrastructure, as well as recruiting and retaining skilled healthcare professionals.

- *Dependency on oil revenue*: Nigeria's economy heavily relies on oil revenue, and fluctuations in oil prices can impact the government's ability to sustain adequate funding for healthcare. Fluctuations in oil prices can impact the government's ability to sustain adequate funding for the health sector.

- *Out-of-pocket expenses*: A significant portion of healthcare financing comes from out-of-pocket expenses by individuals, leading to financial barriers that limit access to essential health services, especially for low-income individuals.

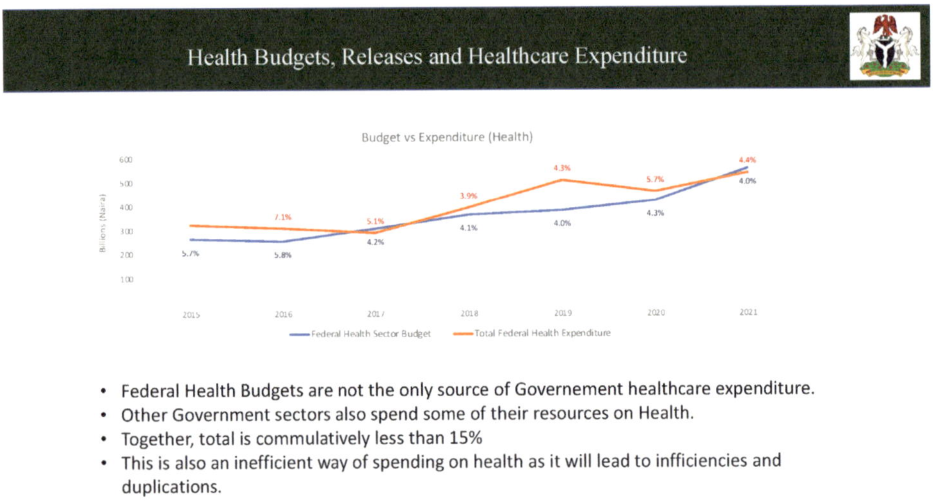

Figure 2.
Health budget, releases, and health care expenditure trend – 2015–2021. Source: FMOH 4-point Agenda Conference presentation, p. 12. November 2023. Available from: https://data.worldbank.org/indicator/SH.XPD.CHEX.GD.ZS?locations=NG [20].

- *Allocation challenges and inequitable distribution*: There are challenges in the effective allocation of healthcare funds, leading to issues such as delayed or incomplete health projects, inadequate procurement of medical supplies, and challenges in workforce development. Resource distribution across States and between urban and rural areas is often uneven, resulting in disparities in health-care access and quality.

- *Health insurance challenges:* Health insurance coverage remains low, with a considerable proportion of the population lacking insurance. This contributes to financial barriers and hampers efforts to achieve universal health coverage [18, 21, 23].

- *Disease outbreak response*: Adequate budgeting is crucial for responding to disease outbreaks and health emergencies. Timely allocation of funds is necessary for effective emergency response, including the procurement of medical supplies, vaccination campaigns, and public health awareness initiatives.

3.2.1 Challenges in health budgeting in Nigeria

- *Poor design, implementation, and monitoring:* Despite budgetary allocations, challenges persist in the design, effective implementation, and monitoring of health programs. Poor execution can result from issues such as corruption, inefficient procurement processes, and mismanagement of resources.

- *Infrastructure deficiencies*: The health sector faces infrastructural deficiencies, including inadequate healthcare facilities, equipment, and personnel. This affects the quality and accessibility of healthcare services, particularly in rural areas.

- *Workforce challenges*: There is a shortage of healthcare professionals in critical areas, leading to challenges in service delivery. Inadequate staffing, poor retention strategies, and limited training opportunities contribute to workforce challenges.

- *Disease outbreaks and emergencies*: The country faces recurring challenges from disease outbreaks, including epidemics and pandemics. Responding to these emergencies' strains healthcare resources, necessitating additional funding and resources.

- *Weak health insurance coverage*: Health insurance coverage remains low, resulting in a significant proportion of the population relying on out-of-pocket expenses for medical care. This financial barrier can limit access to essential health services, particularly for low-income individuals [18, 24].

3.2.2 Key stakeholders and their roles

As shown in **Figure 3** in the supplement.

- *Ministry of health*: The Ministry of Health is central in identifying health priorities, formulating policies, and overseeing the implementation of healthcare programs. It plays a critical role in advocating for adequate budgetary allocations.

- *Ministry of finance*: Responsible for budget formulation, allocation, and financial planning, the Ministry of Finance plays a key role in determining the funds available for the health sector.

- *National assembly*: The legislative arm of the government provides oversight during the budget process. Members of the National Assembly review, debate, and approve budgetary allocations for the health sector.

- *Public*: Public participation in the budgeting process is essential. Citizens engage through public hearings and forums, ensuring that the healthcare budget reflects the needs and priorities of the population.

- *Healthcare implementing agencies*: These include health facilities, departments, and agencies responsible for executing healthcare programs. They play a crucial role in translating budgetary allocations into actual health outcomes.

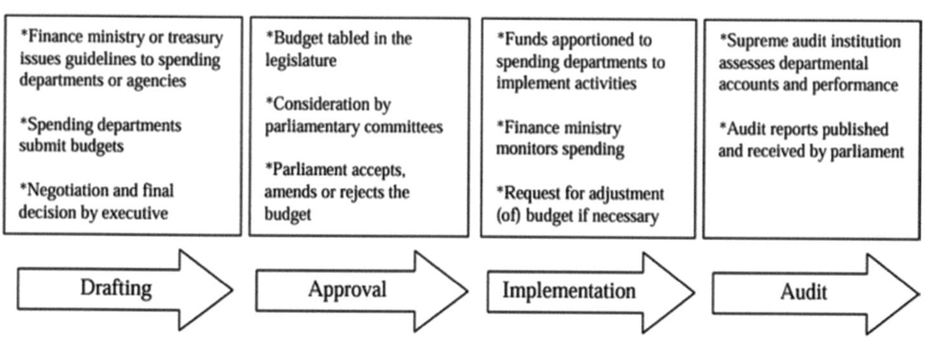

Figure 3.
Stages of Nigeria budget process. Source: Extracted from Parliamentary Centre (2010, p. 11). Available from: https://oidp-afrique.org/wpcontent/uploads/2020/04/Nigeria-Budget_Processes_and_Participatory_Budge.pdf.

- *Development partners and donors*: International organizations and donor agencies contribute funds and technical assistance to support healthcare programs in Nigeria. They play a significant role in complementing government efforts.

- *Private sector and NGOs*: Private healthcare providers and non-governmental organizations (NGOs) are stakeholders in healthcare delivery. Public-private partnerships and NGO initiatives contribute resources and expertise to complement government efforts.

- *Health insurance providers*: Both public and private health insurance providers play a role in expanding health insurance coverage, though challenges in reaching a larger percentage of the population persist.

- *Auditors:* Independent auditors conduct internal budget auditing to ensure accountability and transparency in the utilization of healthcare funds. Their role is crucial in preventing mismanagement and corruption [20, 23, 25].

3.3 Barriers to effective budgeting

3.3.1 Political and economic factors

Political interference is unhealthy for sound planning and budgeting. Limited public awareness and education about healthcare issues contribute to challenges in preventive care and public health initiatives. This affects the overall effectiveness of health programs. Non-inclusion in the budgetary process and not having a voice remains a serious gap. With high rates of multi-dimensional poverty and lack of trust of governments, people are less inclined to participate in town hall meetings and fail to hold their political leaders to account.

3.3.2 Administrative and structural issues

There are gaps in the effective implementation of health policies. These gaps may be attributed to weak governance structures, inconsistent policy execution, and a lack of coordination among relevant stakeholders, including development partners.

3.3.3 Innovative approaches to overcome budgeting challenges

Exploring public-private investment partnerships (PPIPs) in healthcare financing can be a strategy to overcome budgetary constraints. Engaging the private sector and faith-based organizations can contribute to infrastructure development and service delivery. Development partners should be made to have their contributions on budget rather than off budget as the case is now. Streamlining and standardization of the process is as good as the outcome for more aligned and harmonized results-based programme.

3.3.4 Budgeting processes and decentralization for improved health governance

The budgeting process in Nigeria adheres to the internationally accepted cycle, encompassing drafting, legislative approval, implementation, and concluding with monitoring and evaluation. However, a significant challenge arises from the time lag between initiating the process and receiving assent to the Appropriation Bill. The root cause lies in Sections 80 (1–4) and 81(1) of the 1999 Constitution (as amended), which set the timeframe for presenting budget estimates without specifying a concluding timeline. This leads to delays and inefficiencies. To address this, policy recommendations for other Low- and Middle-Income Countries (LMICs) include establishing clear timelines for the entire budgeting process, ensuring swift legislative approval, and emphasizing prompt implementation [20, 21, 23, 25, 26].

Nigeria initially adopted incremental budgeting, but inefficiencies prompted a shift to the zero-based technique for the 2017 budget. However, despite challenges in the budgeting process and performance, Nigeria has witnessed little improvements in certain socio-economic indicators. Notably, these improvements cannot be solely attributed to budget performance, revealing a significant disconnect. LMICs should consider incorporating diverse socio-economic drivers and external factors when evaluating the impact of budgeting on health outcomes [25].

Furthermore, decentralization, if not accompanied by deconcentration, poses challenges in a liberal democracy where health may not be a top executive priority. Inconsistent governance structures and varying typologies of States and Local Government Areas (LGAs) hinder synergies and coherence in policy implementation [20, 25].

Some States outperform others due to differences in technical capacity and assistance. Political interference and the marginalization of technical staff and policy makers are prevalent issues. For LMICs contemplating decentralization, careful consideration must be given to establishing robust governance structures, promoting technical capacity building, and mitigating political interference to ensure effective health policy implementation [20, 22].

3.4 Policy recommendations

- *Clarify budgeting timelines*: LMICs should establish explicit timelines for the entire budgeting process, from drafting to legislative approval, to reduce delays and enhance efficiency.

- *Diversify evaluation metrics*: When assessing the impact of budgeting on socio-economic indicators, LMICs should consider a broader range of drivers beyond the budgeting process itself.

- *Consider budgeting techniques*: LMICs should explore different budgeting techniques, such as zero-based budgeting, to overcome inefficiencies and enhance the scope of budget performance.

- *Integrate decentralization with deconcentration*: For effective health governance, LMICs should pair decentralization efforts with deconcentration to ensure coherent policy implementation and avoid challenges stemming from inconsistent governance structures.

- *Address political interference*: LMICs must actively work to minimize political interference in health policy decisions, fostering an environment where technical staff and policy makers are empowered, respected, and valued.

4. Tanzania's health budgeting landscape

4.1 Overview of health budgeting in Tanzania

- *Political structure:* Tanzania follows a unitary system of governance with a central government and administrative regions. Health services are decentralized to regional and district levels.
- *Budget allocation structure:* Regions and districts have responsibilities for planning and implementing health budgets based on local needs. Central government support is provided through grants and other funding mechanisms.
- *Policy landscape:* Tanzania has a Health Sector Strategic Plan that guides policies and interventions in the health sector. Decentralization allows regions and districts to tailor health budgets to local priorities.
- *Political significance:* Health is a prominent agenda in political discourse and campaigns, reflecting its importance in addressing public health concerns.
- *Challenges in healthcare:* Challenges include variations in resource allocation, healthcare infrastructure, and the need for improved healthcare workforce capacity.
- *Health budgeting process:* Regions and districts engage in a budgeting process involving planning, allocation, and implementation of health resources. The central government provides financial support, and oversight ensures adherence to national health policies [27].

4.1.1 Health services coverage in Tanzania

Health service coverage in Tanzania has made notable progress over the years, driven by government initiatives and partnerships with international donors. However, like many developing countries, Tanzania faces various challenges in achieving comprehensive health service coverage for its population. Tanzania faces significant challenges in its healthcare system, marked by high maternal and child mortality, prevalent diseases like HIV/AIDS, pneumonia, and malaria, and limited access to health personnel. Over 60% of healthcare facilities are government-run, while the rest are faith-based or private. Despite resource constraints, the government is moving towards universal healthcare [27].

4.2 Findings from Tanzania review

- *Health insurance schemes*: Tanzania operates several health insurance schemes, including the National Health Insurance Fund (NHIF) for formal sector employees and the Community Health Fund (CHF) for the rural and informal sector. These schemes aim to improve access to health services and reduce out-of-pocket expenditure.
- *Primary health care*: The country has invested in primary health care as the cornerstone of its health system, focusing on preventive and promotive health services, including vaccination, maternal and child health services, and treatment of common diseases.

- *Infrastructure development*: Efforts have been made to improve health infrastructure, including the construction, and upgrading of health facilities from dispensaries to referral hospitals across the country.

- *Human resources for health*: Despite challenges, Tanzania has worked on increasing the number and skills of healthcare workers, though distribution and retention especially in rural areas remain problematic [28, 29].

4.2.1 Challenges

- *Financial barriers*: Financial constraints are a significant barrier to accessing health services, with many Tanzanians still paying out of pocket for healthcare. Insurance coverage remains low, particularly among the informal sector and rural populations.

- *Geographical disparities*: There are substantial disparities in health service access between urban and rural areas, with remote areas facing shortages of health facilities and healthcare workers.

- *Quality of services*: The quality of healthcare services varies, with issues related to the availability of essential medicines, equipment, and skilled healthcare providers. This affects patient satisfaction and health outcomes.

- *Burden of diseases*: Tanzania is challenged by a dual burden of communicable diseases, such as HIV/AIDS, malaria, and tuberculosis, and a rising prevalence of non-communicable diseases (NCDs) like hypertension and diabetes. This dual burden strains the healthcare system.

- *Health system challenges*: The health system faces challenges in governance, financing, health information systems, and supply chain management, impacting the efficiency and effectiveness of service delivery.

- *Emerging health threats*: Like many countries, Tanzania must contend with emerging health threats, including epidemics and the impacts of climate change on health, requiring a robust health system response [28, 29].

4.2.2 Structure of health financing, stakeholder involvement and coordination

Tanzania's health financing structure involves multiple stakeholders and requires coordinated efforts to ensure adequate funding for the healthcare sector [28].

- *Government funding*: The Tanzanian government allocates a portion of its budget to the health sector, aiming to support healthcare infrastructure, services, and programs. The government budget covers recurrent costs, development projects, and operational expenses within the health sector. In the 2020/2021 fiscal year, Tanzania allocated $387.9 million to the health sector, with $155.5 million designated for development projects. The 2022/2023 budget allocates TZS 1109 billion to the health sector, reflecting a commitment to health improvement initiatives.

The 2022/23 budget highlights key priorities, including strengthening the health system for child vaccinations and enhancing the overall quality of healthcare services. Despite challenges, the government's commitment to addressing these issues signifies a proactive approach to improving the health landscape in Tanzania, as shown in **Table 1** [27].

- *Donor funding:* International donors play a significant role in supporting Tanzania's health system, contributing up to 40% of the health budget. Donors, including organizations like USAID and CDC, provide financial assistance for various health

	Kenya	**Tanzania**	**Nigeria**
Strengths	*Increased health budget*: Kenya has committed to increasing its annual budget in line with the Abuja Declaration, of at least 15% to health. *Innovative financing*: Introducing Health Financing Reforms such as Linda Mama program for free maternity services, has improved access to healthcare services. *Decentralization*: The devolution of healthcare services to county governments aimed at decision-making closer to the communities, improving resource allocation and service delivery	*Community-based health insurance schemes*: The Community Health Fund (CHF) and the improved CHF have enhanced access to healthcare for low-income and rural populations by providing affordable insurance options. *Sector-wide approach*: Tanzania has adopted a sector-wide approach (SWAp) to health financing, improving coordination of resources and interventions across the health sector.	*Large scale programs*: Nigeria has implemented large-scale health programs, such as the National Health Insurance Scheme (NHIS), aimed at increasing access to healthcare services. *Increased investment in public health*: Efforts to increase investment in public health, particularly in response to outbreaks and emergencies, have been notable.
Weaknesses	*Inequitable financing:* Despite increased budget allocations, significant disparities remain in health financing across counties, affecting service delivery in poorer regions. *Dependency on donor funding*: A substantial portion of Kenya's health budget relies on external donors, making it vulnerable to fluctuations in funding. *High out-of-pocket expenditures*: Patients still face high out-of-pocket costs, which can lead to financial hardship and deter people from seeking necessary medical care on time and when necessary.	*Low health budget allocation*: Tanzania's health budget allocation remains below the Abuja Declaration target, limiting resources available for health service improvement. *Fragmented insurance schemes*: The existence of multiple health insurance schemes with varying coverage levels leads to fragmentation and inefficiencies in the health system. *Infrastructure and resource gaps*: Despite efforts, there are still significant gaps in healthcare infrastructure and human resources, especially in rural areas	*Underfunding of health sector*: The health sector is chronically underfunded, with budget allocations consistently falling short of the Abuja Declaration target. *Coverage and accessibility issues*: The PHC and NHIS covers a small fraction of the population, primarily those in formal employment, per-urban and rural areas, leaving a significant portion of the population without insurance coverage. *Corruption and inefficient utilization of resources*: Corruption and inefficiencies in resource allocation and utilization hamper the effectiveness of health expenditures.

Table 1.
Comparative evaluation (SWOT analysis) of each country health expenditure and funding sources.

programs and initiatives. International donors play a crucial role, contributing up to 40% of the health budget. Notably, the US government, through USAID and CDC, provides significant support to Tanzanian healthcare programs.

- *Health insurance:* Health insurance coverage in Tanzania is still low, with only 32% of the population covered as of 2019. Only 1% of Tanzanians are members of private health insurance, indicating limited coverage from the private sector.

- *Private sector contributions:* The private sector, including private health facilities and services, contributes to the overall health financing landscape. Private sector involvement may include out-of-pocket expenses paid by individuals for healthcare services.

- *Coordination mechanisms:* Coordination of health financing involves collaboration between various stakeholders to ensure effective resource allocation and utilization. The Ministry of Health, Community Development, Gender, Elderly, and Children (MOHCDGEC) plays a central role in coordinating health financing activities. The Tanzania Health Financing Strategy provides a framework for coordinating financial resources, with a focus on efficiency, equity, and sustainability.

- *Stakeholder involvement:* The Ministry of Finance, as a key government department, is involved in budget allocation and financial planning for the health sector. Development partners and international organizations actively contribute funds and technical assistance, engaging in collaborative efforts with the Tanzanian government. The private sector, including faith-based organizations, runs a portion of healthcare facilities, contributing to service delivery.

- *Community participation:* Community health funds and community-based health insurance initiatives involve local communities, shown in **Figure 4**, clearly contributes to their healthcare expenses. Community engagement is essential for ensuring that health financing strategies align with the needs and priorities of the population [28].

4.2.3 Budgeting constraints in Tanzania

- *Revenue collection challenges:* Domestic revenue collection can be challenging due to factors such as a large informal economy, tax evasion, and difficulties in expanding the tax base. This limits the government's ability to generate adequate funds for public services.

- *Debt sustainability concerns*: Accumulating public debt can constrain budgetary flexibility. Tanzania, like many other African countries, has faced concerns about the sustainability of its debt levels, which can affect its ability to finance essential services without compromising future fiscal stability.

- *Infrastructure development needs*: Tanzania, as a developing nation, has significant infrastructure development needs. Allocating funds for large-scale infrastructure projects, such as roads, energy, and water, can strain the budget and limit resources available for other critical sectors.

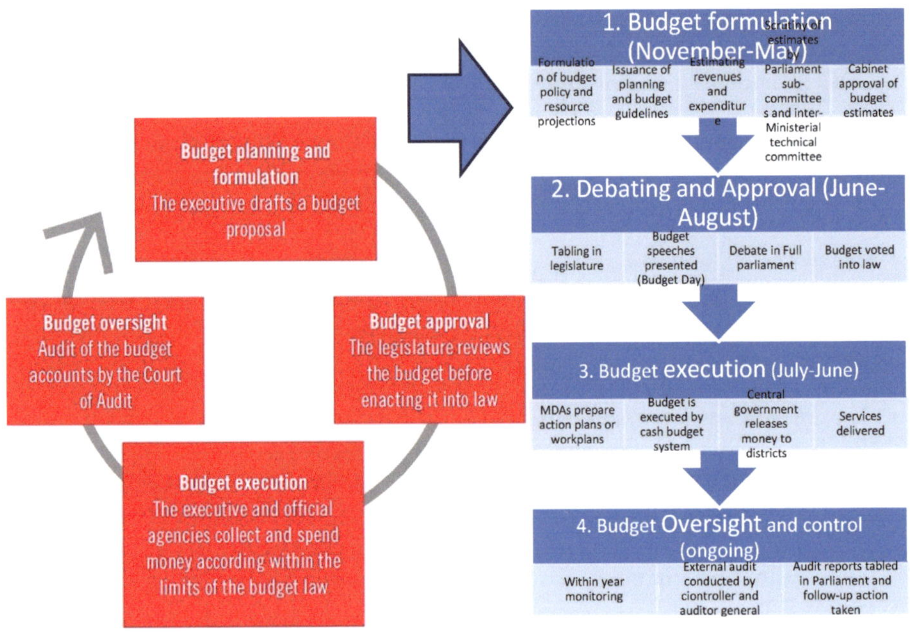

Figure 4.
Tanzania (MOFEA) - stages of budget process and key steps. Source: Ministry of Finance and Economic Affairs (MOFEA), Tanzania. Available at: https://www.policyforum-tz.org/sites/default/files/2021-03/Understanding%20the%20Budget%20Process%20in%20Tanzania%20-%20A%20CSO%20Guide.pdf

- *Social services demands*: The growing population and increasing demand for social services, including healthcare and education, pose budgetary challenges. Meeting the needs of a rapidly growing population requires substantial financial resources.

4.2.3.1 Limited fiscal space for health and issues related to budget execution

- *Limited financial resources*: Tanzania, like many other countries, faces challenges related to limited financial resources. The government struggles to allocate sufficient funds to meet the diverse needs of its population, including healthcare, education, infrastructure, and social services.

- *Dependency on external aid*: Tanzania has historically relied on external aid and donor funding to support its budget. While these funds are crucial for development projects, there is a risk of dependency and vulnerability to changes in donor priorities.

4.3 Success stories

4.3.1 Notable achievements in health budgeting and management

Tanzania willingness to pilot health reforms by WB and WHO, like performance-based pay (PBP) and performance-based results (PBR), and acceptance of external aid has largely influenced the institutionalization of the budget tools, financial management guidelines and governance oversight structures. In the process, the adoption of these initiatives has yielded great dividends in building local capacity, promoted inclusivity and transparency at all levels [27].

4.3.2 Replicability of Tanzania's strategies in other LMICs

There is a strong governance oversight with accountability. The use of MTEF and budget request tools (Dezeko – if translated into Swahili) has been consistently applied across all tiers of government. The strengthening of the coordination mechanisms and enhancing stakeholder collaboration through political and governance oversight have been essential for achieving sustainable and equitable health financing.

4.3.3 Policy recommendations

To address these challenges and improve health service coverage, Tanzania needs to continue investing in health infrastructure, increase the health workforce, enhance the quality of care, and expand health insurance coverage. Strengthening the health system through integrated and comprehensive approaches, focusing on both preventive and curative services, and ensuring equitable access to health services are crucial steps towards achieving universal health coverage.

5. Comparative analysis and cross-country insights

5.1 Political economy analysis (PEA)

In both Kenya and Tanzania, health budgeting is influenced by political priorities, public demands, and the need for efficient resource allocation. Devolution in Kenya and decentralization in Tanzania contribute to localized decision-making in health budgeting; this is yet to be achieved in Nigeria. Challenges in workforce capacity, infrastructure, and resource disparities among regions underscore the complexity of health budgeting in both countries. Political commitment to health issues is evident, reflecting the recognition of health as a critical component of public welfare. Nigeria's health program operates within a complex political and economic landscape characterized by federalism, multi-tiered governance, and diverse socio-economic factors [15, 27].

The political economy of Nigeria significantly influences the formulation, implementation, and outcomes of health policies and programs; hence, a focus on what makes it unique is described below as an in-depth analysis (deep dive).

5.1.1 Key drivers for Nigeria

- *Federal system*: Nigeria's federal structure divides health responsibilities among the federal, state, and local governments. The coordination and alignment of health policies across these levels influence the effectiveness of health programs.

- *Resource allocation*: Resource distribution and fiscal space significantly impact health financing. Competing demands for resources, especially in the context of diverse sectors, influence the prioritization and funding of health programs.

- *Political manifestos*: Health is a crucial element in political campaigns, but government priorities do not often align with political manifestos. This political significance can drive resource allocation and policy focus.

- *Devolution challenges*: The challenges associated with devolution include variations in resource availability, capacity disparities, and differing priorities among States. These factors affect the equitable implementation of health programs.

- *Health act 2014*: The Health Act and the Basic Health Care Provision Fund (BHCPF) provide frameworks for health financing and service delivery. However, challenges related to its implementation, adherence, and political will has impacted their effectiveness [20, 21, 23, 25].

- *Public awareness and advocacy*: The level of public awareness and advocacy influences political will and resource allocation. A strong public demand for health improvements can drive political commitment to health programs.

5.1.2 The implications for Nigeria

- *Resource allocation disparities*: Disparities in resource allocation among states and local governments has resulted in unequal access to healthcare services.

- *Political commitment*: The commitment of political leaders to health programs significantly impacts their success. A sustained commitment to health, beyond political cycles, is crucial.

- *Implementation challenges*: Challenges related to the implementation of health policies and programs may arise due to varying capacities, governance structures, and political will across states.

- *Advocacy and public engagement*: Strengthening advocacy efforts and public engagement can enhance the political will for health improvements and contribute to increased resource allocation.

- *Coordination mechanisms*: Improving coordination mechanisms between federal, state, and local levels is essential for effective health program implementation and resource management.

5.2 Comparative evaluation of health expenditure and sources

See summary in **Table A1** in the annex and supplement.

5.2.1 Comparative analysis

A comparative analysis of health budget expenditure in Kenya, Tanzania, and Nigeria reveals the strengths and weaknesses of their healthcare financing strategies, impacting their ability to achieve universal health coverage (UHC) and improve health outcomes. Each country has its unique approach to healthcare funding, shaped by its economic context, health priorities, and governance structures (**Table 1**).

5.2.2 Comparative analysis of the three countries (Kenya, Tanzania, and Nigeria)

A comparative analysis of health budget expenditure in Kenya, Tanzania, and Nigeria highlights the importance of not just the amount of budget allocated to health but also the efficiency and equity of its use. Strengthening health insurance coverage, ensuring equitable distribution of resources, and focusing on both preventive and curative care are essential steps towards improving health outcomes and achieving UHC in these countries.

5.2.2.1 Comparative insights

- *Funding levels*: All three countries struggle to meet the recommended Abuja Declaration target for health budget allocations, affecting their ability to adequately finance their health systems.

- *Insurance coverage*: Kenya and Tanzania have made strides in expanding insurance coverage through innovative and community-based schemes, whereas Nigeria's insurance scheme has limited reach.

- *Challenges with equity and efficiency*: Inequities in resource distribution and inefficiencies in resource utilization are common challenges across the three countries, impacting the overall effectiveness of their health systems.

- *Dependency on external funding*: Kenya and Tanzania, in particular, face challenges related to dependency on donor funding, which affects the sustainability of health financing.

To enhance their health budget expenditures' effectiveness, Kenya, Tanzania, and Nigeria need to address these weaknesses by increasing domestic health financing, improving efficiency and transparency in fund allocation and utilization, expanding insurance coverage to include vulnerable populations, and strengthening health system infrastructure and human resources.

Strengthening primary health care with appropriate deconcentration putting in place - well motivated and skilled providers in planning and budget management will appropriately guide and develop the bottom-up approaches. Since they remain the first level contact or frontline workers respected by the communities. Their role as duty bearers will be appreciated as interlocutors for the voiceless.

The engagement and involvement of the managerial process – village, community, ward, and district development committees and CSOs need to be revitalized and/or strengthened as part of gate keepers of the communities and people through inclusive and participatory teams that has youths with appropriate gender representation.

5.2.3 Key similarities and differences among Kenya, Nigeria, and Tanzania

The distribution of responsibilities and roles between national and subnational or county governments differ in each country, affecting the efficiency of healthcare service delivery. The emphasis on specific health programs and policies, such as social protection programs and health insurance subsidies, differ among the three countries, although less than 10 per cent of the eligible populations. The level of technical efficiency and governance challenges in health systems vary, affecting their abilities to translate financial resources into improved health outcomes.

Tanzania demonstrates a very strong governance oversight and high political commitment compared to countries like Kenya and Nigeria.

5.2.3.1 Similarities

All three countries are committed to achieving UHC. They also all have similar demographic transition profile, a young population with generic health systems challenges. Government plays a key and major role in their health planning and budgeting with varying degrees of political interference. The adoption of public finance management tools and WHO_WB guidelines is variable and poorly adapted and adopted at the district levels. PHC is foundational in their health for all strategy, however, this is yet to be translated into efficient and effective bottom-up planning and budgeting (**Table 2**).

5.2.3.2 Differences

The differences are that whilst Kenya has an increasing health spending trend, as percentage of GDP, this is not the case with Nigeria and Tanzania. The allocation of health expenditure in Tanzania is focused on PHC whilst Kenya and Nigeria continue to invest heavily on secondary and tertiary care. Staff absenteeism and turnover are common practices noted in Nigeria and Kenya but to a less extent in Tanzania (**Table 3**).

5.2.4 Conclusion

Two countries (Kenya and Tanzania) demonstrate a strong commitment to addressing health challenges through strategic planning, policy frameworks, and political engagement [30]. The political landscape, governance structures, and resource distribution mechanisms shape the health budgeting processes in Kenya and Tanzania.

	Kenya	**Tanzania**	**Nigeria**
UHC Agenda	All three countries, Kenya, Nigeria, and Tanzania, share a commitment to achieving Universal Health Coverage (UHC), as evidenced by efforts to increase access and improve health outcomes.		
Demographic and Epidemiological transitions	They all have a young population. Similar challenges in demographic and epidemiological transitions are observed, necessitating adjustments in service delivery models and healthcare infrastructure		
Government's role in Health financing	All three countries are experiencing a shift towards increased government participation in health financing, with reduced contributions from donors and corporations.		
PFM improvements	There are efforts in all three countries to enhance Public Financial Management (PFM) capacity, although challenges such as delayed fund releases and unspent resources persist.		
Emphasis on PHC	There is recognition of the need to prioritize primary health care for equity and efficiency, although there are challenges in resource allocation and implementation.		
Devolution of the health care system	All three have devolved their health care system with varying capacity, governance, and management oversight.		
Budget cycle, budget tools, budget processes and reviews	All three have legislative Acts, appropriate financial and budgeting tools and clear process for engagement, negotiations, and enactment into law, including the use of MTEF, MTSS and other expenditure tracking tools		

Table 2.
Summary of similarities.

DOI: http://dx.doi.org/10.5772/intechopen.1004996

	Kenya	Tanzania	Nigeria
Health spending as a % of GDP	Increasing trend. Kenya's health spending as a percentage of GDP is higher but relatively lower than the average for LMIC. Increasing government grant and aid	Declining trend. Tanzania has lower ratios, with more external aid funding declining government transfers and out of pocket spending.	Declining trend. Nigeria has lower ratios, with inadequate resource allocation and efficiency. It largely depends on OOP spend with declining government grants and external aid.
Composition of Health expenditure	The allocation of health expenditure across different health sectors varies. Kenya's spending is skewed towards secondary and tertiary care.	Tanzania has a different pattern with focus at the district and primary health care.	The allocation of health expenditure across different health sectors varies. Spending is skewed towards secondary and tertiary care
Devolution and funds flow	Devolution has significantly impacted Kenya's health system, altering the flow of funds between national and county governments	Tanzania has a fully devolved and decentralized system structured along its political system.	The impact of devolution on health in Nigeria has been mixed with more State control over the LGAs - as provided in the 2014 health Act
Role of national and subnational governments	Kenya exerts no influence from the center on the county government. Hence, difficulty for alignment and harmonization of plans.	Tanzania's situation is well aligned with its political system, and it allows a more inclusive and bottom-up approach.	Nigeria's situation is at variance with its national health policy intentions, as the States still maintain a joint account with the local governments (LGAs) with no autonomy for the LGAs to prioritize and budget for its needs.
Efficiency Challenges and Inefficiencies:	High rates of staff absenteeism in Kenya at a high cost	However, this is less of a concern in Tanzania.	Staff absenteeism similar in the case of Nigeria.
Institutional Delivery and Infant Mortality Correlation	There is weak correlation between health financing, outputs, and outcomes, as observed	Tanzania, impacting their ability to achieve optimal returns on health investments	There is no correlation between health financing, outputs and outcomes as stipulated in their strategic plan.
Technical Efficiency and Governance Challenges	Weak technical capacity and efficiency in planning and budgeting with poor governance oversight at the county levels.	Improved technical capacity and adherence to best practices of applying the PFM tools like the MTEF.	Weak technical capacity and efficiency in the planning and budgeting
Specific Health Programs and Policies	Social health insurance coverages less than 10 per cent of the eligible populations in Nigeria, unlike in Kenya and Tanzania where the coverage is more than 32 per cent.		

Table 3.
Summary of differences.

Nigeria's health program, on the other hand, operates within a dynamic political economy, and the success of health policies and programs depends on addressing challenges related to resource allocation, political commitment, and effective implementation mechanisms across the federal structure, especially at the State level. Public awareness and advocacy play pivotal roles in influencing political will and resource prioritization for health improvements. Political commitment to health, as evident in manifestos, and legal frameworks like the Health Act and BHCPF contribute to the complex landscape of health financing in the country. The health budgeting process is a crucial aspect of governance, reflecting the commitment to improving healthcare services across all levels of government [21, 25].

Like Kenya and Tanzania, healthcare budgeting in Nigeria involves collaboration among multiple stakeholders, including government bodies, legislators, the public, and external partners. Engaging these stakeholders is vital for effective and transparent budgeting, leading to improved healthcare outcomes and increased access to services [28, 29].

5.2.5 Common challenges faced by LMICs in health budgeting and management

- *Political interference* – this must be eliminated to ensure transparency and allow full participation of stakeholders and the people. An elitist budgeting process must be avoided in the best interest of the people. No one is more intelligent than everyone.

- *Capacity* of policy makers, programme managers and gate keepers (accountants) at all levels to are improved or upskilled to plan, budget and execute professionally.

- *Governance oversight* – this is necessary to ensure that guidelines and due processes are followed.

- *Accountability* – there must be a regular and institutionalized mutual and social accountability monitoring process at all levels by CSOs and district committees.

- *Inconsistent use of the Medium-Term Expenditure Framework (MTEF) at all levels*: Planning and budgeting document prepared by each Government Ministry, departments, and agencies (MDA). The MTEF helps to make a projection over 3 years and essentially cover: i) programme cost; ii) donors commitments; iii) harmonize all foreign aid; and iv) influence sector strategies. Overall, the MTEF seeks to establish a link between country policies, the budget, and its execution. More from incremental (historical) budgeting to zero budgeting (more of activity-based costing. Most countries still use economic classification with no contingency planning provision. Economic classification is that expenditure classification that provides information on the nature of the expenditure, such as whether funds are being used to pay for wages and salaries, capital projects, and/or social assistance benefits [28].

5.3 Best practices and solutions

5.3.1 Identification of successful strategies from the case studies and recommendations for overcoming common challenges

Better and improved partners coordination, collaboration, alignment and harmonization of plans, budgeting and agreed results – delivering as One (One Plan, One budget, One M&E). Improve coordination and collaboration between the tiers of national and subnational governments to explore potential PFM-related reforms that could be implemented to ensure conditional grants flow directly to health and other frontline facilities (using a DFF mechanism), rather than cascading slowly and irregularly through the different layers of the intergovernmental financing framework [30, 31].

Implementing strategies to continue improving budget execution, absorption of development budget, and disbursement of funds from the exchequer. Budget execution has improved significantly over time. Remaining capacity constraints should be addressed through capacity building on planning, budget preparation, budget management, and execution. Alignment and linking of the project implementation cycle to budgeting process and timely release of funds would contribute to improved budget absorption [29].

Improving monitoring and governance systems to accelerate progress towards greater accountability and agreed health targets. This could further strengthen and institutionalize the annual sector public expenditure and performance review both at the national and the subnational levels through a mutual accountability framework.

Increasing investments in health management skills and information systems to generate timely and useful information for policy review, planning and budgeting, monitoring of performance monitoring, and overall benchmarking.

Consider introducing reforms to accelerate the flow of resources to front line facilities and strengthen the linkages between payment and performance and the achievement of planned results.

6. Global implications and recommendations

6.1 Generalizability of findings

Weak linkages between policies and budgets are related to the absence and inconsistent use of MTEF as seen in Nigeria and Kenya. Tanzania is a gold standard. MTEF is a powerful tool for ensuring government accountability in budgeting. The integration of policy making, planning, and budgeting provides for expenditure programmes to be driven by policy priorities and budget discipline. One of the many benefits of MTEF is that it provides the means to review decisions and make the tradeoffs transparently. This will strengthen institutional processes within government and allow partners access to information by which governments are held to account.

Thus, reforms in budget formulation that transitions to programme-based budgeting can be beneficial to health spending. These reforms widely applied can support better alignment with health sector priorities, provide greater flexibility in the use of funds, and improve transparency and accountability towards expected outputs. These changes can, in turn, support accelerated progress towards universal health coverage by using general budget revenues flexibly to purchase health services [12].

The practice of dual budgeting in Nigeria, where capital expenditure of over 1 m naira (equivalent of USD$1110) goes back to the State governor for approval should be stopped. In Ref. [7], WB in 1998, observed in its report that “dual budgeting may well be the most important culprit in the failure to link planning, policy and budgeting”.

Another limitation of the public expenditure management (PEM)/budget systems is the absence of budget comprehensiveness. The principle is not only a good practice for transparency and accountability [9] but an important feature of a sound budget system that allows for meaningful debate on allocation. OECD, in 2002, proposed zero budgeting with activity-based costing (ABC), as best practice; detailing expenditures by administrative units with supplementary information showing breakdowns by economic and functional categories. This practice is well entrenched in countries like South Africa, Malawi and Ghana [9].

The efficiency of budget implementation and the capacity of ministries, departments, and agencies (MDAs) play also a critical part budget execution into outputs and outcomes. Fozzard, A et al., in their paper, (2002) observe that: "It is no longer assumed that budgetary allocations are automatically transformed into budgetary outcomes. Public sector resource allocation is determined by the criteria and process of decision-making and the process of budget execution" [32]. Therefore, a country's ability to progressively realize economic, social and cultural rights depends on its capacity to formulate and appropriate a good budget based on sound policy and participation, in order to ensure its effective and efficient utilization.

However, evidence from country implementation shows that this transformation does not take place automatically. This book chapter has identified some generic issues, practices, and beliefs that if addressed with key health stakeholders and governments, including CSOs can improve budget formulation, ensure better understanding of the design, implementation, and monitoring of programme-based budgets in the health sector in low- and middle-income countries (LMICs) [31–33].

6.1.1 Applicability to other LMICs and considerations for adapting strategies to diverse contexts

By incorporating these recommendations, LMICs can strengthen their budgeting processes, navigate challenges associated with decentralization, and ultimately contribute to more effective and responsive health governance.

A common budget preparation approach will be useful but not necessarily the same for all context based on WHO 2022 guidance on "how the make a budget work" [12].

Adoption and adaptation of best practices by the United Nations, like the use of HACT and FACE form templates will streamline the different funds requests formats and liquidations of funds [34].

Governance oversight with strong reactions and sanctions of to audit reports.

Build the capacity of MDAs and establish a clear table of authority (TOA).

Strengthen CSOs capacity for advocacy and a voice for the voiceless. Also, it enhances their ability to independently analyze, monitor and report on expenditure as a right issue.

6.1.2 General recommendations for improving health budget management constraints in Kenya

This analysis offers comprehensive recommendations for overcoming health budget management constraints in Kenya, with the goal of enhancing the efficiency and transparency of healthcare spending. Key suggestions include:

- *Strengthening planning and budgeting processes*: Emphasize the importance of meticulous planning and budgeting to address poor financial management. This involves incorporating tools like Public Expenditure Reviews (PERs) and Medium-Term Expenditure Frameworks (MTEF) to foster wider stakeholder participation.

- *Addressing corruption*: Tackle corruption head-on by implementing robust anti-corruption measures within the healthcare system. This may involve strengthening oversight mechanisms and promoting a culture of accountability.

- *Capacity building*: Invest in building the capacity of personnel within Ministries of Health to ensure that they possess the necessary skills for effective budget management. This includes training programs and ongoing professional development.

- *Governance oversight*: Strengthen governance oversight to prevent political interference in the alignment of health sector policies with resource allocation. This can be achieved through legal and legislative processes that safeguard the integrity of budget execution.

- *Enhancing social accountability*: Promote social accountability in program delivery by encouraging the active involvement of communities and civil society organizations. This could be facilitated through open government collaboration, ensuring that key stakeholders have a voice in the decision-making processes.

- *Community and civil society ownership*: Increase community and civil society ownership by involving them in the decision-making processes. This can be achieved through transparent and inclusive practices, allowing these stakeholders to actively contribute to the healthcare budgeting and management.

Overall, these recommendations aim to provide a roadmap for policymakers, practitioners, and stakeholders in Kenya to overcome budget management constraints and work towards achieving universal health coverage.

6.1.3 General recommendations for improving budget management constraints in Nigeria

The book chapter outlines several overarching recommendations to address health budget management constraints in Nigeria, aiming to enhance efficiency, transparency, and ultimately contribute to the achievement of universal health coverage. The key recommendations include:

- *Enhanced planning and budgeting processes*: Strengthen planning and budgeting processes by incorporating internationally recognized tools such as Public Expenditure Reviews (PERs) and Medium-Term Expenditure Frameworks (MTEF). This facilitates more accurate forecasting and wider stakeholder participation in the budgeting process.

- *Anti-corruption measures*: Implement robust anti-corruption measures within the healthcare system to mitigate financial mismanagement. This involves creating and enforcing policies that foster transparency, accountability, and ethical behavior among healthcare officials.

- *Capacity building*: Invest in the capacity building of personnel within health-related government agencies. This includes providing training programs to enhance the skills and knowledge of individuals involved in health budget management.

- *Governance oversight*: Strengthen governance oversight to prevent political interference in the alignment of health sector policies with resource allocation.

Legislative and institutional reforms may be necessary to ensure autonomy and effectiveness in budget execution.

- *Social accountability*: Promote social accountability in healthcare program delivery by involving communities and civil society organizations. This can be achieved through mechanisms that encourage open dialog, feedback, and active participation in decision-making processes.
- *Community and civil society ownership*: Foster community and civil society ownership by actively involving these stakeholders in health budget management. This includes creating platforms for engagement, information dissemination, and collaboration to ensure that diverse perspectives are considered.
- *Open government collaboration*: Encourage open government collaboration in health budgeting processes to enhance transparency and inclusivity. This involves making relevant information accessible to the public and engaging in dialog with various stakeholders.
- *Enhanced monitoring and accountability*: Strengthen mechanisms for monitoring budget implementation and holding stakeholders accountable to improve transparency and curb corruption.
- *Public awareness campaigns*: Launch public awareness campaigns to educate the population on preventive healthcare measures, disease management, and the importance of health insurance.
- *Policy implementation reforms*: Strengthen governance structures and improve the coordination of health policies to enhance their effective implementation.

These recommendations collectively aim to provide a comprehensive framework for addressing health budget management constraints in Nigeria, empowering the government, healthcare professionals, communities, and civil society to work collaboratively towards improving the nation's healthcare system.

Addressing these challenges requires a multi-stakeholder approach, involving collaboration between the government, healthcare professionals, civil society, and international partners. Regular evaluations and adjustments to the strategies will be necessary to ensure sustained improvements in Nigeria's health budgeting and healthcare delivery.

6.1.4 General recommendations to address health budgeting management constraints in Tanzania

The analysis proposes several general recommendations to address health budget management constraints in Tanzania, with the overarching goal of improving efficiency, transparency, and the overall healthcare system. The key recommendations include:

- *Strengthening planning and budgeting procedures*: Enhance the effectiveness of planning and budgeting processes by incorporating established tools such as Public Expenditure Reviews (PERs) and Medium-Term Expenditure Frameworks (MTEF). This facilitates better forecasting and encourages wider stakeholder participation in the budgeting process.

- *Anti-corruption measures*: Implement and reinforce anti-corruption measures within the healthcare sector to curb financial mismanagement. Establish and enforce policies that promote transparency, accountability, and ethical conduct among healthcare professionals.

- *Capacity building*: Invest in the capacity building of personnel within health-related government agencies. This involves providing training programs to improve the skills and knowledge of individuals involved in health budget management.

- *Governance oversight*: Strengthen governance oversight to prevent political interference in the alignment of health sector policies with resource allocation. Legislative and institutional reforms may be necessary to ensure autonomy and effective budget execution.

- *Social accountability*: Promote social accountability in healthcare program delivery by actively involving communities and civil society organizations. Establish mechanisms that encourage open dialog, feedback, and active participation in decision-making processes.

- *Community and civil society ownership*: Foster community and civil society ownership by actively engaging these stakeholders in health budget management. Create platforms for collaboration, information dissemination, and inclusion to ensure diverse perspectives are considered.

- *Open government collaboration*: Encourage open government collaboration in health budgeting processes to enhance transparency and inclusivity. Make relevant information accessible to the public and engage in dialog with various stakeholders.

- *Enhance public financial management*: Improving the efficiency and transparency of public financial management systems can enhance accountability and reduce the risk of corruption. Implementing best practices in budgeting, procurement, and financial reporting can contribute to better fiscal outcomes.

- *Continued dialog and cooperation*: Engaging in ongoing dialog with stakeholders, including international partners, civil society, and the private sector, can foster cooperation and support in addressing budgeting constraints.

These recommendations collectively provide a comprehensive framework for addressing health budget management constraints in Tanzania. They aim to empower the government, healthcare professionals, communities, and civil society to collaboratively work towards improving the efficiency and effectiveness of the country's healthcare system.

6.2 Specific policy and programmatic recommendations

6.2.1 Proposals for international organizations, donor agencies and development partners group (DPG)

The Adoption of WHO 2022 "how to make budget for health better" guidelines [12] is a useful starting point. Having a governance oversight committee supported by a project management unit (PMU) within the MDAs is critical for transparency and accountability. Close and regular coordination between the ministry of health (MOH), ministry of finance (MOF) with key stakeholders through the quarterly health partners coordination mechanism will build trust and confidence in the partnership.

The adoption of the One budget UN approach – applying the medium-term expenditure framework (MTEF) and sector wide approach (SwaP) tools [32] will strengthen government institutions and increased investment by donors and development partners. This will foster alignment and harmonization of plans – eventually contributing to agreed results.

A mutual accountability framework operationalized at the national and subnational levels have proven a good mechanism. Building the capacity of institutions and their staffs to improve planning and financial management skills based on a regular institutional capacity assessment at all levels will make governance better and improve bottom-up planning.

Finally, adoption of a simpler and easy to request and account for funds – aka, applying the UN harmonized assisted cash transfer (HACT) and funding authorization and certificate of expenditure (FACE) forms will make the process easier for MDAs. It is used for request for release and accountability of funds earmarked in the workplan. "The FACE Form is a simplified and harmonized form that replaces agency-specific reporting formats and documentation to support implementing partner requests for expenditure" [34, 35].

6.2.2 Advocacy for sustainable improvements in health budgeting and management should include the following

Strengthening CSO's role – as duty bearers to hold government and legislature to account and strengthen the managerial processes (aka, district development committees).

Conduct of operation research and the use of evidence for decision-making. Promote transparency for timely availability and publication of technical and financial reports – online and/or dedicated website regularly.

Translate the public finance management (PFM) Act into operationally feasible process with clear terms of reference (TOA) and reduced transactions cost with undue political influence.

Strengthen programme leadership and management skills at all levels, including planning, budgeting, monitoring using obligation matrix and results-based reporting (output and/or outcome-based programming).

Finally, to urge policy makers and politicians to penalize erring and/or corrupt officers.

7. Summary of findings and conclusions: Tanzania, Nigeria, and Kenya

7.1 Conclusion across the three countries

- *Common themes*: All three countries emphasize a bottom-up approach in budget planning and preparation with top-down budgeting, in alignment with national goals, and involvement of various stakeholders. Challenges, however, include political interference, delays, and varying levels of transparency. The three countries (Kenya, Nigeria, and Tanzania) share common goals and challenges in their health systems; however, differences in economic status, governance structures, and healthcare priorities contribute to variations in health budgeting, management, and expenditure policies and practices. Understanding these similarities and differences is crucial for designing effective health policies and interventions tailored to each country's context. As shown in **Table 1–3**.

7.2 Recommendations

Several recommendations have been described. **Table 4** summarizes a list of potential recommendations in each country and classifies them according to their level of priority.

7.3 Recapitulation of key findings

For Kenya, the emphasis lies in fortifying planning and budgeting processes through tools like Public Expenditure Reviews and Medium-Term Expenditure Frameworks, addressing corruption head-on, investing in capacity building, strengthening governance oversight, promoting social accountability, and fostering community and civil society ownership. These recommendations form a roadmap for policymakers to overcome constraints and achieve universal health coverage.

In Nigeria, the focus is on enhancing planning processes, implementing anti-corruption measures, investing in capacity building, strengthening governance oversight, promoting social accountability, fostering community and civil society

	Kenya	Tanzania	Nigeria
1. **Key immediate actions**			
a. Result based planning	xxx	xxx	xxx
b. Addressing corruption	xxx	x	xxx
c. Capacity building	xxx	xxx	xxx
d. Governance oversight	xx	x	xx
e. Mutual and social accountability	xxx	xx	xxx
2. **Areas for improvements**			
a. Skilled staff shortages	xxx	xxx	xxx
b. Political interference.	xxx	x	xxx
c. Transparency and accountability	xxx	x	xxx
3. **Future focus**			
a. Continue reforms - programme-based budgeting policy implementation	xxx	xxx	xxx
b. Use of PFM tools and resource management practice improvements	xxx	xxx	xxx
c. Enhanced transparency and building trust	xxx	xx	xxx
d. Inclusivity	xxx	xx	xxx

Key: x = low priority; xx = moderate priority; and xxx = high priority.

Table 4.
Summary of key recommendations and priority for country action.

ownership, and encouraging open government collaboration. These recommendations aim to contribute to improved efficiency, transparency, and progress towards universal health coverage.

For Tanzania, the recommendations mirror those for Kenya and Nigeria, encompassing strengthened planning and budgeting processes, anti-corruption measures, capacity building, governance oversight, social accountability, community and civil society ownership, and open government collaboration. Additionally, enhancing public financial management and fostering continued dialog and cooperation are proposed to further refine the efficiency and transparency of Tanzania's healthcare system.

The overarching theme across all three countries is the need for a multi-stakeholder approach, involving collaboration between the government, healthcare professionals, civil society, and international partners. Regular evaluations and adjustments are emphasized to ensure sustained improvements in health budgeting and healthcare delivery across these diverse nations.

7.4 Call to action for LMICs and global stakeholders

7.4.1 Inclusive comprehensive and comprehensible planning and budgeting

Harmonize top-down budgeting with bottom-up planning through negotiated and agreed results (outputs and outcomes) aka results-based management (RBM). Over concentration on macro policy level and the persistent neglect of expenditure management issues at the site of service delivery.

7.4.2 Governance oversight with clear table of authority

In most cases there is good legislative framework but weak implementation. Tendency to rely on friendship, cronyism, party loyalties and to treat accountability as a personal favor to ordinary citizens. Lack of clear separation of powers between the implementation and oversight arms of government. The Executive Branch of the State (President, Cabinet and Public Service) and the Oversight branch (Parliament) are closely linked and in most cases cabinet ministers (for example, in Tanzania) double as Members of Parliament. This is even more acute at the local level.

7.4.3 Strong social monitoring and accountability system

Failure by most CSOs to use their socio-economic rights, existing constitutional and legislative provisions to participate in governance processes and think beyond formalized consultations and workshops. This has not helped reported and anecdotal widespread acts of corruption, conflict of interest and existence and/or failure to deliver improved health services.

7.5 Future directions for research and policy

WB, WHO and governments should, as of priority conduct LMIC institutional capacity assessment of national and subnational levels, down to the health facility level, where feasible before pushing for programmes-based budgeting.

Secondly, the development partners also need to build capacities and nurture these countries over time through embedded technical assistance (TA). This is very important as most donors and partners assume that governments will always act professionally and responsibly. In the face of multi-dimensional poverty and frequent political interference, policy makers and programme managers remain at risk of victimization and may not act professionally and always in good public faith.

Thirdly, the adoption and adaptation of the revised UNDP harmonized assisted cash transfer (HACT) and fund authorization and certificate of expenditure (FACE) framework will provide a shift from assurance for cash transfers derived from project level controls and audits towards a method of assurance derived from risk/system-based assessments and audits. It reaffirms a shift from a control-based to a risk-based management approach [34, 35].

Acknowledgements

I would like to acknowledge my sincere appreciations for the support and cooperation of the following persons: In Nigeria Drs. Hassana Adamu and Akinlawon Oyemakinde of Palladium Nigeria; Ms. Helen Ekpo, Programme Officer with Options; Dr. Nneka Onwu, retired Director, NPHCDA. In Kenya, Dr. Michael Mwaniki, Pediatrician and Public health practitioner; and in Tanzania, Georgiah Kasori, Programme manager with Amref, Tanzania. Others, Dr. Ima Kashim, Programme manager with the Saudi Islamic Development Bank for sharing her work and experience.

Conflict of interest

Declaration of Competing Interest: "The author declares that he has no conflict of interest or known competing financial interests or personal relationships that could have appeared to influence the work reported in this paper".

Notes/thanks/other declarations

Many thanks to Mrs. Judith Ibukunlayo, Mr. Edwin Agbo for hosting and bearing with me over the past 3 months; and Ms. Ruth Anyango Otieno, my valued partner, for her patience, moral support, and sustained encouragement.

Acronyms and abbreviations

AOP	annual operational plan
BHCPF	basic health care provision fund
CCHP	Comprehensive Council Health Plans
CDF	community development fund
CSO	Civil Service Organization
DHPRS	Department of Health planning, Research, and Statistics
DPG	Development Partners Group
FACE	fund authorization and certificate of expenditure
FCDO	Foreign Commonwealth and Development Office
GDP	gross domestic product
HACT	harmonized assisted cash transfer
HCH	Honorable Commissioner of Health

HRH	Human Resource for Health
IGR	internal generated revenue
LGA	local government agency
LMIC	Low Medium Income Country
LTA	long term agreements
M&E	Monitoring and Evaluation
MBFP	Ministry of Budget, Finance and planning
MBP	Ministry of budget and Planning
MDA	Ministries, Departments and Agencies
MDA	Ministry, Department and Agency
MOH	Ministry of Health
MoU	Memorandum of Understanding
MTEF	Medium-Term Expenditure Framework
MTSS	Medium Term Sector Strategy
NCH	National Council on Health
NGO	Nongovernmental Organization
NHA	National Health Accounts
NHIF	National Health Insurance Fund
OOP	out-of-pocket
PBB	program-based budgeting
PBR	payment by result
PEA	political economy analysis
PEM	Public Expenditure Management
PER	Public Expenditure Review
PETS	Public Expenditure Tracking Survey
PFM	Public Financial Management
PHC	Primary Health Care
SWAP	Sector Wide Approach
TA	technical assistance
TOA	table of authority
UHC	Universal Health Coverage
USAID	U.S. Agency for International Development
VfM	value for money
WB	World Bank
WHO	World Health Organization

Annex 1: key Informant Interview guide (Policy makers, programme managers and partners)

Dear Respondent, greetings. I have been invited to contribute to a book chapter on Healtheconomics in LMIC. I have chosen to focus on Kenya, Nigeria and Tanzania as case studies. So, I am seeking your honest, timely and professional feedback on the questions below. My contact details are on page 35 for any queries.

General consultation questions

1. What is your experience with the budgeting process?

2. How do you manage your budget?

3. What are the biggest challenges you face when it comes to budgeting and budget management?

4. In your opinion, what are the most important conclusions to draw from your experience with budgeting and budget management?

5. What recommendations would you give to someone who is just starting out with budgeting and budget management?

Annex 2: Specific questions: (target – MDAs – programme managers, officers, CSOs, Ward committee members). Qualitative Key Informant Interview Questionnaire on Budgeting and Management in LMIC - Case Study

Introduction: Thank you for participating in this key informant interview. The information gathered will contribute to understanding the budgeting and management processes in Low- and Middle-Income Countries (LMICs). Please note that your responses will be kept confidential, and the data will be used for research purposes only. Signed. Dr. Sam Agbo, MD, MPH, MSc, DLSHTM. Email address: agbosam@gmail.com; Tel #: +447716171804.

Demographic and Informant Information

1. Name and Position:

2. Organization/Institution:

3. Number of Years of Experience in Budgeting and Management:

4. Country/Region of Operation:

Section 1: general Overview

1. Can you provide an overview of the budgeting process in your organization or within the health sector in your country?

2. How are budget priorities determined in your organization or within the health sector at the national level?

Section 2: budget Formulation and Allocation

1. What factors influence the allocation of funds to health programs or projects in your country?

2. How does your organization involve stakeholders, including civil society, in the budget formulation process?

3. Can you share any challenges or successes related to the alignment of the health budget with national goals and priorities?

Section 3: budget Implementation and Management

1. Describe the mechanisms in place for executing and managing the health budget. How is accountability ensured?

2. What challenges, if any, have been encountered in the implementation of health budgets, and how were these addressed?

3. How does your organization or country monitor and evaluate the performance of health programs in relation to budgetary allocations?

Section 4: financial Oversight and Transparency

1. How does financial oversight function within your organization or at the national level to prevent misuse or misallocation of funds?

2. In your experience, how transparent is the budgeting and financial reporting process within the health sector in your country?

3. What role does public awareness and advocacy play in influencing budget decisions and resource allocation for health programs?

Section 5: capacity Building and Institutional Strengthening

1. Can you discuss any efforts or initiatives aimed at building the capacity of individuals or institutions involved in health budgeting and management?

2. In your opinion, what are the critical areas where capacity building is needed to enhance the effectiveness of health budgeting and management?

Section 6: future Considerations

1. Considering your experience, what improvements or reforms would you recommend for enhancing the health budgeting and management processes in LMICs?

2. How can international collaborations or partnerships contribute to strengthening health budgeting and management in LMICs?

Conclusion

1. Do you have any additional insights or comments you would like to share regarding health budgeting and management in LMICs?

Annex 2. Country Case Studies – budgeting process & management guide for KII

Background

1. Is health being a political priority and manifesto of the government?

2. Status of Health allocation, is it increasing?

3. Any improvement in terms of spend and efficiency?

Preparation

1. Financial year? – months of the year - when to when?

2. When does budget preparation start? Is it based on a guidance or template? Y/N?

3. How? Is it a bottom-up approach? Y/N, e.g. County to the national level?

4. Any Template applied? Y/N?

5. Who is involved? – key Stakeholders, facilities, HOD, councilors, CSO, NGOs are involved in the process? private sector?

6. Process – budget formulation, reviews, legislation, and approval?

7. Content: Is the budget based on an economic framework of a) running and capital cost using department's guidance. b) is it inclusive of partners inputs and contributions for year. c) Any contingency planning?

8. Alignment – is this aligned with the government annual and/or long-time priorities and any link to the MTSP?

9. Allocation: is it based on previous (historical) allocation? and programme absorption capacity? – any focus on programme results - outputs/outcomes?

Management

1. Request for funds? – How is this done? Is it based on the workplan?

2. Table of authority? – any financial approval ceiling and guidelines (limits)?

3. Accountability – electronic technical and financial utilization reports?

4. What Challenges – list – e.g. delays, inclusivity?

5. Transparency and Integrity – is this still a challenge? Any improvement?

6. Value for money (VfM) – has money been spent wisely and well? Plus, quality of delivery

7. Audit – are internal audits conducted, respected and persons sanctioned?

8. Budget absorption - please provide estimate at the county level and below.

9. Staffs' skills on budgeting and budget management – is there a continuous improvement plan and career development using a dedicated budget line.

Conclusion (qualitative)

1. Health financing, allocation, and expenditure – is improving overall with high value for money expenditure.

2. Health budgeting – inclusive, consultative and has improved based on an agreed.

3. Health budget management – improving with use of standard template and take audit reports.

4. Accountability – there is a TOA, internal audit reviews, PER, PESTS are conducted.

5. Challenges –? shortage of staff, Any government response?

6. Transparency – is it improving?

7. Strong political oversight and interest in the outcome?

Recommendations, if any (perspectives of the respondent)

1. Policy

2. Programme

3. Practice

	Kenya	Tanzania	Nigeria
Health spending US$ per capita	Increased. 95 (2021) from 71 (2015)	Increased. 37 (2021) from 33 in (2015)	Decreased. 84 (2021) from 96 in (2015)
Government Health spending (%)	Increased. 48.7% (2021) from 40.4% (2015)	Decreased. 27.2% (2021) from 34.4% in (2015)	Decreased. 13.3% (2021) from 16.4% in 2015
Out of pocket spending %	Decreased. 22.8% (2021) from 26.9% (2015)	Decreased. 25.6% (2021) from 25.8% in (2015)	Increased. 76.2% (2021) from 71.9% in (2015
External aid and Priority to health	Increased. 9.3% (2021) from 8.1% (2015)	Decreased. 5.1% (2021) from 7.3% in (2015)	Decreased. 4.1% (2021) from 5.3% in (2015)
GDP US$ per capita	Increased, 2082 (2021) from 1497 (2015)	Increased. 1106 (2021) from 902 in (2015)	Decreased. 2057 (2021) from 2688 in (2015)
Sources of Health expenditure	4 major sources: a. Government transfers - increasing, b. External aid (significant) c. Out of pocket spending d. Voluntary prepayment	3 major sources: a. External aid (significant and increasing) b. Government transfers (decreasing) c. Out of pocket spending (decreasing)	3 major sources: a. Out of pocket spending (significant) b. Government transfers (decreasing) c. External aid (decreasing)

Table A1.
Health expenditure analysis.

Author details

Samson Agbo[1,2]

1 Global Public Health Expert, Newcastle Upon Tyne, United Kingdom

2 Solar-Fi Cares, USA

*Address all correspondence to: agbosam@gmail.com

References

[1] Collaborative African Budget Reform Initiative (CABRI). In: Ross RW, editors. Performance and Programme based budgeting in Africa - a status report. Available from: https://www.academia.edu/5979303/Performance_and_programme_based_budgeting_in_Africa_A_status_report [Accessed: November 7, 2023]

[2] McKie K, van de Walle N. Toward an accountable budget process in sub-Saharan Africa: Problems and prospects. Social Research. 2010;77(4):1281-1310. From Impunity to Accountability: Africa's Development in the 21st Century (WINTER 2010), Published by: The Johns Hopkins University Press Stable. Available from: https://www.jstor.org/stable/23347127. Available from: https://www.academia.edu/538699/_Toward_an_Accountable_Budget_Process_in_Sub_Saharan_Africa_Problems_and_Prospects_Social_Research_2010 [Accessed: November 7, 2023]

[3] Kirsten H. African Legislatures Active in the Budget Process?! Emerging Trends and Consequences for Legislative Identity. Thesis Presented for the Degree of DOCTOR OF PHILISOPHY. 2019. Available from: https://www.academia.edu/109404965/African_legislatures_active_in_the_budget_process_Emerging_trends_and_consequences_for_legislative_identity. In the Department of Political Studies UNIVERSITY OF CAPE TOWN (February 2020). Accessed 2023 November 7

[4] Bossert T, Berman PA. A paper prepared for DDM symposium. A Decade of Health Sector Reform in Developing Countries: What Have We Learned? 2000. Available from: https://www.academia.edu/24637098/A_decade_of_health_sector_reform_in_developing_countries_what_have_we_learned [Accessed: November 7, 2023]

[5] Kutzin J. Health financing for universal coverage and health system performance: Concepts and implications for policy. Bulletin of the World Health Organization. 2013;**91**(8):602-611. DOI: 10.2471/BLT.12.113985. Epub 2013 Jun 17

[6] Schick A. A Contemporary Approach to Public Expenditure Management World Bank Institute, Governance, Regulation, and Finance Division. 1998. Available from: https://documents.worldbank.org/en/publication/documents-reports/documentdetail/739061468323718599/a-contemporary-approach-to-public-expenditure-management. © World Bank. License: Creative Commons Attribution CC BY 3.0 IGO [Accessed: November 7, 2023]

[7] World Bank. Public expenditure management handbook. - Stand Alone Books. 1998. Available from: https://elibrary.worldbank.org/doi/book/10.1596/0-8213-4297-5. https://doi.org/10.1596/0-8213-4297-5. ISBN:978-0-8213-4297-8 © World Bank. License: Creative Commons Attribution CC BY 3.0 IGO [Accessed: November 7, 2023]

[8] Public Expenditure Management and Accountability: Evolution and Current Status of World Bank Work. Poverty Reduction and Economic Management Network Operation Policy and Country Services Network. 2001. Available from: https://documents1.worldbank.org/curated/en/419221468763802853/pdf/264910Public0e1nd0accountability028.pdf [Accessed: November 13, 2023]

[9] Barroy H, Kabaniha G, Boudreaux C, Cammack T, Bain N. Leveraging Public Financial Management for 13 November Better Health in Africa: Key Bottlenecks and Opportunities for Reform. Geneva: World Health Organization; 2019. Available from: https://cdn.who.int/media/docs/default-source/searo/who_final_leveraging_pfm_for_better_healthd839eb86-ddbd-4004-b9a3-f87f48b8c841.pdf?sfvrsn=7a2082d8_1 [Accessed: November 13, 2023]

[10] Piatti-Funfkirchen M, Chansa C, Nkhoma D. Public Financial Management in the Health Sector: An Assessment at the Local Government Level in Malawi. Washington, DC: World Bank; 2020. Available from: http://hdl.handle.net/10986/35925 [Accessed: November 13, 2023]

[11] Piatti-Fünfkirchen M, Barroy H, Pivodic F, Marg F. Budget Execution in Health. International Bank for Reconstruction and Development/The World Bank. Budget execution in Health, Concepts, Trends and Policy Issues. 2019. Available from: https://openknowledge.worldbank.org/server/api/core/bitstreams/14df3be6-c563-535d-9768-cb575b011c4f/content [Accessed: November 13, 2023]

[12] WHO. How to make budgets work for health? In: Barroy H, Blecher M, Lakin J, editors. A Practical Guide to Designing, Managing and Monitoring Programme Budgets in the Health Sector. 2022. Available from: https://www.who.int/publications/i/item/9789240049666 [Accessed: November 18, 2023]

[13] Tsofa B, Waweru E, Munywoki J, Soe K, Rodriguez DC, Koon AD. Political economy analysis of sub-national health sector planning and budgeting: A case study of three counties in Kenya. PLOS Global Public Health. 2023;**3**(1):e0001401. Available from https://doi.org/10.1371/journal.pgph.0001401-. https://rdcu.be/dxsIT [Accessed: November 18, 2023]

[14] Tsofa B, Molyneux S, Gilson L, et al. How does decentralization affect health sector planning and financial management? A case study of early effects of devolution in Kilifi County, Kenya. International Journal for Equity in Health. 2016;**16**:151. DOI: 10.1186/s12939-017-0649-0

[15] Di Giorgio L, Yoo KJ, Maina T. Staying ahead of the curve: Challenges and opportunities for future spending on health in Kenya. Kenya Public Expenditure Review for the Health Sector - FY2014/15-FY2019/20 by World Bank, Health, Nutrition, and Population Global Practice. 2022. Available from: https://documents1.worldbank.org/curated/en/099150006242224188/pdf/P175146046aa000170926707583dac4738d.pdf [Accessed: December 12, 2023]

[16] Public Finance Management Act No. 18 of 2012. Revised Edition 2020. Published by the National Council for Law Reporting with the Authority of the Attorney-General. 2012. Available from: https://www.worldbank.org/content/dam/Worldbank/document/Africa/Kenya/Kenay%20Devolution/Public%20Finance%20Management%20Act%20%282012%29.pdf [Accessed: December 12, 2023]

[17] FMOH. National Health Act, 2014. 2014. Available from: https://extranet.who.int/mindbank/item/7388 [Accessed: December 12, 2023]

[18] Yusuff Adebayo Adebisi AY, Umah JO, Olaoye OC, Alaran AJ, Sina-Odunsi AB, Lucero-Prisno DE III. Assessment of health budgetary allocation and expenditure toward achieving universal health coverage

in Nigeria. Journal of Health Reports and Technology. 2020;**6**(2):e102552. DOI: 10.5812/ijhls.102552. Available from: https://brieflands.com/articles/jhrt-102552.pdf and https://www.academia.edu/52098102/Assessment_of_Health_Budgetary_Allocation_and_Expenditure_Toward_Achieving_Universal_Health_Coverage_in_Nigeria [Accessed: December 12, 2023]

[19] Abuja. African Summit on HIV/AIDs, Tuberculosis and Other related Infectious diseases. 2001. Available from: https://au.int/sites/default/files/pages/32894-file-2001-abuja-declaration.pdf [Accessed: December 19, 2023]

[20] Iloh EC, Nwokedi ME. Budget processes and participatory budgeting in Nigeria: Lessons from Latin America. ANSU Journal of Arts and Social Sciences. 2016;**5**(1):135-154 Available from: https://oidp-afrique.org/wp-content/uploads/2020/04/Nigeria-Budget_Processes_and_Participatory_Budge.pdf Accessed: December 17, 2023]

[21] Akanni O, Lawson OO. Health expenditure and health status in northern and southern Nigeria: A comparative analysis using National Health Account Framework. African Journal of Health Economics. 2013;**2**(1):31-46. Available from: https://www.academia.edu/79371400/Health_Expenditure_and_Health_Status_in_Northern_and_Southern_Nigeria_A_Comparative_Analysis_Using_National_Health_Account_Framework [Accessed: December 17, 2023]

[22] World Bank Group. Health, Nutrition & Population. 2018. Available from: https://documents1.worldbank.org/curated/en/782821529683086336/pdf/127519-WP-PUBLIC-add-series-NigeriaHFSAFINAL.pdf [Accessed: December 17, 2023]

[23] Olasehinde N. Budgeting process, budget performance and economic development in Nigeria. In: Book Democratic Practice and Governance in Nigeria. 1st ed. World Bank Group, Health, Nutrition & Population. Imprint Routledge; 2018. p. 20, eBook ISBN9781003029540. Available from: https://www.taylorfrancis.com/chapters/edit/10.4324/9781003029540-11/budgeting-process-budget-performance-economic-development-nigeria-noah-olasehinde [Accessed: December 17, 2023]

[24] Graven I, Ukarin I, Avinyeze PO. The role of legislators and budget process in Nigeria. Macro Management & Public Policies. 2022;**04**(3):5037. DOI: 10.30564/mmpp.v4i3.5037

[25] Hafez R. Health, Nutrition and Population (HNP) Discussion Paper Nigeria Health Financing System Assessment. Washington, DC: The International Bank for Reconstruction and Development/The World Bank; 2018. Available from: https://documents1.worldbank.org/curated/en/782821529683086336/pdf/127519-WP-PUBLIC-add-series-NigeriaHFSAFINAL.pdf [Accessed: December 17, 2023]

[26] Statista. Health budget, releases, and health care expenditure trend – 2015-2021. FMOH 4-point Agenda Conference presentation, pp12, November 2023. 2023. Available from: https://data.worldbank.org/indicator/SH.XPD.CHEX.GD.ZS?locations=NG [Accessed: December 17, 2023]

[27] Ngowi D. ESRF. Effects of budgetary process reforms on economic governance evidence from Tanzania. 2005. Available from: http://www.tzonline.org/pdf/effectsofbudgetaryprocessreformsoneconomic.pdf [Accessed: December 17, 2023]

[28] A Guide to Budget Work for NGOs. Includes Glossary of Key Budget Terms. 2001. Available from: http://www.internationalbudget.org/resources/guide/index.htm [Accessed: December 17, 2023]

[29] © HakiElimu and Policy Forum. Understanding the Budget Process in Tanzania. A Civil Society Guide. 2008. Available from: https://www.policyforum-tz.org/sites/default/files/2021-03/Understanding%20the%20Budget%20Process%20in%20Tanzania%20-%20A%20CSO%20Guide.pdf. info@hakielimu.org., www.policyforum-tz.org, info@policyforum.or.tz [Accessed: December 19, 2023]

[30] Ecorys. Supporting civil service improvements in low- and middle-income countries: lessons from an evaluation of the ODI Fellowship Scheme. 2021. Available from: https://www.ecorys.com/case-studies/supporting-civil-service-improvements-in-low-and-middle-income-countries-lessons-from-an-evaluation-of-the-odi-fellowship-scheme/ [Accessed: December 19, 2023]

[31] Vecchione E, Parkhurst J. The use of evidence within policy evaluation in health in Ghana: Implications for accountability and democratic governance. European Policy Analysis. Bulletin of World Health Organization. 2003;81:95-99. Available from: https://www.academia.edu/16502773/The_use_of_evidence_within_policy_evaluation_in_health_in_Ghana_implications_for_accountability_and_democratic_governance [Accessed: December 19, 2023]

[32] Foster M, Fozzard A, Naschold F, Conway T. How, When and Why Does Poverty Get Budget Priority? Poverty Reduction Strategy and Public Expenditure Reform in Five African Countries. 2002. ©OverseasDevelopmentInstitute2002. Available from: https://assets.publishing.service.gov.uk/media/57a08d47e5274a27b2001759/R76091.pdf [Accessed: December 19, 2023]

[33] Bossert T, Larranaga O, Giedion U, Arbelaez J, Bowser M. Decentralization and equity of resource allocation: Evidence from Colombia and Chile. 2003. Available from: https://www.academia.edu/1332427/Decentralization_and_Equity_of_Resource_Allocation_Evidence_From_Colombia_and_Chile&nav_from=c5399625-9206-461f-9e62-0f2ce6731d4f&rw_pos=0 [Accessed: December 19, 2023]

[34] UNDP. HACT and FACE forms introduction. 2005. Available from: https://open.undp.org/assets/Training/face-form/story_html5.html [Accessed: December 19, 2023]

[35] UNDP. 2021. Available from: https://popp.undp.org/document/harmonized-approach-cash-transfers-hact. https://agora.unicef.org/course/info.php?id=1949 [Accessed: December 19, 2023]

Chapter 6

Perspective Chapter: Healthcare Economics in the Wake of Trauma – Navigating Costs and Care for the Injured

Avinash Bhandary

Abstract

"Healthcare Economics in the Wake of Trauma: Navigating Costs and Care for the Injured," delves into the intricate relationship between healthcare economics and the management of traumatic injuries. It offers an insightful analysis of medical cost implications, highlighting the financial challenges faced by traumatically injured patients. The chapter examines the spectrum of post-injury care, from immediate medical interventions to long-term rehabilitation, emphasizing the economic aspects of each phase. It also explores the broader impact of traumatic injuries on healthcare financing and policy, providing a comprehensive understanding of the economic ramifications for both individuals and the healthcare system. The focus is on presenting a balanced view that integrates economic considerations with the critical need for effective and compassionate care for the injured.

Keywords: economics, cost, healthcare, injury, trauma

1. Introduction

Traumatic injuries impact the economics of healthcare at a speed that consistently outpaces our ability to understand the true depth of this issue. As traumatic injuries continue to test the resilience and efficiency of well-resourced healthcare systems in developed nations, the challenge of navigating the costs and care for the injured is not due to an inability to appreciate this crisis or from a lack of structure within existing theoretical frameworks. Rather, the gaps in our ability to address these challenges arise from economic models and outcomes-based research that are unable to fully articulate the experience of the injured and capture the consequential nature of traumatic injuries.

The economic impact of traumatic injuries exceeds the structured provisions of Ogden tables[1] in tort systems[2] in the United Kingdom and extends beyond the rigorous debate that lead tort reform[3] efforts in the United States. The complexity of economic and medical issues that coalesce around traumatic injuries overshadows our ability to calculate damages with uniformity and predictability and supports the notion of why as a society we collectively remain reluctant when it comes to adopting a "going monetary rate" for injuries.

In "Healthcare Economics in the Wake of Trauma: Navigating Costs and Care for the Injured," we provide an overview of the economic underpinnings of trauma care and its broader implications. The backdrop of this discussion is the substantial economic burden that traumatic injuries impose and the factors that complicate the ability of economic models to find a balanced resolution. The objective of this chapter is not to depreciate the nuance and rigor of our current systems but to elevate acknowledgment of where and why gaps in knowledge may exist.

2. The economic burden of injury

Economic burden manifests through direct costs such as emergency care, surgical treatments, hospital stays, and rehabilitation, alongside indirect costs such as diminished productivity, enduring disability, and the emotional toll on patients and their relatives. The methodologies and models used to calculate economic damages in personal injury cases aim to consider both non-pecuniary damages and the labor effects of disability. To reach a fair and balanced resolution, a multidisciplinary approach is required, which involves contributions from medical physicians and subject matter experts.

The complexity of these economic implications is due to the varying capacities of healthcare institutions, payers, and providers to accommodate traumatically injured individuals. The funding mechanisms for trauma care can have a significant impact on the availability and quality of medical treatment provided. This discussion examines the stages of traumatic injury from both a medical and economic perspective and analyzes the benchmarks that contribute to and limit the current understanding of the financial impact of traumatic injury.

The calculation of economic damages in personal injury cases is a complex and multifaceted process that aims to account for the non-pecuniary damages and the labor effects of disability. A fair and balanced resolution can only be reached through a multidisciplinary approach that involves contributions from medical physicians and subject matter experts.

The economic implications of traumatic injury are significant and vary depending on the capacities of healthcare institutions, payers, and providers to accommodate traumatically injured individuals. The funding mechanisms for trauma care can profoundly influence both the availability and the quality of medical treatment provided.

[1] Ogden tables, prepared by the Actuary Department of the Government of the United Kingdom, set out multipliers to aid those assessing lump sum damages for future pecuniary loss in personal injury and fatal accident cases.

[2] A Tort is an act or omission that causes legally cognizable harm to persons or property. The tort system, in turn, represents the body of rules concerned with remedying harms caused by a person's wrongful or injurious actions.

[3] Tort reform comprises proposals aimed at modifying civil justice laws to decrease tort litigation and limit damages.

To better understand the financial impact of traumatic injury, it is essential to examine the stages of traumatic injury from both a medical and economic perspective. By analyzing the benchmarks that contribute to and limit our current understanding of these impacts, we can gain a deeper insight into the true cost of traumatic injury and advocate for better funding and support for those affected by it.

3. Current models and methodologies

Economic damages are calculated through a combination of actuarial, life care planning, econometric, and finance-based models designed to estimate the financial impact of an injury over a lifetime. These economic models consider a range of variables, including lost earnings, cost of care, and life expectancy. The Ogden tables, utilized primarily within the UK, offer a standardized means to calculate lump sum damages for personal injury and wrongful death claims based on actuarial assessments of life expectancy and discount rates applied to future losses.

The Ogden tables provide a structured framework for damage calculation in the United Kingdom. However, these frameworks are not free from limitations. Though structured frameworks aim to align with population changes and preserve equal representation, changing population dynamics and the equitability of healthcare accessibility impose limitations that alter the accuracy of conclusions drawn.

One drawback of generalized population-based data is the ability to accurately measure medical outcomes of the injured and estimate the economic impact of opportunity cost that is lost in traumatic injury. When pursuing legal remedies to pacify the multidimensional impact of traumatic injuries, the injured are often stigmatized which shifts attention away from the potentially compounding effects of their individual circumstance, and potential loss in career progression [1]. Second, the inability to access medical care, and barriers that arise from the lack of an adequate support system further clouds the perception of their commitment to receiving medical attention for injuries they are dealing with. The inability of the injured to access healthcare, and the place of the setting which the medical care is obtained leads to analytical gaps in outcomes-based research. These gaps in data challenge the sufficiency of population-based assumptions in adjudicating a resolution. Additionally, the arbitrary nature of end-points within the study design of outcomes based research bears significant weight on the effectiveness of the research in reflecting the reality of the injured.

In the United States, a diversified approach to this debate is utilized. Economists and life care planners use present value calculations that factor in projected earnings growth, inflation, and the probability of employment, but without a singular, universally applied set of tables akin to the Ogden tables. These methodologies are supplemented by expert opinion to explain the interconnectedness of the financial impacts to a jury.

The utility of rigorous debate is an essential component to establishing the economic value of the injury. The monetary value of an injury is as significant to the injured as it is to the vested stakeholders of liability insurers seeking mitigate the verdicts perceived as ruinous. Tort reform represents the deliberate modification of the legal system that governs civil wrongs and damages and rationalizes the process of litigation and compensation of those who suffer injuries as the result of civil wrongs.

Through Tort reform, various jurisdictions aim to limit damages through caps on compensation, arguing that this is necessary to prevent insurance premium inflation and ensure the sustainability of liability insurance. However, in some instances, such reforms may proceed without adequate assessment of the accounting principles and special risk considerations employed by companies that provide liability insurance. The procession and implementation of reforms in the US are heavily debated because of the reforms effect on limiting compensation in order strike a balance between civil wrongs and damages, the need to provide just remedies to those wronged, and the necessity to prevent the exploitation of the legal system.

4. The role of non-pecuniary damages, labor effects of disability, healthcare inflation and hospital based care

Non-pecuniary damages represent compensations for intangible losses such as pain and suffering and loss of enjoyment of life. They are crucial in economically valuing damages. A nuanced approach that goes beyond financial metrics is required to appreciate the pernicious nature in which these losses play out. Psychological and sociological assessments should be integrated to arrive at a compensation figure that reflects the full scope of an individual's loss. When it comes to disabilities, the labor effects of lost futures are critical considerations. They include reduced earning capacity and the need for vocational rehabilitation. Economic models and expert opinions must account for how disabilities affect a person's ability to work. This involves considering sector-specific employment probabilities, the potential for retraining, and trends in labor market dynamics over time.

Healthcare inflation is a significant factor that complicates the calculation of economic damages. Medical care costs rise faster than general inflation, which make acknowledgement of medical cost inflation critical to accurately forecast healthcare cost trends. Recognition of healthcare inflation helps ensure that awarded sums remain adequate over time and contribute to a forward-looking analysis that considers trends in healthcare technology, and trends that affect the provision of healthcare.

To understand how the trend of consolidation of the healthcare market into large hospital systems contributes to cost inflation, charge-to-cost ratio is a key metric. The charge-to-cost ratio (CCR) in hospitals is a financial metric used to compare the total charges billed to patients (or insurers) for services rendered against the actual cost of providing those services. Mathematically, the CCR is calculated as the total charges divided by the total costs for a given period or for specific services or departments within a hospital. What is unclear is how much administrative charges within hospitals factor into CCR. To shed light on this lack of clarity, price-transparency acts have been mandated in the US to encourage Hospitals to share cost-data. The CCR can significantly vary between hospitals, and even between hospitals within the same hospital system due to differences in pricing strategies, cost structures, and patient demographics [2]. Variability in fee structures and lack of transparency in how charges are determined can lead to confusion and inefficiencies in the healthcare market, potentially driving up overall healthcare costs as patients and insurers who may not have clear benchmarks for comparison. Hospitals may use CCR as a level to compensate for underpayments from certain payers (e.g., Medicaid, Medicare) by charging more to private insurers or self-paying patients. This cost-shifting dynamic can contribute to healthcare inflation, as it leads to higher insurance premiums and out-of-pocket expenses for a segment of the population, reflecting a redistribution of healthcare costs rather than a reduction.

For-profit and non-for-profit Hospital systems in the United States have grown into multi-billion dollar entities that span multiple states and extend outside the country with satellite campuses in some instances. The shift toward healthcare consumerism is a stark contrast from the faith-based charitable missions from which hospitals originated. As large-scale healthcare systems increasingly represent the setting in which healthcare is rendered, attention will focus on facility fees, site-neutrality payments and the tax-exempt status of hospitals in an attempt to stem the tide of financial costs shouldered by patients [3].

American taxpayers footed the bill for at least $1.8 trillion in federal and state health care expenditures in 2022 compared to $1.6 trillion in individual income taxes collected the same year by the government, as reported in the latest data released by the Internal Revenue Service (IRS) [4, 5]. Despite financial commitment to health, life expectancy has gone down and quality of care has declined and health-care related debt remains the leading cause of bankruptcy. It is not hyperbole to conclude that our health care system, has transformed from caring for the poor to creating the poor and is now on pace to threaten the primacy of American economy.

Our current understanding of economic damages following traumatic injuries is characterized by disparate approaches and a pressing demand for methodological consistency. The search for solutions is lost in broader systemic inequalities, and the decline of quality becomes entrenched. While existing models offer a basis for dialog, mere descriptive statistics fail to capture the full scope.

Decisions that account for non-pecuniary damages, the impact of disability on work, and the rising healthcare costs will prove to be a more balanced representation of current arguments as opposed to debates based solely on snapshots of population data where proper discussion of metrics that matter is not had. As the economic landscape evolves, socioeconomic lines deepen, reinforcing the need for multi-dimensional economic models to bridge the gaps within economic damage calculation. Lastly, the relational trends that develop between payer policies for trauma patients, risk pool considerations of liability insurance companies, and patient outcomes may foster an understanding where limitations are acknowledged, and insights are gained.

5. Medical care and the cost of help

The road that emerges after a traumatic injury is paved with uncertainty and irrevocably re-routes the injured's life plans in seconds. Aspirations and the ability to prioritize physical and financial well-being are abruptly paused before reality becomes audible again. Emergency medical services then arrive, performing basic life support measures before an ambulance ushers the patient into a world that was utterly unfamiliar to them moments before they were injured. Hospital-level medical attention, diagnostic testing, and specialist consultation follow the patient's arrival at the hospital and quickly become foundational elements of the care team. As the patient progresses toward recovery, each phase of post-injury care involves unique medical needs and potential barriers to rehabilitation goals. The economic impact of the care required shapes the path of recovery for the patient and affects their family's long-term trajectory and ability to preserve financial well-being.

5.1 Acute phase

The period following a traumatic event is crucial and involves resource-intensive care, a wide range of diagnostic tests, and medical support designed to stabilize the patient, treat critical injuries, and triage the patient appropriately. To analyze the financial impact of care for traumatic injuries, health care claims are organized based on when they occur during the patient's treatment. This often results in the evaluation of hospital-based claims, primarily because these claims are more readily available.

Health service utilization categories in the immediate aftermath of a traumatic injury include: Trauma activation services associated with the designated Trauma center, Inpatient, outpatient, Emergency department, surgery, administered medications, radiology, durable medical equipment and supplies, prescriptions, diagnostic testing, and laboratory services. Patients with life-threatening injuries often require immediate surgical interventions to repair or stabilize vital organ functions. Acute injuries are allocated to different trauma centers based on the ability of the accepting hospital to accommodate the patient's medical condition. If operative intervention is required, patient transportability, operating room usage, radiology technician, surgical team, and anesthesia team formation must be readily available. The mobilization of medical professionals that make up the trauma team represents a fee called the trauma activation fee.

The margin of error for trauma-based medical care in the acute phase of an injury is minimal; trauma activation fees ensure that the services required in the rapid response phase are readily available and that a low margin for error is preserved. Trauma activation fees remain a growing area of debate due to large costs and price variability between the not-for-profit and for-profit designation of the hospital employing the trauma activation team [6]. Fees associated with trauma activation have a trickle-down effect on the consumer in the form of surprise bills. In the United States, surprise bills refer to residual fees that patients are financially responsible for. Surprise bills occur as a result of healthcare provider participation with the network of the insurance plan held by the patient. The end result is an in-network versus out-of-network classification; care rendered by providers designated as out-of-network results in fees that lead to substantial patient liability.

The price of care varies with each medical service provided, the charges vary based on the financial liability of the patient, not the value of the care provided. Claims related to ground ambulance services show significant differences based on geographic location, the impact of taxpayer subsidies which affect localities unevenly, and the various ownership models of the ambulance services. These ownership structures range from public sector and private equity to publicly traded companies, independents, and nonprofit organizations. The process of deciding to transport a patient with traumatic injuries to a suitably equipped hospital triggers what is known as trauma activation. This activation adheres to guidelines set by the American College of Surgeons (ACS) and is widely practiced across the United States. Furthermore, trauma centers are classified according to the level of resources they offer, a designation determined by specific criteria laid out in state legislation or regulations, ensuring a standardized approach to trauma care on a state-by-state basis.

Emergency medical services (EMS) represent the first line of care in the field and are critical decision-making personnel who correspond with hospital personnel when it comes to identifying seriously injured patients for transport to major trauma centers. Adhering to field triage guidelines matches patient needs with hospital resources and minimizes over triage of patients with less severe injuries to major trauma centers. Care offered at non-trauma centers is cheaper than major trauma centers, therefore the initial decision of where the provision of care should occur comes with cost implications. However, despite downstream sequelae that universally affects all parties, data suggests more than one-third of patients brought to major trauma centers do not meet field triage guidelines for transport resulting in a cost of $136.7 million dollars annually [7].

When seriously injured patients are brought to trauma centers that meet their needs, they are still subject to disproportionately high trauma activation fees depending on the trauma center to which they are brought. Research has shown a price variation in activation fees of tier one trauma centers in the United States from $1000 to $61,734 with a median of $9,500.

Despite the significance of major trauma centers to the societies they provide care for, financial stability of these centers is an issue of focus. Approximately one-fourth of major trauma centers in the United States are at high risk for financial vulnerability. The financial vulnerability of trauma centers is largely attributed to uncompensated care and negative operating margins [8]. Why major trauma centers operate at negative margins, despite their ability to bolster the healthcare safety net of the public and their inclusion into the expanse of larger hospital systems, is outside the scope of this chapter. Standardization of traumatic activation fees is a reasonable solution however these fees are affected by numerous factors including cost of living within the geographic region, hospital characteristics and availability of chargemaster data of hospitals. Standardization of trauma activation fees would require overarching legislation that remains sensitive to the balance between the rising costs of providing medical care and ensuring the availability of resources required by trauma centers for the acuity of care they provide.

5.2 Post-acute phase

While immediate medical interventions are crucial for survival, long-term rehabilitation plays an equally vital role in maximizing functional recovery and helping trauma survivors regain independence. The phase of care in which rehabilitation occurs is regarded as the post-acute phase of care and is where the burden of injury and the extent of disability is understood. An aging population and advances in healthcare are likely to contribute to an increasing need for rehabilitation services.

The scope and duration of rehabilitation vary widely depending on the nature and severity of injuries. Key medical components of rehabilitation include but are not limited to Physical and Occupational therapy, Speech therapy, cognitive rehabilitation, psychological counseling, continued specialist consultation and care, durable medical equipment, and home modifications.

The economic implications of long-term rehabilitation are unique to the individual circumstances of each patient. Cost-influencing factors such as the care setting, the length of the rehabilitation period, and the presence of a supportive network play a critical role; in cases of traumatic injuries, these elements must be promptly and efficiently addressed.

Rehabilitation can occur in inpatient rehab facilities, outpatient clinics, skilled nursing homes, or in the patient's home, each with varying cost structures. The length of rehabilitation can be extensive, particularly with severe injuries. Costs accumulate over time, leading to financial stress for patients and their families. Growing recognition-implications of Lost Income and Caregiver Burden often go underestimated due to poor follow-up with respect to research participation. Prolonged rehabilitation can further reduce income or require family members to act as caregivers, resulting in lost economic opportunities for both the patient and caregivers. The principle of rehabilitation is focused primarily on the restoration of functional mobility which provides the injured party with the potential to return to a pre-injury work status.

Evaluation of return to work/study in patients involved in major trauma involving pelvic fractures in Australia revealed 59% of the patients had reached the benchmark of returning to work 24 months after injury. Of those who had returned to work, the proportion returning to their pre-injury workplace declined 15% over the following 24 months [9]. In Canada, severe traumatic injury was associated with a return to work 79.3% 36 months after injury, with a resultant mean earnings loss of 19%. Additionally, Physical and mental challenges persisted at month 36 for these patients [10]. Research on return to work rates in the United States of America revealed that among 500 trauma patients at a level 1 trauma center between 2009 and 2011 followed prospectively for 12 months in the United States found that 64% reported a decrease in monthly income, 58% reported unemployment as a result of their injuries, 30% reported a job change related to their injury, and 85% reported financial problems as a direct result of their injury [10, 11].

6. Insured and in debt

Two terms embedded in the ethos of the injured and required for understanding the depth of what is endured by these patients are "financial toxicity" and "catastrophic health expenditures." Financial toxicity is defined as the financial hardship the patient experiences as a side effect of his or her illness and medical treatment for that illness [12, 13].

Applying the concept of Financial Toxicity to patients who require medical care because of injury reveals the post-discharge burden of injury among working-age survivors in the United States extends beyond the capacity for work. Food insecurity, difficulty accessing and affording health care, forced unemployment and forgone medical care due to cost, were also associated with traumatic injury sequelae in the US [14]. After being discharged from the hospital, large medical bills result in out-of-pocket expenses. Expenses may stem from uncovered services, out-of-network providers, owed deductibles, and co-pays. Often, these costs are converted to medical debt, which is then sold to debt collection agencies, re-packaged and, saddled with additional interest rates of up to 27% that compound annually [15]. Debt may impact credit scores when they exceed $400, impact the patient's ability to obtain future loans, and, in some instances, lead non-profit hospitals to displace the patients from their homes [16]. If the injured party returns to work, expectations of their pre-injury physical capacity are uncertain, and the potential loss of employer-sponsored benefits or segmentation into a level of coverage commensurate with their new healthcare risks is an expected outcome. Declines in physical health, and mental health may affect the ability to generate income. New medical debt compounded by the loss of work-related income can cause significant financial hardship that threatens subsistence spending on food, housing, and other health care needs [14]. Financial sequelae cascades until bankruptcy is filed. Financial and Physical well-being is consumed in this process; often, musculoskeletal pathology persists in the form of permanent injury, and psychological symptoms such as depression exist as an under diagnosed byproduct of the traumatic injury.

As more attention is paid to the burden of this crisis, the magnitude of impact is better served by the metrics that fall under Catastrophic Health expenditures (CHE). Catastrophic Health expenditures are defined as any charges or out-of-pocket expenses greater than or equal to 40% of annual post-subsistence income (income after paying for food). When applying the metric of CHE to uninsured patients admitted for trauma, 70.8% were at risk [17].

When the criteria of CHE are extended beyond hospital visit-based claims to charges accrued in post-acute care, the extent of economic impact that occurs from traumatic injuries is viewed with higher resolution and indicates that 70–90% of all uninsured trauma patients are at risk of financial hardship as a result of their injuries. To stem the crisis that skyrocketed health care costs imposed on individuals and families, the Affordable Care Act (ACA) became law in January 2010, with the main provisions of the law enacted in January 2014. The ACA intended to expand healthcare access and mitigate the impact of injury and disease on the uninsured. In achieving this feat, the ACA created new opportunities for insurance companies by subsidizing the purchase of health insurance.

A decade later, trauma-related expenses have proven insurance expansion to be an insufficient safety net. In 2016, in the US, 53% of adults between the ages of 18 and 64 without insurance reported difficulties with paying medical bills, and 20% of patients within the same age cohort who possessed health insurance with insurance deductibles between $1,500 and $3,000 and above for a family reported difficulties paying medical bills. Of the medical bills studied, 66% were attributed to a short-term medical stay or one-time medical expense such as an injury [18]. Health insurance deductibles are the amount you pay for covered healthcare services before your insurance plan contributes payment to a portion of your bills. Out-of-pocket (OOP) maximums include deductible payments but do not include out-of-network charges accrued by providers with the insurance plan. Out-of-pocket maximum limits represent the maximum out-of-pocket costs before the insurance plan covers medical bills. In 2024, OOP Maximums for an individual were $9,450 and were $18,000 for a family. In 2030, the estimated OOP limit for single coverage is $14,100. Comparing trends between wage increases using projections provided by the Congressional Budget Office (CBO) and Centers for Medicare and Medicaid Services (CMS) National Health Expenditure Accounts and OOP limits through the Affordable Care Act, OOP limits are outpacing wage growth. Between 2014 and 2023, the ACA OOP limit increased by 43% compared to a 31% increase in wage and salary growth. Between 2014 and 2033, the CBO expects wages to grow by 83%, and the ACA's maximum OOP limit is expected to grow by 122% over the same period. As the statistical disparities widen, the distortion of the market continues, less protection is offered to the insured, and higher premiums owed to Insurance companies will invariably be handled through federal premium subsidies [19]. Paradoxically, after specific provisions of the ACA came into effect, the net income of large health insurance companies increased by 8.7% between 2017 and 2018. The gain in net insurer profits was more than doubled by increases in Health Insurance stock prices in the S&P 500 since the law took effect in January 2014 [20].

The socioeconomic status of the traumatically injured compounds the financial burden, with patients of lower economic standing being disproportionally affected despite access to government-funded programs. A 2021 report published in the Journal of the American Medical Association found that people in states that did not expand Medicaid in 2014 were 34% more likely to incur medical debt and had more medical debt than Medicaid participants in states where Medicaid expanded [21].

Moving away from public sector funding mechanisms for traumatic injuries toward private health insurance in the United States has not proven to be a financial safeguard for the injured. In 2021, credit reports of patients who were admitted to the hospital between July 2020 and December 2020 for traumatic injuries and who held private insurance during their care were 70% more likely to incur medical debt. Additionally, insured patients who were traumatically injured had a 110% higher bankruptcy rate compared with patient cohorts admitted to the hospital for reasons unrelated to trauma [22, 23].

Uncovering data that clarifies the financial impact of traumatic injuries remains challenging. The accuracy of our assessments are uniquely limited by the availability of data for a problem that is so pervasive for society. To obtain information on injuries, the focus has been primarily on out-of-pocket payments for inpatient admission and extracting information from credit reports. Longitudinal studies following patients post-discharge are consistently limited due to the varying factors that impede follow-up. Of the factors that impeded follow-up, cost and lack of provider-patient communication are paramount. As of 2022, data suggests 47% of Americans who have health insurance find the cost of health care difficult to afford, with 21% of insured patients delaying health care and 61% of uninsured delaying health care due to costs [18], leading one to conclude that the cost of care in the US continues to undermine the ability to use the healthcare-related services. In the United States, a unique aspect of the public health crisis is the increasing administrative costs in healthcare, which are bundled into the high cost of labor. To address the issue of rising market-based administrative service cost, it is essential to balance the savings generated by these services and their impact on benefit designs against the potential productivity losses of those who cannot afford but need care. Evaluating improvements to the market-based healthcare system must include recognizing the cost increases caused by the consolidation of hospitals and insurance companies. Although larger health systems and insurance providers may necessitate more administrative services, this expansion also risks leaving more people, especially those affected by trauma, without adequate care.

When traumatic injuries occur due to civil wrongs, ensuing litigation influences not only the accessibility of care but also the extent of economic impact the injured absorbs, which is quantifiable. As previously mentioned, the data analyzed to measure the depth of financial burden experienced by injured patients is fragmented by the availability of hospital-based claims and relies on patient-reported surveys and credit reports.

The majority of medical care received by traumatic injury survivors is performed in independently owned outpatient settings, often through the private practice sector. Health care provided through independent medical practices fragments data used in research due to the need for more standardization, limiting practical data availability. As the private practice sector of medicine atrophies due to the lack of inflation-adjusted payment and hospital acquisitions of medical practices expand, the path of medical care for the injured bifurcates. In the author's experience, hospital-based care, in either inpatient or outpatient settings, an aversion exists to providing medical care for traumatically injured patients after the acute phase of care has ended. This aversion is mainly attributed to ongoing litigation. It occurs due to the unwillingness of hospital managers to allow their medical providers to be removed from work to participate in the process of litigation and the uncertainty over potential payment for the medical care rendered due to the ambiguous position of collateral source payer liability when an accident is on file for the insured.

A 2021 survey of forensic experts, their methods, estimates, and perspectives did not acknowledge the potential of how actuarial risk premiums impact the reliability of their predictions [24]. Actuarial risk is proportional to the reliability of assumptions implemented in pricing models used by insurance companies to set premiums and factors into risk segmentation. Risk segmentation reflects the redistribution of groups of insureds into risk tiers, ultimately affecting coverage and cost.

The reliance on Medicare rates as an acceptable unit of account for payment for establishing future payment is another deeply flawed approach that fails to acknowledge that Medicare rates do not accurately account for operational shifts in labor and cost. The replacement of payer networks with Medicare reference-based pricing improves provider access; however, this pricing model leaves patients vulnerable to costs due to a lack of facility fee coverage. Additionally, current Medicare rates to the private practice sector are 39% behind inflation [25].

7. Conclusion

In navigating the costs and care for the injured, the methodological quality of our approaches must move beyond the threshold of reproducibility if they are to adjudicate the future care of the injured to methods that acknowledge the complexity of the tasks at hand with unreserved confidence while incorporating practicality into the logic for determining future amounts. Utilizing a multidisciplinary approach that acknowledges limitations in the practicality of our knowledge rather than obscuring those limitations with population-based assumptions is essential. If not, those responsible for establishing the reasonable value of recovery for medical expenses of the traumatically injured will rely on methodologies unable to cope with the problem they are trying to confront.

Thanks

To my Mother, Riaan, Ahalya and Jedica. Every endeavor starts and ends with my love for you.

Author details

Avinash Bhandary
Strata Medical, Orlando, Florida, United States of America

*Address all correspondence to: info@stratalifeplan.com

References

[1] Spearing NM, Gyrd-Hansen D, Pobereskin LH, Rowell DS, Connelly LB. Are people who claim compensation "cured by a verdict"? A longitudinal study of health outcomes after whiplash. Journal of Law and Medicine. 2012;**20**(1):82-92

[2] Levinson Z, Qureshi N, Liu JL, Whaley CM. Trends in hospital prices paid by private health plans varied substantially across the US: Study examines trends in hospital prices paid by private health plans. Health Affairs. 2022;**41**(4):516-522

[3] Bai G, Zare H, Eisenberg MD, Polsky D, Anderson GF. Analysis suggests government and nonprofit hospitals' charity care is not aligned with their favorable tax treatment: Study examines government and nonprofit hospital charity care expenses compared to charity care obligations arising from the organizations' favorable tax treatment. Health Affairs. 2021;**40**(4):629-636

[4] Tax Foundation. Summary of the Latest Federal Income Tax Data: 2022 Update. n.d. Available from: https://taxfoundation.org/data/all/federal/summary-latest-federal-income-tax-data-2022-update/ [Accessed: January 26, 2024]

[5] STAT. US Healthcare Costs: Government Covers 41 Percent of Total. 2023. Available from: https://www.statnews.com/2023/12/19/us-healthcare-costs-government-covers-41-percent-of-total/ [Accessed: March 21, 2024]

[6] Zitek T, Pagano K, Mechanic OJ, Farcy DA. Assessment of trauma team activation fees by US region and hospital ownership. JAMA Network Open. 2023;**6**(1):e2252520

[7] Newgard CD, Staudenmayer K, Hsia RY, Mann NC, Bulger EM, Holmes JF, et al. The cost of overtriage: More than one-third of low-risk injured patients were taken to major trauma centers. Health Affairs. 2013;**32**(9):1591-1599

[8] Marrotte A, Calvo RY, Capacio B, Goljan C, Rooney AS, Carroll AN, et al. Financial vulnerability of trauma centers: A national analysis. Journal of Trauma and Acute Care Surgery. 2023;**94**(5):637-642

[9] Gabbe BJ, Hofstee DJ, Esser M, Bucknill A, Russ MK, Cameron PA, et al. Functional and return to work outcomes following major trauma involving severe pelvic ring fracture. ANZ Journal of Surgery. 2015;**85**(10):749-754

[10] Haas B, Jeon SH, Rotermann M, Stepner M, Fransoo R, Sanmartin C, et al. Association of severe trauma with work and earnings in a national cohort in Canada. JAMA Surgery. 2021;**156**(1):51-59

[11] Murphy PB, Severance S, Savage S, Obeng-Gyasi S, Timsina LR, Zarzaur BL. Financial toxicity is associated with worse physical and emotional long-term outcomes after traumatic injury. Journal of Trauma and Acute Care Surgery. 2019;**87**(5):1189-1196

[12] Scott JW, Knowlton LM, Murphy P, Neiman PU, Martin RS, Staudenmayer K, et al. Financial toxicity after trauma and acute care surgery: From understanding to action. Journal of Trauma and Acute Care Surgery. 2023;**95**(5):800-805

[13] Chan RJ, Gordon LG, Tan CJ, Chan A, Bradford NK, Yates P, et al. Relationships between financial

toxicity and symptom burden in cancer survivors: A systematic review. Journal of Pain and Symptom Management. 2019;**57**(3):646-660

[14] Neiman PU, Taylor KK, Sinco B, Anderson GA, Sangji NF, Hemmila MR, et al. Insult to injury: National analysis of return to work and financial outcomes of trauma patients. Journal of Trauma and Acute Care Surgery. 2021;**91**(1):121-129

[15] NPR. Medical Debt Is Fueling a Boom in High-Interest Credit Cards. Hospitals Reap the Rewards. 2022. Available from: https://www.npr.org/sections/health-shots/2022/11/17/1136201685/medical-debt-high-interest-credit-cards-hospitals-profit [Accessed: January 20, 2024]

[16] RevCycle Intelligence. NY Hospitals Place Liens Against Patient Homes Over Medical Debt. n.d. Available from: https://revcycleintelligence.com/news/ny-hospitals-place-liens-against-patient-homes-over-medical-debt [Accessed: January 28, 2024]

[17] Scott JW, Raykar NP, Rose JA, Tsai TC, Zogg CK, Haider AH, et al. Cured into destitution: Catastrophic health expenditure risk among uninsured trauma patients in the United States. Annals of Surgery. 2018;**267**(6):1093-1099. DOI: 10.1097/SLA.0000000000002254

[18] Kaiser Family Foundation. KFF Health Care Debt Survey. n.d. Available from: https://www.kff.org/health-costs/report/kff-health-care-debt-survey/ [Accessed: February 24, 2024]

[19] Health System Tracker. The Burden of Medical Debt in the United States. n.d. Available from: https://www.healthsystemtracker.org/brief/the-burden-of-medical-debt-in-the-united-states/#Share%20of%20adults%20who%20have%20medical%20debt,%20by%20demographics,%202021 [Accessed: February 20, 2024]

[20] White House. The Profitability of Health Insurance Companies [PDF]. 2018. Available from: https://www.whitehouse.gov/wp-content/uploads/2018/03/The-Profitability-of-Health-Insurance-Companies.pdf [Accessed: March 3, 2024]

[21] Himmelstein DU, Dickman SL, McCormick D, Bor DH, Gaffney A, Woolhandler S. Prevalence and risk factors for medical debt and subsequent changes in social determinants of health in the US. JAMA Network Open. 2022;**5**(9):e2231898. DOI: 10.1001/jamanetworkopen.2022.31898

[22] Consumer Financial Protection Bureau. Medical Debt Burden in the United States. 2022

[23] Scott JW, Scott KW, Moniz M, Carlton EF, Tipirneni R, Becker N. Financial outcomes after traumatic injury among working-age US adults with commercial insurance. JAMA Health Forum. 2022;**3**(11):e224105. DOI: 10.1001/jamahealthforum.2022.4105

[24] Garagulagian R, Rosenbaum DI, Schap D. A 2021 survey of forensic experts: Their methods, estimates, and perspectives. Journal of Legal Economics. 2022;**28**(2):3-27. Available from: https:www.proquest.com/scholarly-journals/2021-survey-forensic-experts-their-methods/docview2886078770/se-2

[25] American Medical Association. Economic and Health Policy Research. 2021

Chapter 7

Perspective Chapter: Shifting toward Value-Based Healthcare – Lessons Learned in the Context of Breast Cancer Treatment

Ieva Bikava, Aiga Balode and Reičela Heinrihsone

Abstract

Latvia, an EU member state, is characterized by one of the lowest healthcare funding levels within the union. This circumstance, coupled with the increasing demands of an aging population, necessitates a reassessment of healthcare funding principles. This paper evaluates, overviews, and analyses the implementation of a value-based healthcare (VBHC) model, widely regarded in contemporary practice as the optimal strategy for delivering effective, efficient, high-quality, patient-centered healthcare services. The study covers the main theoretical aspects of VBHC concept, explores the main lessons learned from various countries and institutions that have attempted to implement VBHC, and delves into the challenges encountered during the implementation of VBHC in breast cancer treatment in Latvia. It focuses on the launch of transition from a pay-for-service model to a VBHC, emphasizing the paradigm shift toward integrated patient-centered healthcare delivery. Furthermore, it examines the pivotal role of data and digital transformation in facilitating this transition as well as the open discussion with the stakeholders.

Keywords: VBHC, breast cancer, effective healthcare, PROM, PREM, digital transformation

1. Introduction

Latvia is an EU member state located in Northern Europe, with approximately 1.88 million inhabitants. It is considered a middle-income country with one of the lowest levels of healthcare funding, totaling 1.888 billion euros in 2024, constituting approximately 12% of the total government budget spending allocated to healthcare.

Oncology ranks as the second leading cause of death among the population in Latvia, accounting for 310.37 death cases from oncological diseases (ICD-10: C00-D48) out of a total of 1611.97 deaths per 100,000 population in 2022. The primary cause of death in oncology among women is breast cancer, with 40.4 cases per 100,000 women in 2022. According to the latest available data from 2021, there were approximately 58.5 newly diagnosed cases of breast cancer per 100,000 population. Of these cases, 30.6% were diagnosed at an early stage (Stage I), 37.5% at Stage II, and unfortunately, a significant portion, 17.7%, were diagnosed at Stage III, with 9.6% diagnosed at stage IV [1].

To enhance the healthcare services aimed at increasing prevention, screening, and early diagnostics in oncology, several political initiatives have been outlined in the National Plan to Improve the Care of Oncological Patients for the years 2017–2020 and subsequently for the period 2022–2024. The primary objectives in the field of breast cancer remain constant: to enhance responsiveness for breast screening services and to improve the quality of diagnostics and treatment. The initial tasks include collaborating with oncology professionals to develop algorithms and patient pathways, as well as adopting quality indicators based on international best practices. Additionally, there is a need to review the existing diagnostic and treatment guidelines and clinical pathways. Furthermore, to enhance patient satisfaction and amplify the patient's voice, the implementation of patient-reported outcome measurements (PROM) will supplement the existing patient-reported experience (PREM) [2].

This chapter consists of four sections and covers the following topics: section one introduces the concept of value-based healthcare, describing the historical background of the approach and the problems it aims to solve, mainly focusing on the development of the concept in the United States. The second section covers the further development of the VBHC approach, which was transferred from the United States with the privately funded healthcare system to European countries and systems related to universal health coverage. This section ends with more practical elements, including recommendations and guidelines for implementing the VBHC for breast cancer treatment. The third section provides an overview of examples of VBHC implementation and reveals shifts in implementation practices compared to its original theoretical approach. The fourth section analyzes the main takeaways from the implementation of VBHC in Latvia, in accordance with the theoretical concept and in comparison to the experiences of other countries. The last section provides conclusions on the existing practice of VBHC implementation and recommendations for other countries aiming to implement the VBHC approach.

2. Initial development of value-based healthcare concept

The concept of value-based healthcare (VBHC) originally emerged in the United States in the early 2000s. Michael E. Porter and Elizabeth O. Teisberg proposed it at a time when the US healthcare system was in crisis, characterized by a dysfunctional competition system, and in 2007 published the first book on this subject "Redefining Healthcare: Creating Value-Based Competition on Results." Avinandan Mukherjee, referring to M.E. Porter, highlighted that the issue with the US healthcare system was not its private nature or the level of competition it faced compared to other countries. Rather, the problem lies in the fact that the competition has not resulted in the anticipated reductions in costs and improvements in quality. The root of the problem lies in a dysfunctional system that facilitated the "shifting of costs, accumulation of bargaining power, and restriction of services." This situation meant that all actors in the system shared responsibility for the problem. Consequently, competition did not occur at the level of medical conditions or over the entire care cycle. Therefore, as concluded by A. Mukherjee, those circumstances led to increased costs and insurance premiums, lack of quality, patient satisfaction, and equitable access to healthcare [3].

Another point made by Willard C. Harill and David E. Melon, which characterizes the problems in the US healthcare at the time, was that the concept of VBHC was initially coined by Porter in 2007 in reaction to the third-party cost transfer and fee-for-service expenditure mitigation tactics employed by Health Maintenance Organizations (HMOs), which were impeding physicians' capacity to allocate sufficient time to patient care [4].

M.E. Porter and E.O. Teiseberg overall characterized 11 problems in the existing US healthcare system: starting from commodity mindset of healthcare, followed by incomplete service planning and delivery strategies and wrong attitudes and incentives, as well as wrong responses to the needs. The idea to cope with this problem was to truly reform healthcare by changing competition nature from "zero-to-positive sum competition" and introducing the concept of value. According to those authors "Value-based competition is based on results and centered on medical conditions over the full cycle of care." As the M.E. Porter and E.O. Teiseberg concluded throughout their research, the premise that superior healthcare quality necessarily entails higher costs is unwarranted; instead, "better" healthcare providers typically exhibit greater efficiency. Enhanced quality is inherently less expensive due to precise diagnostics, diminished treatment errors, reduced complication rates, accelerated recovery, minimally invasive interventions, and a decreased necessity for extensive treatment modalities [3].

In the elucidation by W.C. Harrill and D.E. Melon regarding the healthcare reform and value paradigm in the United States, "value" is delineated as contingent upon the viewpoint of each stakeholder, encompassing "quality, service, patient experience, access, outcomes, and cost" as foundational components. The authors underscored that these reforms broadened the scope of value by recognizing patients as pivotal stakeholders, whose healthcare value is evaluated through the entirety of their clinical care journey and associated experiences [4].

Groenewould et al. characterize Porter's reform as a twofold strategy toward high costs and suboptimal quality and safety in healthcare. Pointing out that healthcare services should be organized into "value-based care pathways around patient groups" and those pathways have to be focused on providing the highest possible value and outcome for patient, not on increasing productivity by shifting the cost. And, secondly—"these pathways should compete for the favor of patients and health care purchasers." By this meaning, that patients should actively participate in the development of those pathways and their evaluation, as the critical consumers, but healthcare providers have to focus on the service quality and outcome measurement, purchasers—focus on "best possible health care for the lowest possible costs" [5].

The implementation of a value-based concept significantly changes the perspective of health economics and the way healthcare services are purchased and evaluated. Moving from volume to value requires reconsidering previously existing assumptions about how to organize and provide services, as well as how to measure outcomes and balance the interests of the involved stakeholders. The transformation process of healthcare service evaluation, which focuses more on long-term results and combines clinical and patient-reported outcome perspectives, poses another challenge. This is especially defiant when considering that for decades, practitioners had the leading impact and domination in healthcare service planning and provision, while patients played a passive role as service recipients.

The reform direction toward value-based competency, initiated by Porter in 2007, received significant support and encouragement for implementation. However, after a decade of implementation, significant critique also emerged. As an example, Groenewould et al. [5] specify four critiques toward the value-based competition approach: first: "VBHC's monistic account of 'value' neglects patient's pluralistic, personal values in life"—which is related to monistic and highly fixed outcome hierarchy for all patients of the one disease group and does not take into account patient individual goals and preferences. The second: "VBHC's instrumental perception of healthcare neglects healthcare's intrinsic 'gift value'"—this critique is related to the approach of how value is measured and believing that healthcare value is related to achieving good outcomes for acceptable costs. The authors remind us that there are also "nonmarket motives" and they are valued "as tokens of love, admiration, respect, honor, and so forth," as well as point out the altruistic nature of healthcare, which cannot be measured according to the existing frame of values. The third—"VBHC disproportionately replaces trust in professionals with accountability"—problem is related to standardization, measurements, and auditing activities, which can have a negative impact on healthcare professionals, as "professional values are under pressure, changing professional ethics into business ethics." In those circumstances, healthcare professionals can feel that they are under pressure and a magnifying glass of accountability, and their freedom to choose the best available strategy for the patient or new initiative proposals are undesirable. The fourth and last critique is related to "VBHC may undermine solidarity by favoring exit over voice"—this means that there are several problems: less educated patients are at risk of not receiving the appropriate service due to limited access to information, and middle and higher-class patients can escape the state-ensured system by receiving private services that are not accessible for the less fortunate. Considering the observed problems, the authors conclude that VBHC's focus on "target and performance management" means measuring service outcomes using standardized measurements and on patients' choice as well as exit or "voting with your feet" in cases when the patient's choice does not comply with standardized guidelines for care. This, in turn, may threaten the concepts of "trust in professionals respectively solidarity." To overcome those problems, the authors recommend implementing the new concept "Values Driven Health Care," this approach, in addition, would take into account patient's personal values and intrinsic values, encourage more to trust healthcare professionals, giving them more space and freedom, and encourage patients to raise their voice [5].

So, we come to the question—"What is Value in Healthcare?" M.E. Porter, in an article from 2010, points out that "Value in health care remains largely unmeasured and misunderstood." Value should consistently be defined from the customer's perspective. In a well-functioning healthcare system, the rewards for all other actors should be determined by the creation of value for patients. And as it is quite clear how to measure effectiveness by dividing costs into outcomes, the challenges lie in the outcome and cost definition. As Porter specifies, "Cost, the equation's denominator, refers to the total costs of the full cycle of care for patient's medical condition, not the cost of individual services" [6].

This implies that it is not solely about cutting costs in isolated services but rather about reorganizing services and redistributing resources, possibly even adding extra resources to some, ultimately resulting in the best possible outcomes with lower expenses in the long term. Yet, it all needs to be data-based decisions that stem from clearly defined and measurable service quality criteria.

An approach that involves analysis of the outcome of all medical services that patient's condition requires and all the costs of those services in a full care cycle, especially in fragmented healthcare system, where each provider serves only some services and is not related and not cooperating with other service providers is kind of "mission impossible" and requires a total mindset change, as well as organizational changes. Also, the possibility of measuring the outcomes is not an easy task, as the value for patients is frequently unveiled gradually and is evidenced by enduring outcomes such as sustainable recuperation, ongoing intervention requirements, or instances of treatment-induced ailments. In the context of outcome measurement, M.E. Porter advocates for the adoption of a three-tier measurement hierarchy. The first tier pertains to the attained or maintained health status, encompassing metrics such as survival rates and the extent of health or recuperation. The second tier focuses on the recovery process, measuring factors such as time to recovery and resumption of normal activities, while also accounting for the disutility associated with care or treatment processes, including diagnostic inaccuracies, inefficacious care, treatment-related discomfort, complications, and adverse effects. The third tier is related to the sustainability of health or recovery and nature of recurrences, measuring long-term consequences of therapy, for example, are-induced illness [6].

Thus, the VBHC concept is complicated and should be evaluated considering several aspects, not using it as a catchy slogan to attract attention to the undoubtable need for value in healthcare.

3. Evaluation of the VBHC concept in the European Union

Issues related to value in healthcare, including but not limited to the lack of resilience, efficiency, and effectiveness in healthcare provision, have been identified and analyzed in many countries. To tackle these challenges, the European Commission established Expert Panel on effective ways of investing in Health (EXPH) and worked on strategy to increase value of healthcare. The new strategy should continue the previously approved improvement process in four directions: (1) prevention, (2) improving outcomes by providing only cost-effective interventions, (3) improving outcomes by increasing quality and safety of process, and (4) increasing productivity.

As delineated in the EXPH report, despite the implementation of enhancements, three overarching issues have surfaced, persisted, or intensified universally. Firstly, there exists unwarranted variation, characterized by fluctuations in investment, access, activity, or outcomes that cannot be rationalized by discrepancies in necessity or the explicit preferences of the served population. The second predicament, interrelated with the first, involves the underutilization of efficacious interventions, leading to (1) a failure to identify, address, or preempt diseases and disabilities within the scope of healthcare capabilities, potentially exacerbating their severity and (2) disparities among patients with comparable functional statuses but dissimilar diagnoses, particularly evident in cases where diagnosis predicates reimbursement for interventions.

The third problem—"overuse which always results in waste," this means paying for activities that do not provide value to outcomes for patients or even cause patient harm in terms of over-diagnosis, over-treatment, and side effects [7].

EXPH report has dedicated a significant amount to discussion on intrinsic and extrinsic values in healthcare and in conclusion, provides the definition of VBHC for the systems with universal health coverage (UHC). EXPH defines VBHC as a "Comprehensive concept built on four value-pillars": (1) personal value— this means care to achieve patients' personal goals, (2) technical value—or best possible outcome with available resources, (3) allocative value—which means equitable resource distribution across all patient groups, and (4) societal value—or providing healthcare services, which encourage social participation and connectedness [7].

EXPH report also provides framework and offers initiatives to increase value in health—reallocation resources from low-value care toward high-value care. Concurrently, it underscores that the embracement of such reallocation necessitates a cultural shift prioritizing patient-centered considerations, inclusive of their preferences and objectives. The initiative is around patient-centered service delivery or change from disease-centered to person-centered services and is defined as "care at all levels needs to be driven by patients' needs, goals, priorities and preferences." These changes imply greater patient involvement and empowerment in all activities—starting from the planning of the service allocation to the assessment of the provided service and new initiative steering. The second initiative is related to quantifying and categorizing loss of value or identifying and minimizing waste of three categories: (a) wasteful clinical care—duplicate services, medically unnecessary services, preventable adverse effects, and patient's psychological suffering; (b) operational wastes—in cases when care could be provided using fewer resources and (c) governance-related waste—which means unneeded administrative procedures, fraud, abuse, and corruption. The third initiative provides approach that deals with unwarranted variation, overuse, and under-use of services, which also leads to value loseses in healthcare. Among theoverall nine initiatives, the last to be mentioned is related to policies for better value—and discusses three examples mentioning its benefits and risks: pay-for-performance, use of cost-effectiveness thresholds, and value-based healthcare. Unfortunately, there is no one ideal payment model suggested for implementation. Significant recognition from EXPH report is that a cultural paradigm shift is imperative to enable the inquiry not merely into the feasibility of a treatment or procedure but rather into its capacity to confer tangible value upon the patient, thereby authentically enhancing their quality of life or fostering prospects for recovery [7].

The third term that arise after "value-based competency" originally coming from US healthcare system, followed by "value-based health care" that came latter and was more related to the care cycle and patient needs and values; the third is "value-based health services (VBHS)." VBHS approach was introduced by WHO with the aim "to help countries achieve UHC by making evidence-informed decisions to use resources efficiently and effectively." The WHO report highlights that value-based health systems (VBHS) extend beyond the singular assessment of value for money during selection processes. Instead, they ensure that the ascertained value is effectively delivered to patients and aligns with their perception of value. Similarly, as the EXPH report points out the need for cultural changes to implement VBHC, the WHO emphasizes that authentic comprehension of value demands a shift in focus from "what is the matter with people" to "what matters to people," thereby prioritizing individuals at the core of care provision [8].

WHO proposes to use a 3D approach in policy formation: data, dialog, and decision-making process and points out that it is crucial to establish robust connections between the 3D approach and a nation's legal framework, as well as to develop strong institutional arrangements and governance mechanisms to bolster the decision-making process. The practical recommendation to provide a policy that could lead to value-based healthcare services is to ensure value through strategic purchasing and an integrated people-centered healthcare service approach. According to the implementation of the VBHS approach, the WHO underscores the critical importance of data and information management, along with ensuring effective governance, in the various approaches outlined that contribute to and establish VBHS [8].

In addition to the policy initiatives outlined by the WHO, another policy brief presents a spectrum of policy instruments that can be utilized to augment value within healthcare systems. These include: (1) fostering collaboration across sectors for health, (2) implementing fiscal and regulatory measures to promote health and prevent diseases; (3) bolstering primary care services, (4) ensuring funding for universal access to healthcare, (5) defining a comprehensive health benefits package, (6) employing strategic purchasing strategies to maximize health gains, (7) incentivizing high-quality care through payment mechanisms, (8) establishing integrated, person-centered health services, (9) promoting evidence-based care practices, (10) accelerating the adoption of eHealth and digital health solutions, (11) engaging patients in their own care, and (12) involving citizens in decision-making processes. The authors of these principles, Peter C. Smith et al., underscore the importance of safeguarding all dimensions of value, as these principles typically emphasize specific aspects. However, they caution that the diverse approaches advocated thus far have addressed facets of healthcare within specific contexts, falling short of achieving the broad performance transformation envisioned by proponents. At the same time, the authors underline the importance of adopting a value-based approach and suggest implementing this concept in stages as experience unfolds [9].

Focusing on the application of VBHC within the context of cancer care, particularly in breast cancer, numerous publications have delved into its implementation. Nuh Z. Canturk and Bahadir M. Gulluogly assert that the objective of value-based cancer care (VBCC) is to ensure consistent and sustainable health outcomes for patients, achievable through the establishment of sustainable healthcare systems. Drawing upon insights from the American Society of Clinical Oncology, the authors delineate four principal domains of VBCC: (1) clinical outcomes encompassing survival rates, quality of life, adverse events, tumor response, and time to progression; (2) cost considerations; (3) elements of care delivery, including "access, quality, communication, and social equity, alongside patient-centered care," which embodies compassion and respect, among other attributes; (4) opportunity for innovation for treatment benefit. The authors propose a new term—value-based quality care (VBQC) that consists of three levels: (1) health state and its degree, (2) duration of recovery and anxiety due to therapy, and (3) continuity of recovery and long-term effects of treatment [10].

Although the authors used the new term—VBQC, according to the content of the model, it is similar to M.E. Porter's (2010) three-tier approach for treatment outcome measurement, described at the end of section one of this chapter. N.Z. Canturk and B.M. Gullology suggest evaluating the value-based outcome metrics for breast cancer using several indicators, based on the European Society of Mastology. As those outcome measurements are similar to M.E. Porter (2010) model, a comparison of both models in relation to breast cancer is provided in **Table 1** [6, 10].

Nowadays, the complete set of measurement variables to assess the quality of breast cancer treatment is provided in the European Quality Assurance Scheme for Breast Cancer (2021), which is planned to be used in the certification process for cancer center accreditation and consists of 86 requirements divided into the following categories: general (20), screening (10), diagnosis (25), treatment (25), rehabilitation (2), follow-up (3), and palliative care (1) [11].

Specific sets of measurable indicators are available for non-metastatic breast cancer that are provided in EUSOMA quality indicators (2023) and contain 56 indicators that are grouped into several categories: pathway indicators (6), diagnosis (6), loco-regional treatment: surgery (14), radiation therapy (6), systemic therapy (14), staging (1), supportive care (2), follow-up and survivorship (3), outcomes (2), and patient-reported outcomes (2) [12].

M.E. Porter (2010)	N.Z. Canturuk, B.M. Gullology (2021)
1. Health status achieved or retained	1. Health state
1.1. Survival: survival rate (1-year, 3-year, 5-year, and longer)	1.1. Expectancy of life: survival rate/survival
1.2. Degree of health recovery: remission, functional status, breast preservation, breast-conservation –surgery outcomes	1.2. Health condition: degree of pain, period without disease, performance quality upon return to work
2. Process of recovery	2. Recovery
2.1. Time to recovery and time to return to normal activities: time to remission, time to achievement of functional and cosmetic status	2.1. Time to recovery: start of treatment
2.2. Disutility of care or treatment process: nosocomial infection, nausea or vomiting, febrile neutropenia, limitation of motion, breast reconstruction discomfort or complications, depression	2.2. Inconvenience and anxiety due to treatment: hospitalization rate, delay and anxiety, pain during treatment, nosocomial infections, deep-vein thrombosis, time to physical activity and to work, redo surgery, lack of consciousness, medical errors
3. Sustainability of health	3. Continuity of health
3.1. Sustainability of health or recovery and nature or recurrences: cancer recurrence, consequences of recurrence, sustainability of functional status	3.1. Continuation of health: recurrence rate
3.2. Long-term consequences of therapy: incidence of second primary cancers, brachial plexopathy, premature osteoporosis	3.2. Long-term effects of treatments: degree of performance, necessity for revisions, insufficient rehabilitation, results of adverse effect, chronic pain

Table 1.
Value-based outcome metrics for breast cancer—level, dimension, and variables used for assessment of the dimension [6, 10].

Due to the fact that the VBHC concept does not consist only of the assessment of the quality of services but also includes patients' perspectives to a large extent, the other sets of variables to assess the healthcare toward VBHC are related to patient-reported measurements. The richest source of measurements that should be collected from patients treated for non-metastatic breast cancer is available in ICHOM (2023) data collection reference guide [13]. Apart from the evaluation criteria, it is important to see practical implementations and effects of the VBHC in practice. That is considered in the next section of this chapter.

4. Global practice of value-based healthcare implementation

There are several publications on guidelines and recommendations on how to practically implement VBHC, including articles on the topic of breast cancer. van Egdom et al. [14], in reference to Erasmus University Medical Centre Academic Breast Cancer Center, developed a strategy for the VBHC implementation blueprint and suggested five methods and practical steps that should be taken. First, institutional dedication, as the authors pointed out—"is pivotal to enable transformation of the current healthcare systems towards a VBHC—system." Second, dedicated multidisciplinary teams consisting of oncological (breast) surgeons, medical oncologists, radiologists, pathologists, clinical geneticists, nurses with specialization in breast cancer, psychologists, gynecologists, plastic and reconstructive surgeons, as well as thoracic surgeons should be formed, and involved in the process. Third—the development of care pathways, that ensure service alignment according to patient needs and the agreed-upon standards. Fourth, determination of a breast cancer outcome set containing specific patient-reported outcome measurement sets (PROMs), as well as outcomes such as patient, tumor, and treatment characteristics, survival rates, and others, in details already described in the previous section. Fifth, the development of a data collection tool provides the possibility to combine and analyze all the necessary data to evaluate different aspects related to VBHC [14].

According to M.E. Porter's findings in 2010, the existing organizational framework and information systems within healthcare delivery present formidable obstacles to the accurate quantification and provision of value. Consequently, a significant portion of providers neglect to effectively gauge value. Instead, providers often limit their measurements to elements directly under their control within a given intervention and those that lend themselves to easy quantification, rather than focusing on parameters crucial for desired outcomes [6].

EXPH report from 2019 indicates that "discourses about value in healthcare tend to focus on reducing costs, increasing efficiency and, more recently, minimizing unwarranted variation in healthcare utilization" [7]. As authors point out, if we really want to understand value, we need to analyze not only "technical value," but have deeper insight into what really matters to patients and clinicians, and what are the value for the citizens and society.

The practical experience of the VBHC implementation for breast cancer in the University Medical Center of Rotterdam in the Netherlands, according to van Egdom and colleagues [14], took about 3 years and consisted of three steps: (1) development of standardized care pathways by the dedicated multidisciplinary team; (2) development of outcome data set in collaboration with breast cancer patients and patient NGOs and (3) integration of data set in clinical practice and linkage to patient electronic health record. After the approach was implemented in Rotterdam, collaboration with eight other hospitals in the Netherlands was initiated, and that provided the possibility to ensure transparency between hospitals with the aim of improving the quality and benchmarking outcomes. In relation to the payment model authors point out that "although VBHC-initiatives are hard to translate to a fee-for-service model, it is expected that all stakeholders will benefit from such a transition to longer term bundles" [14].

Another review on the existing practice of VBHC implementation provided by van Staalduinen and colleagues [15], by screening 1729 publications and 62 of them used for data extraction, have observed the main trends in implementing VBHC. The study showed that the most frequently implemented VBHC component was to measure outcomes and costs for every patient, generally using PROMs. The second most implemented component was to organize care in integrated care units (IPU), and "often, these studies described the implementation of care pathways." The third most popular approach was "building an enabling information technology platform," which means an application to collect patient experiences. Only few studies were about "move to bundled payments for care cycles." The authors observe that their investigation reveals hospitals' apparent lack of comprehensive adoption of value-based healthcare (VBHC) as an integrative management paradigm. Instead, hospitals frequently opt to implement only selected components of VBHC, notably focusing on outcome and cost measurement for individual patients and structuring care delivery around IPUs. The authors draw the conclusion that VBHC may risk being perceived as a transient management trend, leading hospitals to selectively embrace components aligned with their existing management approaches. This selective adoption may, in turn, contribute to the fragmentation of VBHC as a cohesive strategic framework [15].

As highlighted by the WHO, there is an increasing consensus surrounding the necessity for a more proactive or strategic approach to the procurement of healthcare services, particularly in the context of countries striving toward the UHC and endeavoring to attain value in the provision of health services [8]. It only stresses the need for each country to review strategically its approach to financing of health services in order to build more resilient healthcare system.

5. Case study: implementing a VBHC model for breast cancer in Latvia

As mentioned in the introduction, the population in Latvia is 1.888 million and oncology ranks as the second leading cause of death among the population in Latvia. In women population, the primary cause of death in oncology is breast cancer. To cope with this problem, and promote more timely diagnosis and better treatment, there are several state-provided services, including "green corridor" for the services for oncology patients.

Since 2009, the screening service as a state-paid mammography is provided to women starting from 50 years of age, with recurrence after every 2 years until the age of 68 years. Invitation letter is sent to the place of residence of the woman, approximately 3 months after the person has reached the age of 50, 52, 54, 56, 58, 60, 62, 64, 66, or 68 years, if the person had not had the mammography in last year before the date of invitation letter preparation. Invitation is valid for 2 years. Invited women can receive mammography service in any ambulatory care service that provides it, or use the service of mobile mammography, which as a service was implemented to promote its availability to persons living in rural regions with limited service provision [16].

Unfortunately, despite all the activities aimed at increasing engagement, the response rate in 2023 was, on average, 36%, with the highest rate in region Kurzeme—47%, and lowest in Riga region—31% (in 2022—average response rate 30.2%, 2021—30.8%, 2020—29.9%). Screening results in 2023 were as follows: complies with the norm—58.09%, potentially non-malignant changes—38.24%, suspicion of malignancy—0.71%, very suspicious for malignancy—0.12% and cases with incomplete investigation—2.8% [17].

According to the statistics on breast cancer diagnostics distribution by stage (the latest data available is of the year 2021)—significant part of cases unfortunately is revealed in last stages: stage III—195 cases or 17.7%, and stage IV—106 cases or 9.6%. The most diagnosed cases are in stage II—413 or 37.5% cases in 2021. In the early stage I—there were 337 or 30.6% cases [1].

Later diagnosis means that the treatment will cost more, patient prognosis is worse, and the sufferings and disabilities patient will face will be more severe than if it was diagnosed in the early stages. Those problems have been identified already for several years, and healthcare authorities are trying to implement different initiatives to change this outcome, with the aim to diagnose more cases at stage one and, if possible—in the pre-cancer stage.

One of the improvements to provide earlier diagnostics and to shorten the path for patients from first symptoms to diagnosis was the implementation of the "Green Corridor" program in 2016. The aim of this program is to ensure that all patients with a suspected oncological disease have priority access to diagnostic services in 10 days and beyond the quota for the diagnostic services and consultation of an oncologist within 1 month [18].

Another program for oncology patients, implemented in 2022, is the "Yellow Corridor" program, which is aimed to provide diagnostic and consultation services for oncology patients in case of a suspected tumor recurrence. Programs provide the same services as "Green Corridor" but are intended not for the primary cases but for the cases of tumor recurrence [19].

Access to early diagnostic and treatment services for oncology patients, as well as an available range of treatment services, especially medication, has been an issue in Latvia for several years. Under the Parliament Committees, there is a special sub-committee related to oncology. Established in 2017, the Parliament group provides political priority to oncology sector, is still in operation, and regularly organizes meetings with the responsible institutions and patient organizations.

According to the results of a revision by the State Audit Office in 2023, there are several problems in oncology sector: (1) early detection—an underestimated and underutilized tool that can ensure more successful treatment, but it critically depends on patient engagement; (2) the "Green Corridor" program is not functioning because only 25% of patients received service within 10 days, and the average duration from inclusion in the program and diagnosis date is 195 days instead of the planned 65 days to determine the diagnosis; (3) medication, that should be used according to international guidelines, is fully available only for ovarian and non-metastatic bowel cancer [20].

According to the outlined problems and to improve the process of cancer screening, Latvia, in 2022, took part in the project provided by the International Agency for Research "Improving Cancer Care Coordination and Screening in Latvia and Slovakia (ICCCS) project" [21].

Another significant step to mention, performed by Latvia to improve the diagnostic and treatment services, is the development of specialized centers for breast cancer patients. Currently, diagnostic services can be performed in private, state, or municipality-owned healthcare institutions that have a contract to provide those state-paid services. However, the treatment is provided in five hospitals: for adults—two clinical university hospitals in Riga, and two regional hospitals—in Daugavpils and Liepaja; for pediatric cases—Children Clinical University Hospital. Patients can also receive some services related to oncology in private clinics, but the proportion of these patients is estimated to be very small, and there is no data on the oncology services provided by the private sector. In both clinical university hospitals for adults—Pauls Stradins Clinical University Hospital (PSCUH) and Riga East Clinical University Hospital (RECUH) there are specialized breast cancer centers. PSCUH "Breast Disease Center" was established in 2019; it has a multidisciplinary team of specialists, nurses, and patient coordinators and provides all kind of services related to the diagnosis and treatment of breast diseases. The unit is also a member of the European Reference Network Unity for Hereditary Breast Ovarian Cancer. In 2023, PSCUH participated in a pilot project for accreditation provided by the European Commission Initiative on Breast Cancer (ECIBC) [22].

In 2020, the renovation of the Breast Health Center was initiated in RECUH. After the significant improvements providing contemporary diagnostic equipment and renovating premises, in 2023, the new "Breast Health Center" was opened in RECUH [23]. At present, RECUH is also going through the accreditation process to become National Cancer Centre and National methodological center for cancer treatment [24].

Specialists and experts of both leading clinical university hospitals in breast cancer diagnostics and treatment, are cooperating and collaborating to promote the best practice, and have developed patient pathways and adopted clinical guidelines for diagnostics and treatment. All these materials are also provided for public use and are available on the homepage of the Center for Disease Prevention and Control [25]. In addition, to provide more information that is written from the patient's perspective, since April 2024, there has been a special portal called "Patient Academy." The portal was developed by the Patient NGO and provides all the information that can be relevant to cancer patients or their relatives. All materials provided in the portal were developed in cooperation and collaboration with specialists and patients. For example, for breast cancer, there is specific information about the symptoms, causes and risk factors, diagnostics, staging, survival, treatment, and prophylaxis [26].

In the field of patient involvement and reporting of patient-reported outcomes, significant progress has been reached with the implementation of patient-reported experience. Those measurements are provided in all five hospitals providing breast cancer treatment for adults and children. Implementation of PREM reports started in Latvia as pilots in 2020, and in 2023 already 40% of all hospitals are providing PREM reports for the patients. The response rate is the following—11% of all patients have been hospitalized agreed to receive invitation to fill out the PREM report, and from those—32% have filled the questionnaires [27].

Another significant improvement related to patient well-being and recovery is the breast reconstruction surgery. This service has been provided as a new state-paid service since 2022, and provides state-financed breast reconstruction surgery for approximately 300 women annually with breast tumors who have undergone breast removal surgery [28].

The intention to work toward VBHC was approved within one of the National Health Service directions to be addressed in 2023. As expressed in the action plan for the year 2023: Action No.2 is "To develop value-based healthcare services in Latvia" and to "develop a project for the implementation of the value-based service in the treatment of breast cancer" [29].

An evaluation of breast cancer services according to VBHC implementation approaches provided in the theoretical and implementation practice overview in the previous sections is represented in **Table 2**. Assessment is based on three approaches: Twelve concepts of policy levers provided by WHO [9], followed by the WHO "3D model" approach [8], and using Erasmus MC Academic Breast Cancer Center's five-step strategy [14].

As the evaluation shows, several significant steps have been taken toward improving the care of breast cancer patients, and several initiatives are on the agenda. The most hindering factor in providing better treatment and outcomes for Latvia breast cancer patients is the limited funding that prevents reaching the goal of providing treatment according to evidence-based decisions—or according to the existing international clinical guidelines. Funding is also the limiting factor to improving primary health, which triggers other problems—human resource availability, which leads to long waiting lists and belated diagnostics and treatments. There is also a narrative related to the unavailability of treatment and medications, as well as stigma related to oncological diseases and lack of mental support, and those are factors that impact the patients to go for diagnostics and treatment.

Besides the underfunding, there are other directions of action to improve the care toward VBHC. As prevention and early diagnostics are some of the most effective approaches, there is a need to improve the screening programs in two directions: (1) to engage more patients to receive service and (2) to provide better management

Assessment criteria	Evaluation of VBVA for breast cancer in Latvia
WHO Policy Brief No.37. Building on value-based healthcare [9]	
(1) Working across sectors for health	Implementation of the concept "Health in all policies" in Latvia is weak. The promoters of Oncology sector are represented in Parliament as working group of Parliament members, and Oncology has been set as priority TOP subject in health care. Unfortunately, results published of the State Audit Office review concluded that "Oncology—priority without results" [20].
(2) Fiscal and regulatory measures for health promotion and disease prevention	There are some initiatives provided in Latvia, to increase prevention and reduce risk factors. For example, the changes in regulation to raise taxes on tobacco and sweetened drinks, and redirect in addition collected taxes to oncology programs. Also there are discussions on tighter regulation on alcohol selling, to cope with alcohol as one of the risk factors. In the field of prevention, as was outlined in this chapter, the screening programs are not as effective as they should be, so there are activities provided to work toward improvement of the screening in cooperation with IARC.
(3) Strengthening primary health	Strengthening primary health has been a political priority in healthcare sector in Latvia, for decades. Unfortunately, initiatives implemented cannot provide all the necessary needs. The main problem with primary health is the service availability that is related to scarce funding of healthcare, insufficient human resources, and aging population, especially in the sector of family medicine or GPs. As outlined in the OECD review: "The number of health workers remains among the lowest in the EU," and "the proportion of Latvian people with unmet health needs is above the EU average"—and to solve those problems "Latvia is planning a reform of primary healthcare to streamline and improve care provision" [30].
(4) Funding healthcare for universal access	In Latvia healthcare is funded according to universal access and provided for all citizens as state insurance. But, due to insufficient funding, services that are needed for cancer patients, especially innovative and expensive medication, are not included in the reimbursed medication list. That puts a huge burden on patients, as they either have no possibility to receive care according to international clinical guidelines, or should ask for donations, to receive the treatment. As outlined in the OECD review: "Population coverage in Latvia is universal, but some services are excluded," and Health expenditure in Latvia is far below the EU average—so the availability of healthcare services is restricted by annual quotas, out-of-pocket payments represent more than quarter of total health spending [30].
(5) Setting a health benefit package	Health benefit package is not a common practice in Latvia, although some kind of health technology assessment initiatives exist. For example, to include medication in the reimbursed list, there are specific procedures containing cost-effectiveness analysis. But, due to insufficient funding, there already exists "waiting list" for the medications that have been recognized as cost-effective but are not included due to lack of finance.
(6) Strategic purchasing for health gain	The concept of strategic purchasing has been implemented in Latvia for contracting several services paid for by the state. For the oncology sector, strategic purchasing is not yet fully implemented, but there are additional procedures over the control of quality that are used to measure and taken into account, when making a decision to prolong existing contract of services.
(7) Paying for quality	Concept of paying for quality is not implemented yet in Latvia in any sector of healthcare. This is one of the political directions that are outlined in several strategies for health. National Health Service of Latvia, according to their action plan for 2023, held several sessions and work groups on those topics named after "VBHC," to identify measurements that can be used for this model. To implement such a model—there is a need to (1) have agreement on indicators measured by healthcare providers, (2) implement patient reporting outcome measurements PROM, (3) develop and negotiate the funding model and payment system for such "pay for quality" approach,

Assessment criteria	Evaluation of VBVA for breast cancer in Latvia
(8) Integrated people-centered health services	To provide integrated people-centered health services for breast cancer in Latvia—several activities have been done: developed patient pathways, established specialized centers for breast cancer in both leading breast cancer hospitals—PSCUH and RECUH, and improved patient management by introducing patient coordinators. In cooperation with patient NGOs, education and useful information are provided in the specialized patient portal. The weakest part of integrated people-centered services is the ability to receive services that are not the PSCUH and RECUH services—for example, physical and social rehabilitation and services for disabled persons.
(9) Evidence-based care	The diagnostic and treatment services provided by the state are evidence-based care, as there is no reimbursement for alternative treatment or so. Clinical pathways and diagnostic and treatment guidelines are used by clinicians, but due to funding restrictions, they are "adjusted" to financial possibilities. Thus, the patients cannot receive the treatment (mostly innovative medication) that is approved in international guidelines and available in other countries. Another significant obstacle to implementing evidence-based care is related to very limited data that are available and can be analyzed to evaluate diagnostics and treatment.
(10) Stepping up the introduction of eHealth and digital health	Unfortunately, eHealth and digital health are some of the weakest points in the implementation of VBHC, pay for quality, and patient-reported outcomes in Latvia. The hope of improving those processes exists as there are already some initiatives toward systemized data management in eHealth and Digital Health. As of July 2023, the Digital Health strategy of Latvia was approved and outlines aims to reach, as well as there are funds available for digitalization and digital transformation for healthcare institutions. As outlined in the OECD report: "The Strategy sets out plans for digitization of patient medical records; digitalization of healthcare data at facility level; and interoperability of data systems in different facilities, regardless of ownership." This aims to facilitate healthcare professionals' access to comprehensive medical records for their patients [30]. On 23 April 2024, the Government of Latvia made a decision for establishment of a specific Digital health data management institution [31].
(11) Involving patients in their own care	Involvement of patients can be evaluated as very successive, as there are several patient NGOs that are working individually related to the type of oncology, as well as have cooperated and established root organization or alliance. The patient NGOs are involved in different activities and are present in development of new political initiatives, in promoting implementation, as well as supporting patients and raising public awareness on those topics. Cooperation among oncology specialists, patient NGOs, and supporters also persists and can be noticed in different activities—public events dedicated to special oncology topics are well covered by media, as well as development of information for patients that is available online and in printed forms. Patients also can evaluate their treatment by filling in the PREM questionnaires and, hopefully, in the future—also by filling out PROM questionnaires, when those will be provided.
(12) Involving citizens in decision making	Involvement of citizens in decision-making in Latvia persists and, in the case of breast cancer, is provided mainly by engaging related stakeholders—patient NGOs, specialist NGOs, as well as experts in the field.
WHO Policy Brief. 3D approach for ensuring value through health benefits package [8]	
Data—search for reliable data	Unfortunately, reliable data to provide analyses is not available in Latvia. As the existing healthcare-related data are fragmented, analysis of the data needed for breast cancer services, according to existing quality assurance measurement variables [11, 12], cannot be provided. There is a need for improvements in all aspects—in primary care, in hospital information systems, as well as in the interoperability services. However, if taking into account also the patient perspective, at first there is a need to implement a platform where patients can report their results by using PROM questionnaires.

Assessment criteria	Evaluation of VBVA for breast cancer in Latvia
Dialog—start a dialog with partners	As the 3D approach foresees, the first stage is available data. In the case of breast cancer in Latvia, there is a good platform to form the dialog as all involved stakeholders are well organized and have previous experience in cooperation and collaborations, where the data will be available.
Decisions—inform evidence-based decisions	To provide evidence-based decisions, the lack of data is the hindering factor, again.
Erasmus MC Academic Breast Cancer Center five-step strategy [14]	
(1) Institutional dedication	In Latvia, the institutional dedication to implementing VBHC in breast cancer is outlined as one of the several ways of action for the National Health Service. As the role of this institution is to provide institutional leadership, the possibility of implementing the VBHC approach in breast cancer relies on the other actions and their priorities. Theoretically, the institution is provided and, in the year 2023, provided several working group sessions on this topic.
(2) Dedicated multidisciplinary team	In both leading clinical university hospitals providing services for breast cancer patients—PSCUH and RECUH, there are special divisions consisting of multidisciplinary teams of practitioners, nurses, and coordinators. In those clinics, there have already been some pilot projects where PROM questionnaires were used, but mainly manually.
(3) Care pathways	Patient pathways, as well as clinical pathways, have been developed in Latvia for breast cancer patients; they are reviewed during the accreditation process of cancer centers in 2022 and 2023.
(4) Breast cancer outcome set	At this moment, there is no reconciled set of outcomes that has to be measured for breast cancer patient treatment outcomes in Latvia. There are initiatives to analyze and implement measurements provided in breast cancer quality assurance and EUSOMA guidelines, but that is only at the discussion phase. On the subject of implementation and use of PROM questionnaires, there are also only discussions that consider the restrictions of the financial resources for the responsible authority.
(5) Data collection tool	Data collection tools that can be used to obtain, combine, and analyze all the variables for the implementation of VBHC have not yet been on the agenda. As in the current circumstances, when a lot of data that has to be used is not available electronically and is either written on patient paper cards or is missing all, the possibility of providing necessary data digitally—is the first topic to resolve.

Table 2.
Evaluation of VBHC approach for breast cancer implementation in Latvia.

for the patients, who are screenings result indicates the need for further diagnostic services. The holistic approach to screening is on the agenda, currently drafting the new National Oncology Plan and nudged by the doctors to continually raise public awareness on this issue.

The second challenge is related to data-based decisions and all the activities related to data management—starting from the data set that has to be used, then—entrance of data into healthcare institution IT tool or patient portal, then providing interoperability and data collection and combining, then the analyses, data interpretation, dialog on findings, and all of that can lead to data-based evidence and decisions. Partially each medical treatment provider does it individually, but it is not being integrated into a unified platform, thus kept in a silos format.

According to different evaluation approaches used in **Table 2**, in general, one can assess that Latvia is on the right path toward VBHC implementation in breast cancer, considering (1) the aim to implement it and state institutions that have this on their action plan, (2) there are special centers for the breast cancer services, consisting of multidisciplinary teams and dedicated professionals, who works to provide best possible and patient-centered services, and (3) there are patient pathways and clinical guidelines, as well as desire to provide quality assurance and become accredited cancer centers. Those initiatives, if followed by the data collection tools to collect and analyze data on different aspects, can lead to better quality of care, provide evidence for service evaluation, and lead the system toward "pay for quality."

To implement the VBHC, of course, there is a need for emphasis on the activation of one of the most used practices—the use of PROM questionnaires, to provide treatment results from a patient perspective. And then to have the IT platform or data analysis tool where all the data can be combined and analyzed. Data visibility is another issue that should be further utilized to make the outcomes of the VBHC more vivid and communicated across other sectors.

According to evaluation results and research practice, the possibility of implementing VBHC approach, as was originally stated by M.E. Porter "Value-based competition is based on results and centered on medical conditions over the full cycle of care" [3] and measure results of full cycle—at this moment, it seems a "Mission impossible" due to existing lack of data, the overly fragmented services in healthcare, and unpredictable situations with healthcare providers in the future.

6. Conclusions

From the descriptions provided in the introduction sections of this chapter, it can be concluded that there is a divergent understanding of the concept of VBHC worldwide. Although the initial approach advocated by M.E. Porter suggests that value should be determined for the entire care cycle and the effectiveness of services should be assessed by analyzing the entire process from initial suspicions to complete recovery or palliative care, in practice, implementing such an approach has not been successful. As inferred from this concept, further development in European countries, where predominantly healthcare, especially in oncology, based on state-funded services and progress toward universal health coverage, to implement and introduce the VBHC concept requires actions across 12 distinct policy pillars [9], which substantially transcend the boundaries of a single institution and must be a national priority in healthcare with long-term strategy and leadership.

International organizations, pooling their experience and expertise, have also developed practical implementation recommendations and guidelines that have already been applied and tested for the fragmented implementation of such models. As outlined in the third section of this chapter, the most used and implemented components of VBHC are patient-reported outcome measurements or PROM and PREM, followed by the implementation of quality indicators to assess the services and move toward the concept of "pay for performance." Only a few articles are related to the change in the payment model, such as the payment for the whole cycle of care and measurement quality and values of the whole care process cycle. From the practical perspective, as G. Steinman et al. have characterized in the analysis of VBHC implementation in the Netherlands—there are four discourses on the VBHC in healthcare: patient empowerment; governance—as a mechanism to steer and incentivize toward better outcomes; professionalism—as intrinsic motivation of medical professionals to be aligned with the interests of patient, to deliver best possible care, and fourth—Critique—that is related to standardized outcome measurements, and other aspects [32]. At the same time, the

WHO calls for such an approach to be considered by all countries, including in the context of limited funding "the shift from value for money alone to VBHS is fundamental to achieving the UHC objectives of quality health care" [8].

As outlined in the WHO Policy Brief to provide the possibility to develop a health benefit package that is used to identify the most valuable or effective healthcare services, there is a "3D model"—data, dialog, and decisions [8], which highlights, in particular, the need for a coherent view of data and data collection and analysis tools. For Latvia, one of the crucial aspects is the data management issue that has its sprouts but has to be further developed in order to provide all the necessary information for the treatment. To achieve this goal, there will be special methodological centers established that overall will monitor the treatment quality and data availability. For oncology, it is foreseen to have one methodological center that would unite all five hospitals involved in the treatment of cancer.

Although the commitment to introduce the concept of VBHC in breast cancer treatment in Latvia is documented only in 2022, as the research showed three of five main steps suggested by Erasmus MC Academic Breast Cancer Center's five-step strategy [14]—by establishing institutions, organizing dedicated multidisciplinary teams, and developing patient pathways, has been already done. The next step in introducing breast cancer data set has been started in the scope of the accreditation of cancer centers and during the workshops organized by the National Health Service. One of the most challenging factors hindering the implementation of VBHC in breast cancer is related to digitalization of healthcare and successful implementation of activities outlined in the Digital health strategy and implementation of the Digital Competence Centre for the Health Sector.

Latvia has all the institutional and normative elements in place for the advancement of VBHC, yet availability of financing might hinder both the adequate progress of health data management and treatment options. However, the strong NGO network of cancer patients and the zealous ambitions of doctors in university clinics keep nudging the healthcare system in Latvia to get ready and adjust to change that includes also greater patient empowerment.

To summarize, quite a lot has already been done in line with the global concept of VBHC, although it has been done under different titles rather than the implementation of VBHC. The work that has been done in the breast cancer domain and is planned to develop further with outcome set measurements is in accordance with international guidelines and practice, although it is not relevant to VBHC's understanding of the best possible value in the full cycle of care.

Considering moving toward an initial understanding of the VBHC concept, provided by M.E. Porters, and analyzing the full cycle of care, the problem lies in creating a unified understanding and developing a global strategy for establishing a unified approach starting from screening or early signs and ending with reconstructive breast surgery and rehabilitation or palliative care. However, this is a politically strategic decision that constitutes global state policy and cannot be implemented by individual institutions providing specific stages.

Acknowledgements

We express our gratitude for the support and advice provided by Arvīds Irmejs, the enthusiast of quality services in breast cancer treatment and VBHC implementation for breast cancer in Latvia—Breast surgeon, Supervisor of the Breast Disease Center in PSCUH, and professor of oncology in Riga Stradins University.

Author details

Ieva Bikava*, Aiga Balode and Reičela Heinrihsone
Riga Stradins University, Riga, Latvia

*Address all correspondence to: ieva.bikava@rsu.lv

References

[1] Health Statistics DataBase of Latvia. Data sets: (1) MOR10. Death causes by month; (2) MOR20. Deaths and death rates by gender; (3) ONKO021. New cases of malignant neoplasms by site and region; (4) ONKO040. Number and percentage distribution of malignant neoplasms by stage (without cases registered form death certificate) and (5) Available from: https://statistika.spkc.gov.lv/pxweb/en/Health/ [Accessed: April 27, 2024]

[2] Cabinet of Ministers of Latvia. About the Plan for the Improvement of Health Care Services in the Field of Oncology 2022-2024. Adopted in 06.07.2022. Available at: https://likumi.lv/ta/id/333775-par-veselibas-aprupes-pakalpojumu-uzlabosanas-planu-onkologijas-joma-2022-2024-gadam [Accessed: April 27, 2024]

[3] Mukherjee A. Redefining health care: Creating value-based competition on results. International Journal of Pharmaceutical and Healthcare Marketing. 2008;**2**(1):76-76. DOI: 10.1108/17506120810865442

[4] Harrill WC, Melon DE. A field guide to U.S. healthcare reform: The evolution to value-based healthcare. Laryngoscope Investigateive Otolaringology. 2021;**6**:590-599. DOI: 10.1002/lio2.575

[5] Groenewould AS, Westert GP, Kremer JA. Value based competition in health care's ethical drawbacks and the need for a values-driven approach. BMC Health Services Research. 2019;**19**:256. DOI: 10.1186/s12913-019-4081-6

[6] Porter ME. What is value in health care? The New England Journal of Medicine. 2010;**363**(26):2477-2481. DOI: 10.1056/NEJMp1011024

[7] European Commission. Defining Value in "Value-Based Healthcare". Report of the Expert Panel on Effective Ways of Investing in Health (EXPH). Publishing Office of the European Union; 2019. DOI: 10.2875/872343

[8] WHO. WHO Policy Brief. From Value for Money to Value-Based Health Services: A Twenty-First Century Shift. World Health Organization; 2021. ISBN: 978-92-4-02034-4

[9] Smith PC et al. Policy Brief 37. Building on Value-Based Health Care. Towards a Health System Perspective. WHO Regional Office for Europe; 2020. ISSN: 1997-8073

[10] Canturuk NZ, Gulluoglu BM. Value-based quality care for breast cancer: More than guidelines. European Journal of Breast Health. 2021;**17**(4):297-301. DOI: 10.427/ejbh.galenos.2021.6333

[11] European Commission Initiative on Breast Cancer. Manual for breast cancer services. European Quality Assurance Scheme for Breast Cancer Services. 2021;**Version 1**:22-284. DOI: 10.2760/155701

[12] Rubio IT et al. EUSOMA quality indicators for non-metastatic breast cancer. An update. European Journal of Cancer. 2024;**198**:113500. DOI: 10.1016/j.ejca.2023.113500

[13] International Consortium for Health Outcomes Measurement. Non-metastatic Breast Cancer data collection reference guide. Version 5.1.0. 2023. Available from: https://www.ichom.org/patient-centered-outcome-measure/non-metastatic-breast-cancer/ [Accessed: April 27, 2024]

[14] LSE E et al. Implementation of value based breast cancer care.

European Journal of Surgical Oncology. 2019;**45**:1163-1170. DOI: 10.1016/j.ejso.2019.01.007

[15] Van Staalduinen DJ et al. The implementation of value-based healthcare: A scoping review. BMC Health Services Research. 2022;**22**:270. DOI: 10.1186/s12913-022-07489-2

[16] National Health Service of Latvia. Preventive Examinations of the Cervix and Breasts Cancer. Available from: https://www.vmnvd.gov.lv/lv/dzemdes-kakla-un-krusu-profilaktiskas-parbaudes [Accessed: April 27, 2024]

[17] National Health Service of Latvia. Program Results of State Paid Services for Breast Cancer Screening. Available from: https://www.vmnvd.gov.lv/lv/programmas-rezultati [Accessed: April 27, 2024]

[18] National Health Service of Latvia. State Paid Healthcare Services. Green Corridor in Oncology. Available from: https://www.vmnvd.gov.lv/lv/onkologijas-zalais-koridors [Accessed: April 27, 2024]

[19] National Health Service of Latvia. State Paid Healthcare Services. Yellow Corridor in Oncology. Available from: https://www.vmnvd.gov.lv/lv/onkologijas-dzeltenais-koridors-jeb-laundabigo-audzeju-recidivu-diagnostika [Accessed: April 27, 2024]

[20] The State Audit Office of the Republic of Latvia. Press Release on the Results of the Performed Revision of Oncology Services. 2023. Available from: https://www.lrvk.gov.lv/lv/aktualitates/paslaik-nenodrosinam-agrinu-onkologisko-slimibu-atklasanu-un-pacientiem-nepieciesamo-zalu-kompensaciju [Accessed: April 27, 2024]

[21] International Agency for Research on Cancer. IARC News. IARC Launches the Improving Cancer Care Coordination and Screening in Latvia and Slovakia (ICCCS) Project. 2022. Available from: https://www.iarc.who.int/news-events/icccs_project/ [Accessed: April 27, 2024]

[22] Pauls Stradins Clinical University Hospital. Clinics and Centers. Breast Disease Center. Available from: https://www.stradini.lv/lv/content/kruts-slimibu-centrs-0#department-services [Accessed: April 27, 2024]

[23] Riga East Clinical University Hospital. Breast Health Center. Available from: https://aslimnica.lv/kruts-veselibas-centrs/ [Accessed: April 27, 2024]

[24] Riga East Clinical University Hospital. The Accreditation Working Group of the Cancer Centre at East Hospital Continues Its Work, Developing a Methodology and Finalizing the Design of Patient Pathways. Available from: https://aslimnica.lv/the-accreditation-working-group-of-the-cancer-centre-at-the-east-hospital-continues-its-work-developing-a-methodology-and-finalising-the-design-of-patient-pathways/ [Accessed: April 27, 2024]

[25] Centre of Disease Prevention and Control of Latvia. Clinical Algorithms and Patient Pathways. Oncology. Available from: https://www.spkc.gov.lv/lv/kliniskie-algoritmi-pacientu-celi-indikatori-esf-projekts [Accessed: April 27, 2024]

[26] Cancer Patient NGO "Onkoalianse". Portal for Patients "Patient academy". Available from: https://onkoalianse-pacientu-akademija.webflow.io/ [Accessed: April 27, 2024]

[27] Centre of Disease Prevention and Control of Latvia. Patient Experience. 2024. Available from: https://www.spkc.gov.lv/lv/jaunums/pacientu-pieredze [Accessed: April 27, 2024]

[28] Ministry of Health of Latvia. Press Release. Improvements for Oncology Patients. 2022. Available from: https://www.vm.gov.lv/lv/jaunums/kruts-rekonstrukcijas-operacijas-dzeltenais-koridors-jauni-inovativie-medikamenti-ieguvumi-pacientiem-no-onkologijai-papildu-pieskirtajiem-lidzekliem-2022gada [Accessed: April 27, 2024]

[29] National Health Service of Latvia. Action Plans. Action Plan for 2023. Available from: https://www.vmnvd.gov.lv/lv/darbibas-plans [Accessed: April 27, 2024]

[30] European Commission. State of Health in the EU. Country Health Profile: Latvia; 2023. Available from: https://eurohealthobservatory.who.int/publications/m/latvia-country-health-profile-2023 [Accessed: April 27, 2024]

[31] Cabinet of Ministers of Latvia. Conceptual Report on the Establishment of the Digital Competence Centre for the Health Sector. 2024. Available from: https://tapportals.mk.gov.lv/legal_acts/8e898e12-2172-4073-9c5f-df7acb208247 [Accessed: April 27, 2024]

[32] Steinmann G et al. Redefining value: A discourse analysis on value-based health care. BMC Health Services Research. 2020;**20**:862. DOI: 10.1186/s12913-020-05614-7

Chapter 8

Perspective Chapter: Unravelling the Policy Paradox – A Critical Examination of Post-Apartheid South Africa's Healthcare Development in the Context of Developmental State Goals

Kiera Lander

Abstract

Post-apartheid South Africa has had economic development goals aligned with that of a developmental state (DS). However, almost three decades later, persistent rates of high inequality, poverty, and unemployment prove that not only has the African National Congress (ANC) been unsuccessful in achieving its development goals; but the reality of its macroeconomic policy has not been that of a developmental state. While the presented policy on healthcare in South Africa appears, prima facie, to be committed to deep developmental goals, other policies thwart the intentions of this legislation. These policies entrench and perpetuate inequalities in health outcomes between rural and urban, private, and public, as well as racial profiles of citizens. The policies that undo the developmental spending on healthcare include cadre deployment which ensures weak civil service management and conflicting messages in policy decisions as they develop. Further, this mixed policy approach towards healthcare has undermined South Africa's development goals. Although the ANC may have to combat the apartheid legacies of inequality, poverty, and unemployment, its failure in achieving meaningful development can be largely attributed to its misdirected policy approach to both its macroeconomic environment and basic healthcare.

Keywords: developmental, healthcare, inequality, poverty, development, corruption

1. Introduction

South Africa has, under the leadership of the African National Congress (ANC), long promoted becoming a democratic developmental state (DS) to combat persistent levels of unemployment, poverty, and inequality. Since the explicit commitment to becoming a DS in 2011, the ANC has not translated its policy promises into reality. South Africa has taken a neo-liberal character across its economy and institutional fabric, which has effectively thwarted its ability to first, become a developmental state and second, to achieve the level of economic development it so desired. Whilst this paper does not intend to focus on why there has been stark economic underdevelopment since 1994, it wishes to prove that the ANC has effectively failed to embody the developmental state it so envisioned. Defining the developmental state, its ideal characteristics, and specifically the ideal approach to education will help cross-compare the relative experience in South Africa. The state of its economic underdevelopment signifies the ANC's failure to effectively realise not just its developmental goals, but for the scope of this paper, its embodiment of a DS. An evaluation of macroeconomic policy and health outcomes shall illustrate the ANC's incapacity to effectively realise a DS, contrary to its policy promises.

2. An overview of the developmental state

A DS has the potential to stimulate rapid economic development. In a historically underdeveloped country; applying the DS framework to South Africa seems to be a worthwhile trajectory to adopt. Even though the ANC committed itself to becoming a DS in 2011, it effectively failed to realise their policy promises. I first define the DS and discuss the key ingredients of a successful DS according to Chang. This allows us to make a cross-comparison of the socio-economic reality of the DS in SA. I then distinguish that the failure of the DS in SA is not to be attributed to a lack of capacity. Instead, the ANC's failure to realise a DS is a product of its policy incoherence, corrupt bureaucracy, and its inability to dismantle the neoliberal character of the state, which consequently stifles the development of an underperforming healthcare sector.

2.1 Defining the developmental state (DS)

Best illustrated by the East Asia miracle economies, the developmental state broadly refers to one that stimulates economic development through deliberate state intervention. The East Asian miracle economies centred the *nature* of their state intervention around achieving rapid economic development through selective industrial policy; and the level of development achieved determined its political success. A successful DS tactfully intervenes to promote rapid and holistic economic development. Development in these states was to be signified by a combination of structural change in terms of policy thinking and welfare enhancement through policy implementation [1].

DS literature is known for directly opposing the Washington Consensus (WC) policies that were popular at the time [2]. The WC, supported by the World Bank and the International Monetary Fund (IMF), promised country's rapid economic growth should they adopt the neoliberal policy framework. The role of the state itself was to be minimal and should in no way be involved in the allocation or distribution of resources. Instead, the market forces would stimulate a competitive macroeconomic environment that through the product of neoliberal policies like financialisation, deregulation, and privatisation [3, 4]. The DS instead promoted state intervention, and deemed the 'invisible hand' as an ineffective measure to achieve economic development. DSs saw the need to stimulate and strengthen the institutional framework to dismantle historical economic fragmentation; this would ultimately reinforce the "embedded autonomy" of the state [3, 4].

2.1.1 The 'ingredients' of a DS

The 'ingredients' of a DS can be divided into *two* streams. First, there are three key 'features' that are foundational for any state attempting to transition into a DS. Second, outside of these features, there are 'tools' that help guide the effective strategy of state-led economic development. This section will explore these defining mechanisms.

2.1.2 The 'key features'

Developmental state literature is adapted to suit the specific economic needs of a country. However, there are key 'ingredients' that form the foundational framework of a successful DS. These features can almost be understood as 'pre-requisites' for a state trying to adopt a DS approach. First, a state needs to be run by a highly organised, well-educated bureaucracy [1]. By having a reliable, well-resourced bureaucracy that can carry out effective decisions that improve the socio-economic environment of the country, citizens will develop a sense of trust in their government. This leads to the second key feature of a DS, which is a sense of national unity. Namely, successful implementation of macroeconomic policies relies on their being a cohesive relationship between the state and its citizens. This cohesive state-citizen relationship helps foster the third key feature: a unified developmental vision. Having a common developmental vision, along with a sense of national unity, ensures the internal and external social cohesion that is necessary for effective policy absorption. Cohesion, internally, between state actors and externally, between the citizen and the state, is a vital mechanism for any DS. For example, Johnson emphasises cross-sector cohesion for the sustainable maintenance of long-term, holistic economic development[1] [5].

2.1.3 Tools of a successful developmental state (DS)

Chang [1] stresses that economic development theories guide us, and thus following a step-by-step blueprint in applying the DS theory is unnecessary. Instead, the development thinking of successful DSs is to be assimilated and adapted to the needs of a particular state. For example, Singapore's DS was more flexible in that they used the combination of a strong State-Owned Enterprises (SOE) sector, free trade and Foreign Direct Investment (FDI) to promote economic growth. Japan embodied a more classical and rigid approach to the DS agenda through the aggressive use of SOEs that helped the state shape policies and remain ever-present in the guidance of economic development. Hence, besides the abovementioned 'ingredients', Chang outlines a framework of socio-economic tools that successful developmental states have applied [1].

The experiences of the East-Asian Tigers serve as proof that the same 'tools' of a DS can be designed and implemented in different ways and yet still yield rapid economic growth. Thus, DS tools or further 'ingredients' should ideally:

1. Meet the development needs of the particular country.

2. Make use of the state's strengths and resources.

[1] Holistic economic development refers to development across sectors and institutions. Some examples include a combination welfare enhancement, human capital development and a promotion of economic growth.

There are six core tools[2] that have been identified as significant contributors to implementing a successful DS. First, the South Korean DS, for example, used *export-led industrialisation* patterns to achieve a high level of domestic economic growth; but also to incentivise their producers to align with the political agenda of the state [6]. Producers received aid from the Korean DS so that their firms could keep up with the competitive market and enhance their productivity. In return, the firms were incentivised politically to align themselves with the state, and ensure they maintained a high-performing industrial sector [6].

Redistributive social policies highly depend on a capable bureaucracy and a strong institutional base. These policies are pertinent to welfare development. Examples include egalitarian wage structures, implemented to reduce inequality and a progressive taxation system [1].

SOEs and Central Planning Agencies are both instrumental in coordinating policy-thinking and the implementation thereof. These organisational vehicles help orientate the state and its institutional frameworks. Public-private partnerships (PPP) further promote cross-sector cohesion by creating an environment in which both the private and public sectors work together to maximise resources, productivity and, thus, economic performance. Sweden, for example, achieved a durable industrial policy and improved economic performance through the use of strategic PPPs, further explained in Section 4 [1].

Last, *human capital development* is one of the most *crucial* tools of a DS. Having a well-educated bureaucracy is necessary for effective planning and decision-making, which drives economic growth [7]. This allows the state to impress the development vision and national identity on the population. Educational opportunities are *aligned* to industrial policy so that the education system produces a human capital base for the specific jobs the state wanted to endorse, as seen in South Korea [6]. These 6 tools help DSs realise rapid, state-led economic growth. Therefore, as this essay seeks to explore the prospects of the South African DS, it is important to note that these tools are intended to work together so that sustainable, *holistic* economic development is stimulated.

3. The rhetoric of a developmental state

South Africa's development challenges are not unfamiliar to the average citizen, or even the international community. This section intends to contextualise the country's developmental challenges as foregrounding information. Although this is a minor point to my argument, it applies to understanding the root of the ANC's policy motivation. Further, this section serves as evidence that the development commitments made by the ANC have not translated into reality. This signifies the ANC's failure to not only realise its promises as a developmental state but to also achieve the rapid economic growth that would ideally come with it.

The African National Congress's development discourse has promised to uplift and transform the state and create a "better life for all", at least in its policy-thinking and socio-economic goals [8]. Preceding the New Growth Path, the ANC approached the abovementioned development obstacles through a series of different economic frameworks. After the failure of AGISA to effectively realise the development promises it had

[2] These tools consist of (1) export-led industrial policy, (2) redistributive socio-economic policies, (3) the use of SOEs, (4) central planning agencies, (5) amalgamated public-private partnerships, and (6) human capital development.

made, the ANC switched its economic policy framework. In its attempt to stimulate the economy and improve citizenry welfare, the ANC began identifying with the ingredients of a *developmental state* as the backbone of its macroeconomic policy goals. The developmental state dream was coined to improve upon the failures of the initial post-apartheid policy frameworks. However, the implementation and outcome of ANC's developmental state policy promises seem to be misaligned with the reality of South Africa's present economic fabric. Although the ANC has alluded to being a DS in its development policy, the definition of what being a developmental state means to South Africa is still unclear.

3.1 The complexities of South Africa's political economy: a background

The Republic of South Africa battles not just present socio-economic fragilities but has inherited the apartheid regime's uniquely unequal and fragmented political economy. South Africa's history has been one of the central causes of its current underdevelopment and a motivating reason for the ANC's push for rapid economic growth and development. The consequences of the apartheid regime on South Africa's current democratic framework have raised controversy on what the best way forward is.

Post-apartheid South Africa experiences some of the highest rates of inequality, poverty, and unemployment; whilst simultaneously upholding one of the best constitutional frameworks in the world [9].

The rates of inequality, poverty, and employment are indicators of South Africa's economic development failures. The National Treasury declared these three determinants as the primary reason for the economic unsustainability of the state. Whether it is unemployment causally reinforcing poverty and inequality, or the structural legacies of apartheid have become too huge for the government to effectively dismantle—development in South Africa needs rapid, meaningful, and sustainable solutions.

3.2 Unemployment, poverty, and inequality: indicators of underdevelopment

The transition into a democracy promised economic transformation of the state. The ANC acknowledged that revitalising the economy would include diversification of sectors, macroeconomic stability and a series of other economic development promises that are discussed in Section 3. However, the bureaucratic regime in the South African state entrusted its economic transformation is plagued by patronage, clientelism and corruption [10]. The reality of the average South African citizen is economically dismal, contrary to the hope we started the democratic era with. After each policy release, the ANC acknowledges the fiscal unsustainability of South Africa's debt-to-GDP ratio, unaffordable expenditure by State-Owned Enterprises (SOE), and our declining investment rates. Each year, there has been a promise to restructure the state in a "different" way to previous policy attempts. There is a promotion of the necessity of state intervention and the need to transform South Africa into a developmental state in 2011, and then, policies promoted in these documents immediately took on a neoliberal character. The following year, inequality has increased, unemployment has increased, and poverty remains persistently high; and the blame is shifted to the previous fiscal year's austerity measures or lack of coherence between policy thinking and implementation. No matter how you look at it, the trajectory of South Africa's 'triple threat': unemployment, inequality, and poverty signifies the state's failure to actualise its policy promises. Ultimately, this characterises the state as one in crisis, with possibilities of meaningful economic development and becoming a developmental state seeming untenable [11].

One of the headlines in South Africa's policy promises has been dedicated to reducing unemployment. The NDP signifies the causal relationship between unemployment and translation into inequality and poverty. Explicitly stated, the NDP (among other policy documents) claims that increasing employment rates will eliminate poverty and reduce inequality through the enhancement of individual income and overall productivity growth of the state [10]. This narrative has been reproduced from the initial transition into a democratic state in 1994, through to our current socio-economic policy promises in 2020. However, as depicted in **Figure 1**, the official unemployment rate has subsequently increased since 1994, from 20% to 29.2% in 2020. 1995 was the lowest level of unemployment at 16.9% the post-apartheid state has ever achieved. It can thus be concluded; that the employment-orientated policy approach has effectively been unsuccessful [13].

It is no surprise, then, that the high levels of inequality and poverty have not been eliminated, but systematically widened. The bottom 50% of the population has had a decreasing share of pre-tax national income, whilst the top 10% of the population have enjoyed an increasing level of pre-tax income [13]. The top 1% of the population, although account for a lower percentage of national income than the top 10% of the population, still enjoy higher levels of income on average than the bottom 50% [13]. This level of income inequality is, as shown by the graph, only widening with time. Wealth inequality has too been skewed in favour of South Africa's elite few, at the expense of the poor. Wealth has been concentrated in the hands of the top 1% of the population, with the rate of wealth owned by the top 1% of the population increasing over time, since 1994 [13]. The inability of the South African state to effectively diminish the wage and wealth gap means that many South Africans will continue to live below the poverty line. And, although poverty has gradually declined since the 1990s, South Africa's poverty rates are still obstinately high. The persisting structural inequality ensures that the country remains socially fragmented and systematically underdeveloped. Conclusively, despite the ANC's promises to deliver on economic development through a process of eliminating inequality and poverty, via increasing employment opportunities—the realities of the state seem in contradiction with what was outlined on paper.

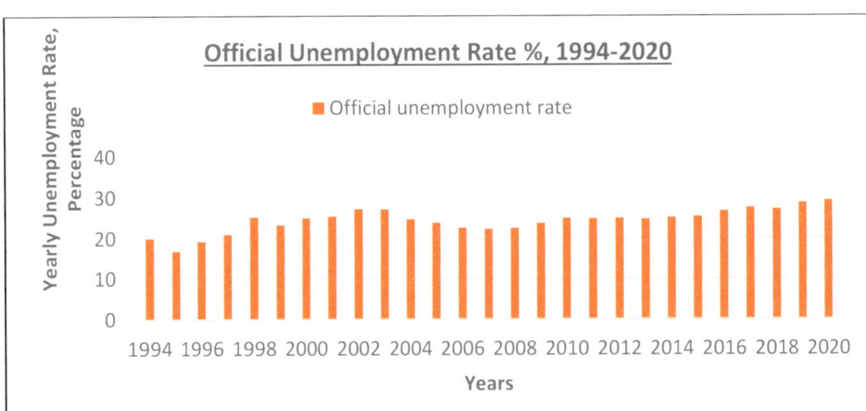

*Data Source 1: *Data sourced from the South African Reserve Bank (1) for the creation of this graph*

Figure 1.
*Official unemployment rate as percentage, South Africa [12]. Data Source 1: *Data sourced from the South African Reserve Bank [12] for the creation of this graph.*

4. A history of the ANC's macroeconomic policy approach

We have seen in the importance a DS places on a coherent policy framework that works in sync with the rest of the economy. However, it was not until the release of the New Growth Path (NGP) in 2011 that the ANC committed to becoming a developmental state. To fully conceptualise the capacity of its bureaucracy, it is helpful to understand the contextual background of the ANC's macroeconomic policy from the time of its leadership in 1994 before its commitment to a developmental state rhetoric. This section discusses the South Africa's macroeconomic patterns and then implores an evaluation of its policies thereof.

One of the flaws in South Africa's development approach can be boiled down to the misdirection in their policies. Before the DS dream, the policy-thinking of the state was internally inconsistent, externally unsuccessful and lacked a sense of coherence from one policy agenda to the next [9]. The ANC seemed to be:

1. Uncertain about its policy approach and

2. In contradiction with its own goals from the onset of its leadership.

This inconsistency and policy uncertainty translated into the developmental state era. Namely: that it promised a commitment to a developmental state framework, yet its policy implementation has contradicted its promises by remaining entrenched in a neoliberal political economy.

Some observe that the state has been the catalyst for development failures through a policy mis-focus on technocratic policy solutions. However, in slight contradiction to *policy implementation,* some argue the failure of the state to address development effectively is a *lack of focus at an institutional level* and a *lack of clarity* regarding macroeconomic policy for correct implementation [14]. Ansari (2021) argues that South Africa's policy pitfalls materialised post-1994 for three reasons. First, he argues there has consistently been a *policy misalignment* between the theoretical aims of the state and its eventual application. Second, he argued that the *lack of coherence within the state and instability* at a government level rendered policy measures ineffective. Third, the policy aims of the government to achieve pro-poor development contradicted with the neoliberal behaviour of the state across macroeconomic frameworks and institutions, such as in education and healthcare. For instance, although the post-apartheid democracy aimed to decrease social inequalities through social interventionist tactics; the policy adjustments introduced by GEAR encouraged the privatisation of education, which effectively contributed to increasing the educational inequality gap between private and public learner outcomes [15]. Thus, it is imperative to further investigate the evolution of the ANC's policy inconsistencies and incoherence.

4.1 The evaluation of SA's policy documents, 1994-2020

The Reconstruction and Development Programme (RDP) was the first policy criteria put forward by the new democratic state. It set the tone for the African National Congress (ANC) as a developmental state, with policy aims outlining six key principles for its development process. "Integration and Sustainability", "Nation Building" and "Assessment and Accountability" are the headlines of three of the set-out principles of the RDP, which align strongly with the focus of a redistributive policy approach [8]. At this point, there was not an explicit commitment to DS goals, but the ANC cemented its commitment to achieving economic development and enhancing the welfare of South African citizens through diminishing the stark inequalities left behind by the apartheid regime. The RDP was an ambitious national policy agenda that emphasised welfare goals, such as employment creation, poverty, and inequality reduction. It further promoted liberalised trade policies, restricting of industries through industrial policy, was compatible with privatisation and was an overall commitment to fiscal and monetary discipline [8, 16]. Two years later, Growth, Employment, and Redistribution (GEAR) was implemented as a response to the insufficient economic growth achieved by RDP.

Although GEAR initially claimed that it would build its framework in line with RDP's redistributive goals, it completely shifted macroeconomic policy-thinking by transferring the state into one characterised by neoliberalism. Favouring the use of the market, and trickle-down economics as the determinant of economic development, neoliberalism promoted free trade, financial deregulation, and privatisation of markets. Neoliberal economists viewed the achievement of economic growth and efficiency, namely by using increased Gross Domestic Product (GDP) as the signifier of economic development. The attachment to free-market fundamentalism rejected the use of state intervention [17]. Neoliberals believed that by allowing rational agents and the markets to behave under their self-interested goals, the economy would naturally stimulate itself.

GEAR streamlined its focus on the liberalisation of markets, a relaxation of exchange controls and an advancement of the private sector role with the assumption that this model would speed up economic growth, employment, and private investment [18, 19]. The focus on *economic growth* as the key mechanism to reduce high levels of unemployment, poverty, and inequality [19]. Some other features of GEAR that aligned with the neoliberal economic model that was popular at the time included monetary policy that used inflation targeting, trade liberalisation, a stringent fiscal deficient and increased competitiveness of industrial sectors [16]. The explicit focus on clearly neoliberal tactics leads to a negative impact on the economy's performance, with heavy social costs. Unemployment skyrocketed, and income inequality immediately widened, as did the wealth inequality gap. The austerity measures introduced by the National Treasury compromised the economy and led to a stark increase in inequality [16]. Therefore, contrary to even the initial promise of GEAR to keep the development goals set out in the RDP, its implementation was conducive to that of the neoliberal state, which negatively affected the economic performance of the state.

In 2006, the Accelerated and Shared Growth Initiative for South Africa (AGISA) was launched in response to the failures of GEAR by committing to the narrative that economic growth was to be a national effort and acknowledged the need for upskilling the population to improve the growth of the employment sector [20]. The commitment to a neoliberal agenda remained with the emphasis on trickle-down economic assumptions and the behaviour of the government was still significantly aligned to a neoliberal economic character. However, internal inconsistencies became apparent as AGISA emphasised trickle-down effect, whilst simultaneously wanting to increase state interventions as a mechanism to improve the welfare of the marginalised. Despite AGISAs promise to effectively halve unemployment and poverty, these economic determinants worsened after its implementation [16]. The mixed and incoherent policy approach of the ANC became apparent: first, the shift from RDP to GEAR and second, the inconsistency internally in the AGISA framework. The important thing to note with RDP, GEAR and AGISA is first, that the ANC exposed its incapacity to remain consistent with its promises set out in its policy frameworks.

It was only with the New Growth Path (NGP) that the commitment to a developmental state became the clear standpoint of the ANC. As previously established, the persistent rates of unemployment, poverty and inequality continued to plague the economy with stringent limitations, effectively stunting development and growth. Thus, the adopting of the developmental state goals became the ANC's response to the failure of its preceding policy attempts. Similarly, to the RDP, GEAR and AGISA, the NGP started off with the acknowledgement of South Africa's "triple threat" that had systematically remained the same, or even worsened since 1994 [21]. The NGP ensured South African citizens they were going to prioritise economic development and optimise the performance of the government in its quest to promote "a more inclusive economy" in line with the DS narrative it had since promised [21].

Chapter 4 of the NGP (2011) titled "*Institutional Drivers: Developmental State*" outlined the ANC's commitment to being a DS as a critical means to stimulate employment opportunities and economic growth thereof. The NGP made an explicit commitment to acknowledging that their DS would not be held "hostage to market forces". Instead, the NGP committed to enhancing the state's efficiency and cohesion with civil society. Economic development was to be stimulated through export-led industrial policy, job-creation, and income distribution. Thus, it was here that the DS rhetoric [21].

A year later, the NDP was launched. Even though there was a commitment to being a developmental state in 2011, the NDP openly criticises the failures of South Africa's (and the world's] neoliberal economic approach. It emphasised the inability of competitive, capitalist neoliberal economical methods to foster meaningful development, especially within South Africa's highly complex economic environment [22]. It was with the release of the NDP that the disparity between the ideological, economic thought and the policy in practice became starkly clear. The incoherence in policy-thinking had now persisted for almost a decade along with the socio-economic complexities of South Africa's civil society. Hence, the ANC was using the promises of being a developmental state as a smokescreen for its failure to properly execute it in practice [23]. The role of economic stability and access to public goods became a predecessor of any other method of economic stimulation. A streamlined focus on improving access to *quality* healthcare, education, housing, electricity, and water was detailed. Alongside the promises made to civil society, and acknowledgement of the need to create an accountable, corruption-free bureaucracy was employed as a central goal of the government at large. The shift in policy-thinking seemed highly committed to a developmental agenda.

However, the NDP was still not internally consistent. We saw with previous policy documents there was an issue of internal inconsistency, as well as external implementation. The failures of South Africa's economic development trajectory have been largely attributed to its poor policy approach and weak civil service. Part of the poor policy approach includes the internal incoherence within the document itself, which is not consistent with the requirements of DS literature that requires an absolute commitment to coherent policy; and another part of it is attributed to its implementation [or lack thereof]. For example, the NDP cements itself to the ideology of becoming a DS as the only meaningful mechanism to combat South Africa's development challenges [22]. The promise to build a capable DS by coordinating government sectors vertically[3] and horizontally,[4] strengthening and stabilising the public service and

[3] Vertical coordination across Government sectors refers to improving relations between national, provincial, and local government tiers.

[4] Horizontal coordination refers to relations in interdepartmental government sectors so that there is an efficient resolution of socio-political issues.

improving the governance of SOEs, is outlined as the primary role of the state [22] . However, the state still preserved a neo-liberal macroeconomic policy. For example, the NDP still maintained a minimalist state role and labour market de-regulation [16]. Despite the NDP critiquing neo-liberalist economic policy and committing itself to being a DS; South Africa remained entrenched in the neoliberal character it had set out for itself in 1996.

Outside of policy inconsistencies, the ANC seemed to forget the pre-requites any successful DS requires. Not only does the NDP negate responsibility for SAs failed development, but it lends it only to the legacies of apartheid. In such, it forgets that the developmental state will fail if there is not an efficient bureaucracy capable of effectively executed the policies outlined. There was a further lack of commitment to detangling the capitalist and neoliberal commitments of the country. Hence, the institutional framework of the country remained largely characterised by capitalist relations and a competitive market-led economy. It thus argued that the NDP committed itself to being a developmental state without adequately adapting the methods and character of its bureaucracy and institutional framework to be aligned to developmental paradigms. For example, the NDP asserted the ANC's commitment to eradicate corruption and embody an accountable bureaucracy aligned to a Confucianist value system, as DS literature encourages [16]. However, as **Figure 2** depicts below, there has been little improvement to the "Corruption Perceptions Index" since 2003. **Figure 2** illustrates that in the years 2011 and 2013, when the NGP and the NDP were released, the country experienced some of its highest corruption rates from 2003 to 2020. It can be concluded that in the same years the ANC declared its commitment to the DS, the country's corruption rates worsened. The stagnant and worsening levels of corruption indicate the ANC's inability to develop an accountable bureaucracy that is needed for a functioning state. This means that the state continued to be characterised by political illegitimacy, and an unaccountable bureaucracy. The lack of state capacity signifies the ANC's inability to effectively realise as DS, as opposed to their policy promises.

In 2019, the policy document: "Economic transformation, inclusive growth, and competitiveness: Towards an Economic Strategy for South Africa" was released [18]. Prior to this, thought, President Cyril Ramaphosa continued to stress the

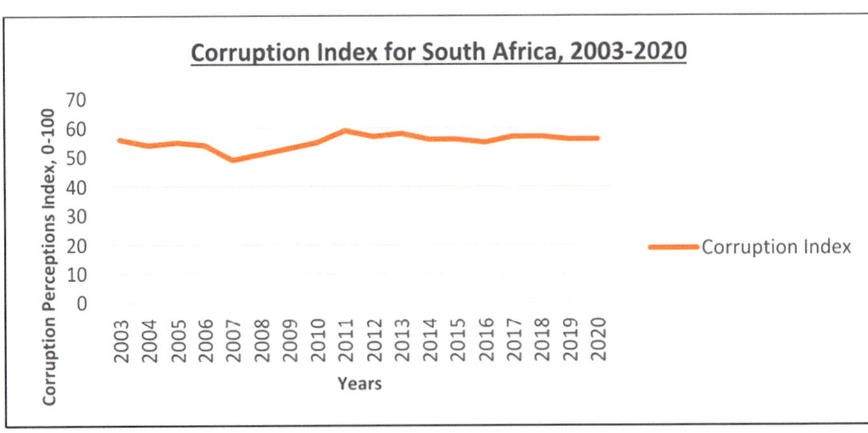

Figure 2.
Corruption perception index, South Africa.

ANC's creation of the developmental state by using the state as a vehicle to drive social, economic, and political transformation. There was a stringent belief in the capability of the Presidency to lead a capable developmental state [24]. The trust in the bureaucratic regime meant that the policy promises of the ANC remained committed to the creation of DS to deliver meaningful economic development to the country. The Reconstruction and Recovery plan, established in 2020, continued to align itself with DS goals by continuing to assert the role of state and planned interventions as the mechanism for economic reconstruction recovery and stimulation post-COVID-19 [25]. However, even when the ANC clamped down on the role of state as the primary means of restoring economic stability to the economic fragility catalysed by COVID-19, the policy promises were not actualised. The austerity measures adopted by the National Treasury, the cadre deployment and Covid-related corruption all worked to dismantle, again, the ability for the state to realise a developmental state to any extent [24]. The macroeconomic character of the state remained obstinately neoliberal with the continued liberalisation of markets and minimal state interference in its institutions [26].

4.2 The ANC's failed developmental state: a consequence of policy incoherence

The previous section analysed the ANC's move towards the DS rhetoric since the release of the NGP in 2011. It showed us that barriers to achieving a DS, is not one of capacity, for South Africa has both the ability and need to become a DS. SA's impossibly detrimental development challenges do not prevent it from implementing the DS agenda successfully. The East-Asian Tigers and successful Latin America DS's were all inherently underdeveloped, battling legacies of structural inefficiency and economic fragility. The DS literature pulls economies out of their "economic rut" and into an era of meaningful, sustainable development patterns. Hence, this chapter has argued that the ANC's failed DS is not because of unfavourable economic conditions, but can be attributed to:

1. An incoherent and inconsistent policy framework,

2. Cadre deployment and rising corruption,

3. A misalignment between DS policy promises and their macroeconomic approach. Although the policy-thinking has been that of a DS, the macroeconomic environment of SA has remained persistently neoliberal [26].

The ANC has tried to deal with South Africa's development issues by adopting a DS. However, this has not been actualised because of policy incoherence between the policy and reality, and the ANC's failure to properly implement the ideal characteristics of a DS. Instead, there has been a neoliberal approach that has undermined the ANC's progress as a DS. This can be more clearly seen in South Africa's healthcare sector.

5. Case study: the ANC's approach to healthcare

In this chapter, we turn our attention to healthcare within the context of a developmental state. Understanding the intricacies of healthcare provision and financing is crucial for assessing a nation's progress towards developmental goals, particularly with South Africa. Before understanding the South African case, the nexus between healthcare and economic development is explored, along with an overview of the South Korean case.

5.1 The nexus between healthcare and economic development

The nexus between healthcare development and economic growth is well-documented in the literature. Health has a vital role in maintaining economic development, as it is essential for and a result of economic progress. A country's health status affects economic development in multiple ways, as it influences human capital accumulation, workforce efficiency, and quality of life. Moreover, the impact of healthcare expenditure on the economy's growth is a subject of extensive study. While some research shows the positive relationship between healthcare expenditure and economic growth, other studies emphasise the need to account for issues such as corruption, bureaucracy, underinvestment, and inefficiency in health-related resource utilisation. This is where the developmental state comes in.

South Korea provides an interesting example of the interplay between economic growth and healthcare development, achieving universal health insurance within 12 years. This achievement has contributed to improving the overall health of the population, which has had a positive impact on the country's economic development, in line with its developmental state goals [27, 28].

5.2 The south Korean healthcare system: a public private partnership (PPP) system in a developmental state (DS)

There are multiple methods by which healthcare service financing and delivery systems can be designed [29], and can include, but are not limited to:

1. Government-led provision (public health centres, dementia centres, public hospitals, local medical centres) in which the government delivers (or entrusts to the private sector) health and medical services using tax resources.

2. Privately led hospitals and clinics that deliver health care services; users freely select and use private hospitals and clinics, and then the Corporation, the public payer, reimburses the user's costs.

3. A private sector delivers healthcare services and private insurance companies provide financing.

4. Communities such as medical cooperatives provide health care services as funders, deliverers, and users.

5. A corporation, a public funder, directly provides health care services with health insurance funds (corporation-operated hospitals and clinics, corporation health promotion projects).

Among the five types above, Korea's health care service delivery system and financing fall into the second type, in which private hospitals and clinics deliver medical services using national health insurance as a resource; otherwise known as a form of PPP [2]. The proportion of public hospitals in Korea is only 6%, and the rest are all private hospitals. This is in comparison to the average proportion of public hospitals in the Organisation for Economic Co-operation and Development (OECD) countries is 51% [29].

Since the National Health Insurance Act was enacted in the 1970s, Korea has aimed to provide medical services through private hospitals and clinics rather than public hospitals. The government at the time needed to minimise national welfare expenditures while making national economic development its top priority, so it did not establish public hospitals but instead used the private industry to maintain efficiency of healthcare provision whilst aligning it with the state, as per DS literature suggests [29]. As a result, instead of establishing a public hospital, the government had private providers provide medical services and raise financial resources through public insurance [29].

Under the policy goal that health insurance finances should not hinder national economic development, the government limited insurance benefits items and applied strong price controls on insurance benefit items and high out-of-pocket ratios [29].

Korea's medical system has become the foundation for all citizens to receive medical services at low prices anytime, anywhere, making it one of the most exemplary healthcare systems worldwide. Understanding South Korea's healthcare system is important as it provides insight into the trade-offs and policy decisions made in balancing economic development goals with the provision of healthcare, quality, and spending. This can provide the reader with an understanding of what should idealistically inform South Africa's endeavours to achieve its developmental state objectives.

5.3 A contextual analysis of South Africa's healthcare sector

The healthcare sector in South Africa is marked by significant inequalities, reflecting the broader social and economic disparities in the country. The South African health system faces systemic and structural challenges, including inefficiencies, staff shortages, and variability in care levels between rural and urban areas [30]. The healthcare system comprises a large poorly funded public sector and a smaller, better-resourced private sector, leading to persistent inequality between the two [31]. This inequality is further exacerbated by high levels of poverty and unemployment, with the public sector being under-funded and overburdened.

Similar to the education sector, where deep inequalities persist, the healthcare sector also experiences disparities along racial and socio-economic lines. For instance, racial inequality is clear in the healthcare sector, with differences in access to quality care and health outcomes [32]. Socio-economic status contributes to disparities in health outcomes, reflecting the wider social determinants of health. These disparities are further compounded by the two-tiered nature of the healthcare system, with significant differences in access and quality of care between the public and private sectors [33].

The healthcare sector in South Africa is characterised by significant disparities. According to the General Household Survey, only 17 out of 100 South Africans have medical insurance, with about 73% of white individuals, 52% of Asian individuals, and only 10% of black Africans being members of a medical scheme [34]. The private health sector in South Africa accounts for the largest share of health expenditures, with about 79% of doctors working privately [35]. This disparity in private coverage reflects the broader inequalities in the healthcare system.

Furthermore, the distribution of healthcare resources is inequitable, with over 120 medical schemes historically excluding black South Africans until the 1970s and still mostly catering to the wealthier population [35]. The public healthcare system, which serves most of the population, faces challenges such as medicine shortages and procurement issues [35]. The country's healthcare system is burdened by the largest HIV/AIDS epidemic in the world, accounting for about 17% of the global burden of HIV infections [30].

The public sector serves roughly 84% of the population without private health insurance, while the private sector caters to the remaining 16% [31]. This unequal distribution of resources has led to significant disparities in the quality of care and patient outcomes between the two sectors.

The public healthcare system faces a range of challenges, including widespread inefficiencies, staff shortages, and suboptimal care levels [36]. Despite being one of the top five African countries in terms of density of medical personnel per 1000 population, the South African public health system is chronically understaffed, particularly in rural and remote areas [36]. About 70% of doctors work only in the private sector, leaving only 30% of physicians available to serve the public sector [36]. This shortage of healthcare workers contributes to the suboptimal care levels and patient management in the public sector, who depend on the under-resourced public sector [37]. This has perpetuated inequality in access to quality health services.

In summary, the two-tiered nature of the healthcare system in South Africa has led to significant disparities in the quality of care and patient outcomes between the public and private sectors. The public sector faces challenges related to inefficiencies, staff shortages, and suboptimal care levels, while the private sector is largely funded through individual contributions to medical aid schemes or health insurance, serving a smaller portion of the population [31]. Addressing these disparities requires comprehensive efforts to strengthen the public healthcare system and reduce inequalities in access to quality health services.

5.4 Misalignment between the developmental state goals and the approach to healthcare in South Africa

5.4.1 The role of policies and thwarting health outcomes

Section 3 outlined the inconsistency, incoherence, and mixed policy approach of the ANC. Should the policy approach be fragmented and misdirected, it is understandable then, that sectors such as education are underperforming. The misdirection of macroeconomic policies creates a foundational base for an inefficient and incapable institutional environment. Health outcomes are compromised. This is like the disparity identified with the release of the NDP. There was a commitment to being a developmental state, but no effort was made to ensure the state could implement the developmental agenda. Further, there was not a meaningful attempt to detangle the neoliberal character of the country inherited from the apartheid regime and maintained by the previous macroeconomic frameworks. The lack of a consistent provision of resources, service delivery, and infrastructure development is a failure on behalf of the macroeconomic promises made within the abovementioned policy documents to achieve universal healthcare, and economic development.

5.4.2 The example of the National Health Insurance (NHI) program, and post-Covid reflections

To improve the healthcare system, the SA government proposed the introduction of an NHI. The NHI, uncoincidentally like that used in South Korea (outlined in Section 4.2.), a well-established developmental state, has the primary goal of improving the health system both in access and quality, for equality of care. Despite the ANC's commitment to the DS paradigm, the reality of its macroeconomic policy diverges from the developmental ethos envisioned. This misalignment is clear in the healthcare sector, where policies ostensibly aimed at advancing developmental goals paradoxically perpetuate inequalities in health outcomes, exacerbating disparities between rural and urban areas, and the public and private sectors.

5.4.2.1 Defining the National Health Insurance

South Africa has been desperately trying to solve its development challenges since the shift to a democratic regime in 1994. One of the ANC's first attempts to improve the welfare of South African citizens was to introduce the NHI Bill in 1994. The primary aim of the NHI was to equalise access to *quality* healthcare for all South Africans. It is important to note that the NHI's primary function is to finance citizens' medical care, and not an organisational vehicle to run the hospitals. The NHI was to be implemented in three stages, a systematic approach characteristic of a developmental state approach [38–40].

1. The first stage was dedicated to improving the quality of health systems by strengthening the overall governance and management of hospitals.

2. The second stage was focussed on cementing how the financing framework of the NHI would operate. In Ghana, implementing an NHI did not effectively combat health inequality primarily because it was not tax-funded and thus 60% of Ghanaians could not afford the premium [41]. This way, persisting income inequality affects the ability to access medical insurance. Thus, to simultaneously target public vs. private sector divisions and income inequality, the design of South Africa's NHI financing would be funded by progressive taxation measures [39].

3. The third stage was to continue the strengthening of the healthcare institutions started in stage one, whilst formalising the payment structures and tax allocations for the NHI; and distributing resources to equalise the quality of healthcare across hospitals.

At the time of the NHI policy proposal, SA was characterised by extreme inequalities, such as unequal access to quality healthcare. It was the intent of the NHI not just to join the global move towards a universal healthcare system, but to deliver on the promises of Section 27 of the Constitution. Section 27 of the Constitution states that one of the fundamental rights of *all* South African citizens, irrespective of race, gender, or class, is the right to equal access to quality healthcare [38]. However, fast-forward 27 years, South Africa's healthcare system is still vastly unequal in both quality and access; distinctly clear between the private and public sectors. Although, theoretically, SA is in its second stage of the NHI, the government could not effectively deliver on its policy promises, leading to public mistrust in the NHI. The implications of the NHI, should it be carried out effectively, will not just dissipate the inequalities persisting in the healthcare sector and relieve the overburdened public sector, but it will also start macroeconomic spill-overs that contribute positively to long-run economic growth [39].

5.4.2.2 *COVID-19, a health crisis, or an opportunity to realise the DS?*

The reality of SA's socio-economic environment battles stubbornly high unemployment rates that have remained above 20% since 1997. This has contributed to the poverty rates, which were sitting at 55.5% in 2015 [9]. From those that are employed, there is stark income inequality clear by the Gini-coefficient of income that has persistently remained above 0.60 [9]. These macroeconomic factors have only been worsened by the pandemic. COVID-19 increased unemployment rates, which consequently aggravated the poverty and inequality rates. Thus, this leaves a large proportion of the population *unable* to meet their own financial needs, let alone pay for amenities such as healthcare. Along with a plethora of other challenges, COVID-19 has harshly affected, and exposed, the inequities present in its healthcare sector.

Before the onset of the pandemic, South Africa's health institutions were already characterised by harsh divisions between the public and private health sectors; inequalities in access between rural and urban areas; and the overall stress of under-resourced and under-managed hospitals nationwide [38]. One of the primary reasons for the inequalities in access to quality healthcare is affordability. Like much of SA's socio-economic environment, its healthcare sector is bifurcated between public and private health sectors. Most South Africans cannot afford medical aid, which allows people to access healthcare of a much higher quality from the private sector. As discussed above, fewer South Africans can afford healthcare as unemployment rates have risen, illustrating the need for universal healthcare in the country.

Some other effects the pandemic had on the health sector included exposing the incapacity of the public health sector. Hospitals, nationwide, could not meet the demands of the care required by ill patients. They were overburdened, under-staffed and under-resourced. Comparatively, the private sector, although also struggled to keep up with the increased healthcare demand, was far more able to deal with the onslaught of the pandemic. This further exacerbates the already concerning and persistent inequality in the country. By deepening the divide between those who can afford private healthcare and those who cannot, this provides additional motivation for the necessity of the NHI.

5.4.2.3 *The increasing need for the NHI*

COVID-19, if anything, has exposed the importance of non-economic factors, such as healthcare, education and climate change, have on the development and basic functioning of global economies [42]. Seeing that healthcare is one of the most pertinent public goods worldwide, it is essential that polices be put forth to protect and promote the quality of that good. The pandemic has sparked a global shift towards including non-economic factors in the framework of international governance [42]. South Africa is no exception, and it is thus essential that the state strengthens its health sector so that citizens may realise their basic human rights, and so the economy can be stimulated effectively.

Recall that the NHI's primary goals are to improve equity and social protection. If the pandemic has only heightened socio-economic inequities, and essentially left many citizens without the security of quality healthcare, then a fortiori, the potential equity gains from implementing the NHI are vital.

5.4.2.4 Necessary, but unfeasible, measure: the reality of SA's bureaucracy

However, it would be ignorant to disregard the fact that SA has not implemented the NHI thus far. As Reid (2020) highlights, the NHI is an idealistic concept that is likely to take a while to be envisioned [43]. The SA government has a track record of being unable to realise its policy thinking in practice. The corrupt bureaucratic regime has historically proved its incapacity to be a capable state-head. With the onset of the pandemic, we saw the bureaucracy engage in further rent-seeking activities. This has proved, especially to the public, that the ANC-led bureaucratic regime is incapable of being the accountable state head that the NHI would rely on. The fear associated with the NHI in SA is that it will simply provide state actors with more rent-seeking opportunities; and thus, civil society will be further disadvantaged.

COVID-19 stimulated cross-sector dependence, and collaboration between the health minister and the scientific community, which are much-required facets for the efficient implementation of the NHI in a DS. This provided the state with the perfect opportunity to re-imagine its attempt at the DS. It provided the evidence needed that perhaps, with the effective management and accountability structures in place, and the correct application of the DS ingredients, Universal Health Care (UHC) is not simply an idealistic dream.

The proposal of the NHI in South Africa reflects the government's ostensible commitment to addressing deep-seated socio-economic disparities [40]. However, despite the kick-start opportunity provided by COVID-19, implementing the NHI has continued to be hindered by bureaucratic inefficiencies, conflicting policy decisions, and cadre deployment practices, which undermine effective civil service management. These systemic challenges not only hinder the realisation of developmental objectives but also perpetuate socio-economic inequalities, particularly clear in health outcomes.

The COVID-19 pandemic further exposed the vulnerabilities within South Africa's healthcare system, amplifying existing inequities and highlighting the urgent need for comprehensive healthcare reforms. While the NHI represents a critical step towards addressing these challenges, its feasibility remains contingent upon addressing the systemic barriers hindering its implementation, particularly within the context of misdirected policy approaches and bureaucratic inefficiencies. The failure of South Africa to attain the status of a DS has had significant repercussions on its healthcare system, as exemplified by the challenges encountered in implementing the NHI. This failure to achieve meaningful development post-apartheid is intricately linked to a misaligned policy approach, particularly clear in healthcare. The discrepancy between policy intent and implementation not only undermines the principles of the DS but also exacerbates existing socio-economic disparities, particularly in access to quality healthcare.

5.4.3 The ANC's healthcare approach: a misfocus on healthcare quality and a note on healthcare spending

South Africa's healthcare spending has seen a stark increase from 1994 to 2022, as shown in **Figure 3**. However, this increased expenditure has not always translated to a proportional improvement in the quality of healthcare. According to a report on public services, government employment, and the budget, South Africa's provincial healthcare spending has shown annual nominal growth over the years. Despite this

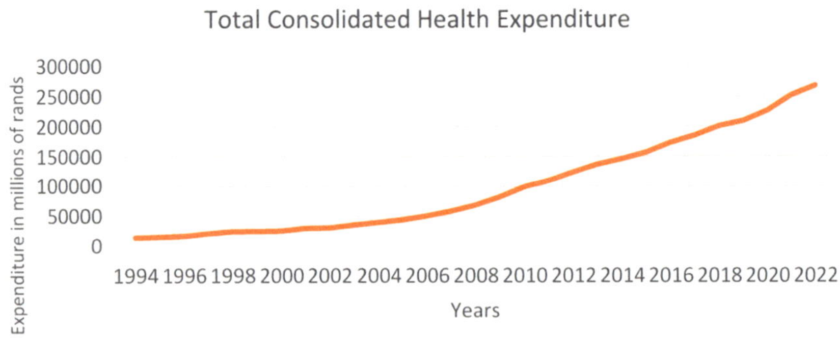

*Data Source 1: *Data sourced from the South African Reserve Bank (1) for the creation of this graph*

Figure 3.
Gross healthcare expenditure, South Africa.

increased spending, the country's health system continues to face systemic and structural challenges, including widespread inefficiencies, staff shortages, and suboptimal care levels. The healthcare system comprises a large, poorly funded public sector and a smaller, better-resourced private sector, leading to persistent inequality in the quality of health service provision.

The disparities in healthcare spending and resource allocation have contributed to the inefficiency and inequity in South Africa's healthcare system. The country's two-tiered, highly unequal healthcare system has perpetuated inequality rather than addressing it, with the public sector being under-funded and overburdened.

Despite the increased healthcare spending, the reality of service provision, infrastructure, and medical resources remains a challenge, with persistent shortages and variability in care levels between different areas.

The ANC has significantly increased healthcare spending in South Africa, with approximately 6–6.5% of the Gross National Product (GNP) being allocated to health services. However, despite this increased funding, the country's healthcare system continues to face challenges related to inefficiency, inequity in service provision, and the misallocation of financial resources [44]. The public sector, which serves most of the population, is under-funded and struggles to provide quality care, while the private sector caters to a smaller portion of the population with well-resourced facilities [45]. This unequal distribution of resources has led to a situation where the high cost of private care has detrimental effects on public health care, perpetuating inequality in access to quality health services [46].

The high cost of private healthcare has led to limited access for most of the population, who depend on the under-resourced public sector, as seen in the Eastern Cape [46]. This has resulted when the public sector cannot meet the healthcare needs of the population effectively, despite increased funding. The disparities in healthcare spending and resource allocation have contributed to inefficiency and inequity in South Africa's healthcare system.

Although South Africa has witnessed a growth in healthcare spending over the years, this increased expenditure has not always translated to a commensurate improvement in the quality of healthcare. The country's two-tiered healthcare system, characterised by disparities between the public and private sectors, has contributed to inefficiencies and inequities in service provision. Addressing these challenges requires comprehensive efforts to strengthen the public healthcare system and reduce inequalities in access to quality health services.

6. Executive summary

South Africa's policy approach to healthcare has undermined its development goals, despite the commitment, prima facie, to deep developmental objectives in healthcare policy. The aspiration to become a developmental state has not been effectively realised, as evidenced by persistent inequalities in health outcomes and shortcomings in the public health infrastructure. While introducing the NHI aimed to ensure access to quality health services for all citizens, other policies have perpetuated disparities in healthcare provision and policy implantation. Issues such as cadre deployment, conflicting policy decisions, and a mixed policy approach have hindered proves towards achieving meaningful development in healthcare; and as a result in economic development.

The well-documented nexus between healthcare development and economic growth. Health plays a crucial role in sustaining economic development, acting both as a determinant and a result of economic progress. A country's health status affects economic development through various channels, including human capital accumulation, workforce productivity, and overall quality of life. This was briefly explored in the DS, South Korea, as one exemplar in healthcare development emphasising that South Africa has not fully realised the potential in this area. The analysis underscores the need to strengthen the health system, improve infrastructure, and address shortages of medical professionals to effectively realise and align with the country's DS development goals in healthcare.

Ultimately, this chapter calls for aligning state policies with the ideals of human development and socio-economic justice to overcome the persistent development deficits in South Africa's healthcare system, so that the dream of becoming a developmental state is not incessantly deferred.

7. Conclusion

Under the leadership of the ANC, South Africa has claimed to be a developmental state in their policy rhetoric since the release of the NGP. However, years later, this rhetoric has not translated into reality. Instead, the state has taken a persistent neo-liberal character which has consequently undermined both the economic development goals of the ANC and, more importantly, their capacity to embody a developmental state. This disparity between policy promises and reality can be seen in healthcare where, despite the ANC's promises to be a DS, they have consistently embodied neoliberalism in their education spending and learning outcomes, undermining the economic development and DS goals of the state. We saw that a combination of other macroeconomic policies and cadre deployment has sufficiently thwarted the country's ability to realise a DS. It can thus be concluded that if the ANC continues its current development trajectory, its policy incoherence, incapable bureaucratic regime, and its ability to coordinate institutional development such as in healthcare, its dream to be a developmental state will be incessantly deferred.

List of abbreviations

ANC	African National Congress
GEAR	Growth, Employment and Redistribution
RDP	Reconstruction and Development Programme
NGP	New Growth Path
NHI	National Health Insurance
DS	developmental state
FDI	Foreign Direct Investment
SOE	State-Owned Enterprise
NDP	National Development Plan
WC	Washington Consensus
IMF	International Monetary Fund
HIV	Human Immunodeficiency Virus
AIDS	Acquired Immunodeficiency Syndrome
AGISA	Accelerated and Shared Growth Initiative for South Africa
PPP	Public-Private Partnership
GDP	Gross Domestic Product
GNP	Gross National Product
OECD	Organisation for Economic Co-operation and Development
SA	South Africa
RSA	Republic of South Africa

Author details

Kiera Lander[1,2,3]

1 Health Economics and Health Policy Analysis, University of Bristol, England

2 Politics, Philosophy, and Economics, University of Cape Town, South Africa

3 Politics, Philosophy, and Economics, University of Witwatersrand, Oxford, United Kingdom

*Address all correspondence to: landerkiera@gmail.com

References

[1] Chang H-J. How to 'do' a developmental state: Political, organisational and human resource requirements for the developmental state. In: Edigheji O, editor. Constructing a Democratic Developmental State in South Africa: Potentials and Challenges. Boulder, USA: Lynne Rienner Publishers; 2011. pp. 82-96. DOI: 10.1515/9780796926531-007

[2] Chang H-J, Grabel I. Reclaiming development from the Washington consensus. Journal of Post Keynesian Economics. 2004;**27**(2):273-291

[3] Wade RH. The developmental state: Dead or alive? Development and Change. 2018;**49**(2):518-546

[4] Campbell JL. Institutional analysis and the role of ideas in political economy. Theory and Society. 1998;**27**(3):377-409

[5] Johnson C. The developmental state: Odyssey of a concept. The Developmental State. 1999;**12**:32-60

[6] Chibber V. The developmental state in retrospect and prospect: Lessons from India and South Korea. In: The End of the Developmental State? Routledge; 2014. pp. 30-54. Available from: https://www.taylorfrancis.com/chapters/edit/10.4324/9781315884363-2/developmental-state-retrospectprospect-vivek-chibber

[7] Chia YT. Education, Culture and the Singapore Developmental State: "World Soul" Lost and Regained?. Basingstoke: Palgrave Macmillan; 2015 A

[8] Republic of South Africa. White paper on Reconstruction and Development In: Office PMo, editor. Parliament: Ministry of Office Republic of South Africa; 1994

[9] Francis D, Webster E. Poverty and inequality in South Africa: Critical reflections. Development Southern Africa. 2019;**36**(6):788-802

[10] Zalk N. Selling off the silver the imperative for productive and jobs-rich investment: South Africa. New Agenda: South African Journal of Social and Economic Policy. 2016;**2016**(63):10-15

[11] Padayachee V, van Niekerk R. " shadows of liberation": ANC economic and social policy from African claims to GEAR. New Agenda: South African Journal of Social and Economic Policy. 2017;**2017**(67):12-18

[12] South African Reserve Bank. Total Expenditure – Consolidated General Government: Health. Republic of South Africa: South African Reserve Bank; 2024. Available from: https://www.resbank.co.za/en/home/what-we-do/statistics/releases/onlinestatistical-query

[13] World Inequality Database. South Africa – World Inequality Database: World Inequality Database. 2023. Available from: https://wid.world/country/south-africa/

[14] Pooe TK. Developmental state No birth right: South Africa's Post-1994 economic development story. Law and Development Review. 2017;**10**(2):361-387

[15] van der Berg S, Gustafsson M. Educational outcomes in post-apartheid South Africa: Signs of progress despite great inequality. In: South African Schooling: The Enigma of Inequality: A Study of the Present Situation and Future Possibilities. 2019. pp. 25-45. Available from: https://link.springer.com/chapter/10.1007/978-3-030-18811-5_2

[16] Mosala S, Venter J, Bain E. South Africa's economic transformation since 1994: What influence has the National Democratic Revolution (NDR) had? The Review of Black Political Economy. 2017;**44**(3-4):327-340

[17] Williamson J. A short history of the Washington consensus. Law & Business Review America. 2009;**15**:7

[18] Sibeko B, Isaacs G. The cost of austerity: Lessons for South Africa. Institute for Economic Justice Working Paper Series. 2019;2

[19] Congress AN. Growth, employment and redistribution: A macroeconomic strategy (South African Government policy document). In: Finance Do, editor; 1996

[20] Republic of South Africa. Accelerated and Shared Growth Initiative for South Africa (AsgiSA). In: Department ED, editor. AsgiSA Pretoria; 2006

[21] Republic of South Africa. The New Growth Path: Framework In: Department ED, editor; 2011

[22] Republic of South Africa. National Development Plan 2030: Our Future - make it work. In: Commission NP, editor.: Republic of South Africa; 2013

[23] Fine B. Across Developmental State and Social Compacting: The Peculiar Case of South Africa. ISER Working Paper No. 2016/1. Grahamstown: Institute of Social and Economic Research, Rhodes University; 2016

[24] Merten M. Budget Votes: Ramaphosa talks governance restructuring — putting the Presidency at the centre of a capable, ethical, developmental state. 2021. Available from: https://www.dailymaverick.co.za/article/2021-06-02-ramaphosa-talks-governance-restructuring-putting-the-presidency-at-the-centre-of-a-capable-ethical-developmental-state/

[25] Republic of South Africa. Economic trasnformation, inclusive growth, and competitiveness: A contribution towards a growth agenda for the South Africa economy. In: Economic Policy Division NT, editor; 2020

[26] Sebake BK. Neoliberalism in the South African post-apartheid regime: Economic policy positions and globalisation impact. International Conference on Public Administration and Development; 2017

[27] Lee JC. Health care reform in South Korea: Success or failure? American Journal of Public Health. 2003;**93**(1):48-51

[28] Ukwandu DC. South Africa as a developmental state-is it a viable idea? African Journal of Public Affairs. 2019;**11**(2):41-62

[29] Lee SY. 한국 보건의료제도 특징이 보건의료성과에 미친 영향에 관한 연구 [The Impact of Health Care System on Health Care Performance in Korea]. Social Sciences Study. 2013;**24**(4):271-293 (Original Article is in Korean)

[30] Ataguba JE-O, Alaba O. Explaining health inequalities in South Africa: A political economy perspective. Development Southern Africa. 2012;**29**(5):756-764

[31] Govender K, Girdwood S, Letswalo D, Long L, Meyer-Rath G, Miot J. Primary healthcare seeking behaviour of low-income patients across the public and private health sectors in South Africa. BMC Public Health. 2021;**21**(1):1649

[32] Africa DSS. Public healthcare: How much per person? 2022. Available from: https://www.statssa.gov.za/?p=10548

[33] Cowling N. Private healthcare in South Africa - statistics & facts: Statista. 2024. Available from: https://www.statista.com/topics/11421/private-healthcare-in-south-africa/#topicOverview

[34] Statista. Distribution of health care choices of households in South Africa in 2022, by type. 2022. Available from: https://www.statista.com/statistics/1412622/distribution-of-health-care-choices-of-households-in-south-africa-by-type/

[35] Center CUIM. South Africa – Summary. 2024. Available from: https://www.publichealth.columbia.edu/research/others/comparative-health-policy-library/south-africa-summary

[36] Andreoni A, Chang H-J. Bringing production and employment back into development: Alice Amsden's legacy for a new developmentalist agenda. Cambridge Journal of Regions, Economy and Society. 2017;**10**(1):173-187

[37] Rensburg R. Healthcare in South Africa: How Inequity Is Contributing to Inefficiency. Johannesburg': University of the Witwatersrand; 2021. Available from: https://www.wits.ac.za/news/latestnews/opinion/2021/2021-07/healthcare-in-south-africa-howinequity-is-contributing-toinefficiency.html

[38] Republic of South Africa. National Health Insurance for South Africa: Towards Universal Health Coverage In: Health Do, editor; 2017

[39] Republic of South Africa. Financing a National Health Insurance for South Africa: For the Minister of Finance. In: Committee DT, editor; 2018

[40] Republic of South Africa. National Health Insurance Bill. In: Africa PoRoS, editor; 2019

[41] Pauw TL. Catching up with the constitution: An analysis of National Health Insurance in South Africa post-apartheid. Development Southern Africa. 2022;**39**(6):921-934

[42] Rodrik D. Globalisation after Covid-19: My plan for a rewired planet. 2020. Available from: https://www.prospectmagazine.co.uk/magazine/dani-rodrik-globalisation-trade-coronavirus-who-imf-world-bank

[43] Reid S. Coronavirus pandemic holds lessons for South Africa's universal health care plans. 2020. Available from: http://theconversation.com/coronavirus-pandemic-holds-lessons-for-south-africas-universal-health-care-plans-137443

[44] Kew J. South Africa's Health Plan Is a Funding Calamity, Discovery Says. 2023. Available from: https://www.bloomberg.com/news/articles/2023-12-11/south-africa-s-health-plan-is-a-funding-calamity-discovery-says

[45] Gordon T, Booysen F, Mbonigaba J. Socio-economic inequalities in the multiple dimensions of access to healthcare: The case of South Africa. BMC Public Health. 2020;**20**(1):1-13

[46] Willie MM, Maqbool M. Access to public health services in South Africa's rural Eastern Cape Province. Available from: SSRN 4405870. 2023

Chapter 9

Perspective Chapter: Open versus Minimally Invasive Surgery Accessibility in Different Economic Level Countries

Abdallah Al Farai, Mohammad Al Farei and Adil Al Zadjali

Abstract

In high-income countries (HIC), minimally invasive surgery (MIS) has become the preferred method for many surgical procedures due to its clinical benefits, which are supported by advanced healthcare systems capable of investing in costly equipment and ongoing surgeon training. Conversely, in low- and middle-income countries (LMICs), the adoption of MIS is limited by several challenges; hence, open surgeries remain the predominant method, especially in public healthcare systems and rural areas where access to sophisticated equipment is restricted. The high cost of procuring and maintaining laparoscopic and robotic tools, along with the need for specialized training, creates significant barriers to the widespread use of MIS in LMICs. This chapter explores the disparities in accessibility to MIS across countries with varying economic levels, highlighting the significant differences in healthcare infrastructure, resources, and training. It examines the ongoing global efforts as well to address these disparities.

Keywords: minimally invasive surgeries, high-income countries, low- and middle-income countries, healthcare systems, economy

1. Introduction

Surgery by itself means any manual or instrumental acts on the body to diagnose, repair, or remove any pathology or injury. It started with simple techniques mainly to treat injuries and wounds and to fix bony fractures. There were reports that trepanation was the first true operation done as early as 12,000 BCE in the Mesolithic or the Middle Stone Age [1, 2]. Subsequently, things evolved progressively and rapidly over the nineteenth and twentieth centuries.

The origin of minimally invasive surgery (MIS) can be traced back to the early nineteenth century with the introduction of the first cystoscope, which is a tube-like instrument or an endoscope used to visualize the urinary bladder. Endoscopes, which were initially used for cystoscopy, later found application in examining other organs and body cavities like thorax and abdomen. Hans Jacobaeus conducted the first endoscopic therapeutic procedure in 1912, performing thoracoscopy. In the 1930s and 1940s, laparoscopy was primarily employed as a diagnostic technique by a small number of internists, including Heinz Kalk in Berlin and John Ruddock in Los Angeles. It was not until the 1940s and 1950s that gynecologists Raoul Palmer in Paris and Hans Frangenheim in Germany began using laparoscopy for diagnosing gynecological conditions and evaluating infertility [3–6]. With time, the quality and complexity of MIS evolved until the first use of robotic systems in human patients in 1985 for neurosurgical biopsies utilizing a robot platform known as Programmable Universal Machine for Assembly 200 (PUMA) [7]. Furthermore, the Robotics Centre at Imperial College modified the device and employed it for standard urologic and prostate treatments [8]. The Robodoc® surgical technology is an image-guided technology that was created in 1992 specifically for prosthetic hip replacement [9]. Similarly, robotic surgery evolved over time involving much complex interventions in the abdomen, thorax, and cardiovascular system.

Open surgery involves large incisions, which often result in longer recovery times, greater pain, and higher risks of infection and scarring. Conversely, MIS, such as laparoscopic or robotic-assisted procedures, uses smaller incisions, leading to reduced pain, shorter hospital stays, faster recovery, and fewer complications [10, 11]. Patients undergoing minimally invasive procedures typically experience quicker returns to normal activities. However, the choice between these methods depends on the complexity of the surgery, with some conditions still requiring open procedures for optimal outcomes.

2. Economic factors and healthcare system

2.1 Overview of healthcare systems in high-, middle-, and low-income countries

Healthcare systems vary significantly across high-, middle-, and low-income countries, reflecting disparities in resources, infrastructure, and access to care.

In high-income countries (HICs) with higher GDP per capita and higher patient awareness and demand for minimally invasive options, healthcare systems are typically well-funded, well-developed, robust health insurance systems and feature advanced infrastructure. They often have universal or near-universal coverage, wide availability of both open and MIS, with higher adoption rates of cutting-edge MIS and better trained surgical staff for advanced procedures, resulting in providing comprehensive services through public or private providers. Countries like the United Kingdom (with the National Health Service) and Germany have government-funded systems, while others, such as the United States, rely on a combination of private insurance and government programs [12]. HICs usually offer cutting-edge technology, specialized care, and robust preventive services but may also face challenges like rising costs and unequal access for some populations.

Low- and middle-income countries (LMICs) with moderate to low GDP per capita often have mixed healthcare systems and face the greatest challenges in healthcare, particularly in surgical accessibility with underfunded healthcare systems, limited medical infrastructure, and shortages of healthcare professionals. 84 percent of the world's population, 90 percent of the global disease burden in 2001, 24 percent of global Gross Domestic Product, and just 13 percent of global health spending are found in LMICs [13, 14].

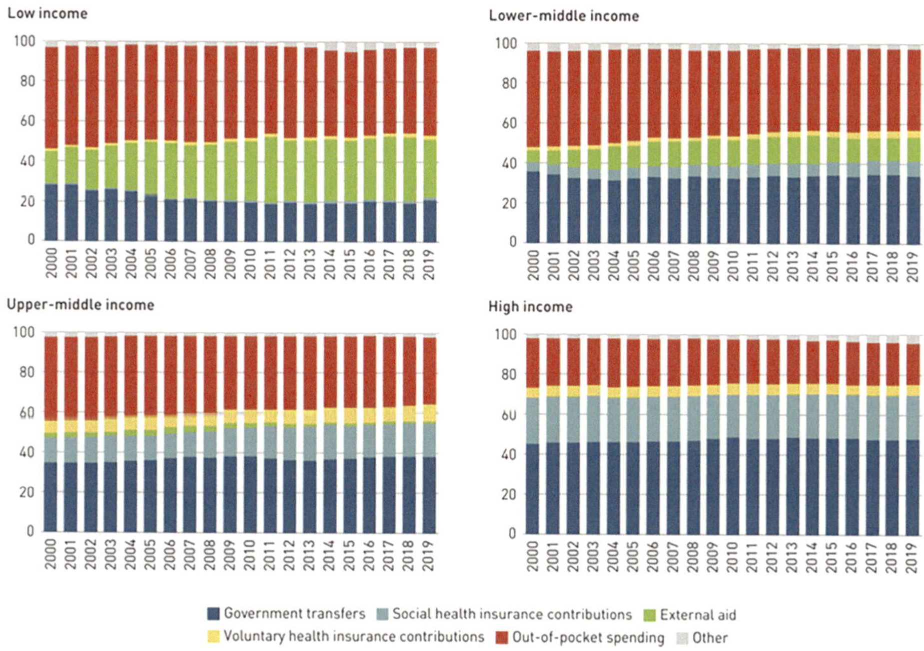

Figure 1.
Funding source share (% of total health spending).

Resources may be more limited, leading to disparities in access between urban and rural areas, and in some scenarios, these resources come from international aid and nongovernmental organizations (NGOs). These countries may still struggle with healthcare infrastructure, but they are increasingly adopting policies to improve accessibility and affordability. Basic healthcare services, including maternal and child health, are often prioritized, though access may remain limited [15, 16].

Between 2000 and 2019, the composition of health spending's funding sources shifted, with all income levels seeing a decrease in out-of-pocket spending as shown in **Figure 1**. In low-income countries, out-of-pocket and external aid combined accounted for over three-quarters of health spending in 2019. Government transfers decreased from 28% to 21% in these countries between 2000 and 2019, while the share of external aid increased from 16% to 29% [17].

2.2 How economic factors influence surgical care accessibility

Economic factors play a pivotal role in shaping access to surgical care, with the impact being particularly pronounced in LMICs. Each year, over 5 billion people cannot access safe and affordable surgical care and anesthesia and up to 2% of economic growth is lost due to untreated surgical conditions in LMICs [18]. In LMICs, chronic underfunding of healthcare systems creates a cascade of challenges. The scarcity of resources manifests in multiple ways: insufficient hospitals and surgical facilities, a dearth of trained surgeons, and a persistent shortage of essential medical supplies. This infrastructure deficit is further exacerbated by systemic issues such as government corruption and inefficient resource allocation, which divert funds away from critical healthcare needs. Where public healthcare funding is inadequate or insurance coverage is limited, patients often face high out-of-pocket expenses, making even lifesaving surgeries inaccessible. Poor health system infrastructure and government corruption are also significant issues in many LMICs [19–21]. The financial burden of surgical care in these regions often falls heavily on patients. With limited public healthcare funding and inadequate insurance coverage, individuals frequently face exorbitant out-of-pocket expenses. This financial strain forces many to make the difficult choice between seeking necessary surgical treatment and meeting other basic needs, leading to delayed or forgone care. Consequently, this contributes to elevated morbidity and mortality rates, creating a vicious cycle of poor health outcomes and economic stagnation.

Even in middle- and high-income countries, economic disparities continue to influence surgical care accessibility. While the overall healthcare infrastructure may be more robust, low-income individuals within these societies often face significant barriers. These can include limited access to elective surgeries, inadequate insurance coverage, high co-pays, and challenges in accessing high-quality postoperative care. The resulting delays in treatment for economically disadvantaged populations frequently lead to worse health outcomes and increased risk of complications, perpetuating health inequities.

The global distribution of healthcare resources further compounds these issues. Surgical care tends to be concentrated in urban centers, leaving rural and underserved areas with inadequate access. The high costs associated with establishing and maintaining surgical facilities, training specialists, and acquiring advanced medical equipment create significant hurdles for economically challenged regions. This results in a persistent gap in surgical access, with many areas struggling to provide consistent and high-quality care. On the other hand, investment in surgical care is lifesaving and strengthens the overall health system, which fosters economic prosperity [18, 22]. Other studies have shown that long waiting times for surgical procedures resulted in a significant loss of economic benefits [23]. Beside the financial barriers, there are other factors affecting the accessibility to a proper surgical care including structural aspects of healthcare and cultural beliefs and attitudes [24].

Addressing these economic barriers requires a multifaceted approach. Strategies may include increasing public healthcare funding, expanding insurance coverage, investing in healthcare infrastructure in underserved areas, and implementing policies to reduce out-of-pocket expenses for essential surgical procedures. Additionally, international cooperation and support can play a crucial role in bridging the resource gap and building capacity in LMICs.

3. Cost of surgical equipment and technology

The costs of open surgery and MIS equipment vary significantly, reflecting differences in technology, resources, and long-term financial implications.

Open surgery generally involves lower upfront equipment costs. Surgeons use basic surgical tools like scalpels, forceps, and retractors, which are relatively inexpensive and reusable. Operating rooms for open surgery require fewer specialized instruments, making initial setup costs lower. However, the long-term costs can be higher due to longer patient recovery times, extended hospital stays, and higher rates of postoperative complications like infections, which increase overall healthcare expenditure [25, 26].

In contrast, MIS, such as laparoscopic or robotic-assisted surgery, requires specialized equipment that is more expensive upfront. Laparoscopic surgeries utilize video cameras, specialized surgical instruments, and sometimes robotic systems, all of which involve significant costs. Robotic-assisted surgeries, in particular, require expensive machines and maintenance. Ng AP et al. found that, for laparoscopic patients, the average hospitalization cost was $16,000 ± 14,800, while for robotically assisted cases, it was $18,300 ± 13,900 ($P < .001$) [27]. As a cost comparison, open prostatectomy disposable materials cost around $212 per patient while robotic prostatectomy costs around $831 per patient [28]. Despite the high initial costs, MIS often results in reduced long-term costs due to shorter hospital stays, quicker recovery times, and fewer complications [25, 26].

While MIS equipment is costlier, it can reduce the financial burden on healthcare systems by improving patient outcomes and minimizing indirect costs, such as reduced time off work and lower rates of rehospitalization. The overall financial impact depends on balancing upfront investments with long-term savings. As an example, Fisher et al. found that minimally invasive distal pancreatectomy was associated with >$8500 in lower cost compared to the open approach [29].

4. Training and expertise in different regions

4.1 Access to specialized training for MIS in high-income versus low-income countries

In high- and low-income nations, access to specialized training for MIS differs significantly. In HICs, surgeons have relatively easy access to advanced training programs, fellowships, and certifications in MIS. Medical institutions in these regions often invest in cutting-edge technology, and continuous professional development is supported through workshops, simulation labs, and international conferences.

In contrast, low-income countries face significant barriers to specialized MIS training. Limited financial resources, inadequate infrastructure, and a lack of access to modern surgical equipment hinder opportunities for advanced training. Many surgeons in these regions may have to travel abroad to receive proper MIS education, which is often cost-prohibitive and they might not repatriate to their original countries due to bigger remuneration and quality of life [30]. Additionally, the absence of local trainers and ongoing mentorship makes it difficult to develop a sustainable training pipeline, leading to a reliance on traditional open surgeries despite the global shift toward MIS [31].

4.2 Impact of skill gaps on the availability of MIS

MIS requires specialized training, technical expertise, and experience with advanced equipment, which many surgeons lack due to limited access to training programs or resources. Without properly trained surgeons, even hospitals equipped with MIS technology may underutilize it, relying instead on traditional open surgeries. Additionally, the availability of trained surgeons without proper MIS equipment may lead to decay in as little as 2 weeks, especially if they are not used for an extended length of time [32].

In HICs, while training is more accessible, skill gaps still exist, especially in rural or underserved areas where surgeons may not have the same exposure to advanced techniques as those in urban centers. These gaps can lead to longer wait times for patients and unequal access to the benefits of MIS.

Addressing these skill gaps through improved training programs, simulation-based learning, and global collaborations is essential for expanding the availability of MIS and ensuring equitable access to advanced surgical care.

5. Healthcare surgical infrastructure and technological MIS adoption

Healthcare surgical infrastructure and the adoption of MIS in LMICs face substantial challenges due to limited resources and systemic gaps. Surgical facilities in many LMICs often lack essential infrastructure, such as fully equipped operating rooms, reliable power supplies, and sterile environments, making it difficult to perform even basic surgeries safely. As an example, an analysis of the anesthetic capability in 22 LMICs revealed that more than one-third of the facilities lacked both anesthetic machines and oxygen supply [33]. The CO_2 gas shortage may play a role in the inability to run MIS services as the medical uses come after the food and beverage industries and the oil and gas industries in utilizing the CO_2 [34]. In addition, the availability of surgical specialists is often concentrated in urban centers, leaving rural areas severely underserved.

Adopting MIS technologies in these regions is especially challenging due to the high costs of laparoscopic and robotic equipment, which are often beyond the financial reach of public hospitals [35]. The need for specialized training further complicates adoption, as many surgeons in LMICs do not have access to the advanced education required to perform MIS. Even when training opportunities are available, the lack of consistent mentorship and practical exposure can limit the ability to sustain such practices.

Despite these barriers, some LMICs are making progress through partnerships with international organizations and NGOs, which help provide both equipment and training. Additionally, innovations like low-cost laparoscopic tools and portable surgical kits are emerging as potential solutions to improve access. However, scaling MIS in LMICs requires sustained investment, infrastructure improvements, and policies focused on building a local healthcare workforce capable of utilizing advanced technologies.

6. Patient accessibility and affordability

6.1 Out-of-pocket costs for patients

In many of LMICs, healthcare systems are underfunded, with limited public health coverage, forcing patients to pay directly for services, medications, and even basic medical supplies. This financial burden can be especially challenging for low-income populations, who may have to choose between healthcare and other essential needs like food or education. For major treatments, such as surgery or chronic disease management, the costs can be catastrophic, pushing families into poverty [17]. Sirag et al. used data from 145 countries and found that there is a threshold impact between poverty and out-of-pocket medical expenses. The degree of poverty was not significantly affected by out-of-pocket health expenses below the cutoff point of roughly 29%. But at the threshold, poverty increased with additional rises in out-of-pocket medical costs relative to overall health spending [36].

The lack of comprehensive insurance systems and subsidies exacerbates this issue, leading many patients to delay or forgo necessary treatments, contributing to worsened health outcomes and higher long-term healthcare costs.

6.2 Insurance coverage and government support for different types of surgeries

The insurance coverage for surgeries is often limited in these countries with many populations relying on out-of-pocket payments for care. Government support for surgeries, particularly complex or elective procedures, is typically inadequate due to underfunded healthcare systems. While some countries provide limited public health coverage for essential surgeries, such as emergency or lifesaving procedures, elective and advanced surgeries like MIS are often not covered. Public hospitals may offer lower cost options, but wait times can be long, and quality varies. Many individuals, especially in rural areas, lack access to both government-supported and insured surgical care, exacerbating healthcare disparities. Additionally, variations in health insurance designs impact not only the kinds of benefits that can be obtained at a lower cost and, thus, the outcomes we may anticipate but also the individuals who are more likely to get affiliated [37].

6.3 Patient accessibility in urban vs. rural areas

In urban areas, patients generally have better access to healthcare facilities, specialized services, and advanced technologies due to the concentration of hospitals, clinics, and medical professionals. Urban populations benefit from shorter travel times and a wider range of healthcare options, including private care.

In contrast, rural areas often face significant barriers to healthcare access. These include fewer medical facilities, a shortage of healthcare professionals, and long travel distances. Rural patients may also experience longer wait times for specialized care, limited access to advanced treatments, and higher costs, contributing to health disparities between urban and rural populations. Even in high-income countries, the differences are present between urban and rural areas. Nuako et al. found that in the US the patients from rural clinics had 22% fewer interactions with the healthcare system on average over the study period in comparison to those from urban clinics [38].

7. Global health initiatives and future trends

Efforts to bridge the gap in access to MIS between low- and high-income countries are gaining momentum through various global initiatives, partnerships, and innovations.

One of the primary strategies has been increasing training and capacity building. International organizations, such as the World Health Organization (WHO), Global Surgery Foundation, and NGOs, are working to train surgeons in LMICs in MIS techniques. This involves hands-on workshops, simulation training, and knowledge-sharing programs, often in collaboration with academic institutions from HICs.

In addition, technology transfer plays a vital role. HICs and private companies are developing low-cost, portable laparoscopic and robotic tools that are tailored to the resource constraints of LMICs. These technologies are more affordable, easier to maintain, and suited for environments with limited surgical infrastructure. For example, simplified laparoscopic systems, like the Gas Insufflation-Less Laparoscopic Surgery (GILLS) system, have been introduced in some regions to enable MIS where traditional laparoscopic setups are impractical [39, 40].

Furthermore, telemedicine and remote support is helping connect surgeons in LMICs with mentors and experts in HICs, enabling remote guidance and consultation during complex MIS procedures.

Policy advocacy through global health organizations, such as the Lancet Commission on Global Surgery, is also pushing for increased investment in MIS as part of universal healthcare goals, aiming to make these advanced surgical techniques accessible to all populations [41].

8. Real-world examples of accessibility challenges and solutions

Real-world examples of MIS accessibility challenges and solutions highlight the diverse efforts to bring advanced surgical care to LMICs. These examples illustrate the obstacles faced and how innovative approaches have begun to address them.

1. Ethiopia: Low-cost laparoscopic tools

   In Ethiopia, a partnership between the University of Gondar and U.S.-based universities helped introduce low-cost laparoscopic tools designed specifically for low-resource settings. Using portable laparoscopic systems, Ethiopian surgeons were able to perform MIS without the high cost of traditional gas insufflation systems [42, 43]. This solution improved access to advanced surgical techniques while being economically feasible for the local healthcare system.

2. Rwanda: Telemedicine and remote training

   Rwanda has made significant strides in using telemedicine to improve surgical care. Through partnerships with international organizations, Rwandan surgeons can receive remote training and guidance from experts in HICs. This model allows Rwandan hospitals to perform complex MIS procedures with real-time support, bridging the skill gap and increasing local surgical capacity [44, 45].

3. Kenya and Ghana: National laparoscopic training programs

   In Kenya and Ghana, a collaboration between the government and international partners led to the establishment of laparoscopic training programs and courses [46, 47]. These aim to build local expertise by training surgeons across the country. With an emphasis on sustainable development, trained surgeons are encouraged to become local trainers, further expanding access to MIS in public hospitals.

These examples demonstrate the ongoing efforts to overcome MIS accessibility challenges through innovative solutions that address both financial and infrastructural barriers. By focusing on affordable technologies, capacity building, and remote support, LMICs are beginning to close the gap in MIS access.

9. Conclusion

Despite the tremendous challenges in adopting MIS in some countries, the ongoing global initiatives—such as capacity building programs, affordable technology innovations, and telemedicine support—are helping bridge the gap between the HICs and LMICs. While progress is being made, sustained efforts are required to make MIS more accessible across all economic levels, ensuring equitable access to high-quality surgical care worldwide.

To note, the intricate relationship between economic factors and surgical care accessibility underscores the need for comprehensive, equity-focused healthcare policies. By addressing these economic disparities, nations can work toward ensuring that lifesaving surgical care is accessible to all, regardless of economic status or geographical location, ultimately contributing to improved health outcomes and economic prosperity on a global scale.

Conflict of interest

The authors declare no conflict of interest.

Author details

Abdallah Al Farai[1*], Mohammad Al Farei[2] and Adil Al Zadjali[3]

1 Sultan Qaboos Comprehensive Cancer Care and Research Centre, University Medical City, Muscat, Oman

2 Zubair Investment, Muscat, Oman

3 Sultan Qaboos University Hospital, University Medical City, Muscat, Oman

*Address all correspondence to: a.alfarai@cccrc.gov.om

References

[1] Henschen F, Thomas S. (Translator). Kraniets Kulturhistoria. The Human Skull: A Cultural History; Translated by Stanley Thomas with an Introduction by Kenneth P Oakley. 1966

[2] Wikipedia Contributors. History of Surgery [Internet]. Wikipedia, Wikimedia Foundation; 2024. Available from: https://en.wikipedia.org/w/index.php?title=History_of_surgery&oldid=1239053017

[3] Nakayama DK. The Minimally Invasive Operations that Transformed Surgery. 2017 by the American College of Surgeons [Internet]. Available from: https://www.facs.org/media/fv0oschd/10_minimally_invasive.pdf

[4] Bush RB, Leonhardt H, Bush IM, Landes RR. Dr. Bozzini's Lichtleiter. Urology. 1974;**3**(1):119-123

[5] Hoksch B, Birken-Bertsch H, Müller JM. Thoracoscopy before Jacobaeus. The Annals of Thoracic Surgery. 2002;**74**(4):1288-1290

[6] Gordon S. Art. VIII.—Clinical reports of rare cases, occurring in the Whitworth and Hardwicke Hospitals. Dublin Quarterly Journal of Medical Science. 1866;**41**(1):83-99

[7] Kwoh YS, Hou J, Jonckheere EA, Hayati S. A robot with improved absolute positioning accuracy for CT guided stereotactic brain surgery. IEEE Transactions on Biomedical Engineering. 1988;**35**(2):153-160. Available from: https://ieeexplore.ieee.org/document/1354

[8] Davies BL, Hibberd RD, Ng WS, Timoney AG, Wickham JEA. The development of a surgeon robot for prostatectomies. Proceedings of the Institution of Mechanical Engineers, Part H: Journal of Engineering in Medicine. 1991;**205**(1):35-38

[9] Paul HA, Bargar WL, Mittlestadt B, Musits B, Taylor RH, Kazanzides P, et al. Development of a surgical robot for cementless total hip arthroplasty. Clinical Orthopaedics and Related Research®. 1992;**285**:57-66

[10] Patil M Jr, Gharde P, Reddy K, Nayak K. Comparative analysis of laparoscopic versus open procedures in specific general surgical interventions. Cureus. 2024;**16**(2)

[11] Horesh N, Emile SH, Garoufalia Z, Gefen R, Zhou P, Wexner SD. Upfront laparotomy versus conversion from minimally invasive surgery to open surgery in colon cancer: Is there a difference in outcomes? Surgery. 2024;**176**(1):69-75

[12] Mounier-Jack S, Mayhew SH, Mays N. Integrated care: Learning between high-income, and low- and middle-income country health systems. Health Policy and Planning. 2017;**32**(suppl_4):iv6-i12

[13] Glied S, Smith PC, editors. The Oxford Handbook of Health Economics. Oxford, England: Oxford University Press; 2013

[14] Lopez AD, Mathers CD, Ezzati M, Jamison DT, Murray CJ. Global and regional burden of disease and risk factors, 2001: Systematic analysis of population health data. The Lancet. 2006;**367**(9524):1747-1757

[15] Mills A. Health care systems in low-and middle-income countries.

New England Journal of Medicine. 2014;**370**(6):552-557

[16] Lewis TP, McConnell M, Aryal A, Irimu G, Mehata S, Mrisho M, et al. Health service quality in 2929 facilities in six low-income and middle-income countries: A positive deviance analysis. The Lancet Global Health. 2023;**11**(6):e862-e870

[17] World Health Organization. Global Expenditure on Health: Public Spending on the Rise?. Geneva, Switzerland: Whorl Health Organisation; 2021. [Accessed: September 22, 2024]

[18] Meara JG, Leather AJ, Hagander L, Alkire BC, Alonso N, Ameh EA, et al. Global surgery 2030: Evidence and solutions for achieving health, welfare, and economic development. The Lancet. 2015;**386**(9993):569-624

[19] Kushner AL, Cherian MN, Noel L, Spiegel DA, Groth S, Etienne C. Addressing the millennium development goals from a surgical perspective: Essential surgery and anesthesia in 8 low- and middle-income countries. Archives of Surgery. 2010;**145**(2):154-159

[20] Funk LM, Weiser TG, Berry WR, Lipsitz SR, Merry AF, Enright AC, et al. Global operating theatre distribution and pulse oximetry supply: An estimation from reported data. The Lancet. 2010;**376**(9746):1055-1061

[21] Kruk ME, Wladis A, Mbembati N, Ndao-Brumblay SK, Hsia RY, Galukande M, et al. Human resource and funding constraints for essential surgery in district hospitals in Africa: A retrospective cross-sectional survey. PLoS Medicine. 2010;**7**(3):e1000242

[22] Smith ER, Concepcion TL, Niemeier KJ, Ademuyiwa AO. Is global pediatric surgery a good investment? World Journal of Surgery. 2019;**43**:1450-1455

[23] Poenaru D, Pemberton J, Cameron BH. The burden of waiting: DALYs accrued from delayed access to pediatric surgery in Kenya and Canada. Journal of Pediatric Surgery. 2015;**50**(5):765-770

[24] Grimes CE, Bowman KG, Dodgion CM, Lavy CB. Systematic review of barriers to surgical care in low-income and middle-income countries. World Journal of Surgery. 2011;**35**:941-950

[25] Xu T, Hutfless SM, Cooper MA, Zhou M, Massie AB, Makary MA. Hospital cost implications of increased use of minimally invasive surgery. JAMA Surgery. 2015;**150**(5):489-490

[26] Fitch K, Engel T, Bochner A. Cost differences between open and minimally invasive surgery. Managed Care (Langhorne, Pa.). 2015;**24**(9):40-48

[27] Ng AP, Sanaiha Y, Bakhtiyar SS, Ebrahimian S, Branche C, Benharash P. National analysis of cost disparities in robotic-assisted versus laparoscopic abdominal operations. Surgery. 2023;**173**(6):1340-1345

[28] Ho C, Tsakonas E, Tran K, Cimon K, Severn M, Mierzwinski-Urban M, et al. Robot-Assisted Surgery Compared with Open Surgery and Laparoscopic Surgery: Clinical Effectiveness and Economic Analyses. Ottawa, Canada: Canadian Agency for Drugs & Technologies in Health; 2013

[29] Fisher AV, Fernandes-Taylor S, Schumacher JR, Havlena JA, Wang X, Lawson EH, et al. Analysis of 90-day cost for open versus minimally invasive distal pancreatectomy. HPB. 2019;**21**(1):60-66

[30] Naraynsingh V, BahadurSingh S, Maharaj R, Harnarayan P, Cawich SO. Surgery in the West Indies: A perspective from Trinidad. Current Medicine Research and Practice. 2014;**4**:1126-1129

[31] Klimczuk A, Dovie DA. Bridging Social Inequality Gaps-Concepts, Theories, Methods, and Tools. United Kingdom: IntechOpen; 2024

[32] Kelc R, Vogrin M, Kelc J. Cognitive training for the prevention of skill decay in temporarily non-performing orthopedic surgeons. Acta Orthopaedica. 2020;**91**(5):523-526

[33] Hadler RA, Chawla S, Stewart BT, McCunn MC, Kushner AL. Anesthesia care capacity at health facilities in 22 low-and middle-income countries. World Journal of Surgery. 2016;**40**:1025-1033

[34] O'Neill JT. Carbon Dioxide Shortage Impacts Health Care Surgeries | Health Facilities Management [Internet]. Available from: https://www.hfmmagazine.com/articles/4607-carbon-dioxide-shortage-impacts-health-care-surgeries

[35] Sheetz KH, Claflin J, Dimick JB. Trends in the adoption of robotic surgery for common surgical procedures. JAMA Network Open. 2020;**3**(1):e1918911

[36] Sirag A, Mohamed NN. Out-of-pocket health expenditure and poverty: Evidence from a dynamic panel threshold analysis. Healthcare. 2021;**9**(5):536

[37] Giedion U, Díaz BY. A Review of the Evidence. The Impact of Health Insurance in Low-and Middle-Income Countries. Washington, USA: Brookings Institution Press; 2010. pp. 13-32

[38] Nuako A, Liu J, Pham G, Smock N, James A, Baker T, et al. Quantifying rural disparity in healthcare utilization in the United States: Analysis of a large midwestern healthcare system. PLoS ONE. 2022;**17**(2):e0263718

[39] Webb MM, Bridges P, Aruparayil N, Chugh C, Beacon T, Singh T, et al. The RAIS device for global surgery: Using a participatory design approach to navigate the translational pathway to clinical use. IEEE Journal of Translational Engineering in Health and Medicine. 2022;**10**:1-2

[40] Rangad G, Pandey S, Das JK, Das H, Gnanaraj J, Mishra A, et al. A single centre observational study comparing feasibility of Gas Insufflation Less Laparoscopic (GILLS) cholecystectomy under spinal & general anaesthesia in a low to middle income country using RAIS-abdolift device. HPB. 2024;**26**:S512

[41] Meara JG, Greenberg SL. The Lancet Commission on Global Surgery Global surgery 2030: Evidence and solutions for achieving health, welfare and economic development. Surgery. 2015;**157**(5):834-835

[42] Reynolds CW, Rooney DM, Jeffcoach DR, Barnard M, Snell MJ, El-Hayek K, et al. Evidence supporting performance measures of laparoscopic appendectomy through a novel surgical proficiency assessment tool and low-cost laparoscopic training system. Surgical Endoscopy. 2023;**37**(9):7170-7177

[43] Morrow E, Bekele A, Tegegne A, Kotisso B, Warner E, Kaufman J, et al. Laparoscopic simulation for surgical residents in Ethiopia: Course development and results. The American Journal of Surgery. 2016;**212**(4):645-648

[44] Robertson FC, Mutabazi ZA, Ntakiyiruta G, Musafiri S, Dusabejambo V, Walker T, et al. Barriers to performing minimally invasive surgery in Rwanda: An assessment of national

demand, utilization rates, and perceived challenges. Journal of the American College of Surgeons. 2016;**223**(4):S67

[45] Dworkin M, Cyuzuzo T, de Dieu HJ, Katabogama J, Ntirenganya F, Rickard J. Barriers to surgical care at a tertiary hospital in Kigali, Rwanda. Journal of Surgical Research. 2020;**250**:148-155

[46] Long KL, Spears C, Kenady DE, Roth JS. Implementation of a low-cost laparoscopic skills curriculum in a third-world setting. Journal of Surgical Education. 2014;**71**(6):860-864

[47] Kang MJ, Apea-Kubi KB, Apea-Kubi KA, Adoula NG, Odonkor JN, Ogoe AK. Establishing a sustainable training program for laparoscopy in resource-limited settings: Experience in Ghana. Annals of Global Health. 2020;**86**(1):86-89

Chapter 10

Perspective Chapter: Patient Advocacy – From a Seat at the Table to Equal Stakeholders

Janet L. Wale and Dominique Hamerlijnck

Abstract

Much has changed in individual and policy level patient advocacy in the years since the late 1980s when HIV/AIDS activists challenged the United States medical product regulator and aspects of how randomised controlled trials are conducted. Delays in access to innovative, life-saving medical interventions continue to be a key topic. We provide storylines to explore three interrelated pathways. The first follows the involvement of patients in the medical product lifecycle and clinical trial regulation, where the biopharmaceutical industry is a major stakeholder. The second follows the course of evidence-based practice and patients, the need for outcome measures of patient experience data and patient-relevant outcome measures that incorporate the patient voice into person-centred models of healthcare; and how regulators and HTA bodies are accelerating access to innovative medical products. The third storyline uses the European Union with its public-private funding of medical and healthcare research as a case study to highlight how patient advocacy is changing. Following the maturation of patient advocacy from patients as research subjects to patient involvement and centredness throughout the medical product lifecycle, we suggest possible next steps to continue to evolve patient advocacy into equal stakeholders within healthcare and innovative medical product development.

Keywords: patient involvement and partnership, medical product development, regulation, health technology assessment, patient-relevant outcomes, patient experience data, driving innovation

1. Introduction

1.1 The beginnings

In 1978 the World Health Organisation (WHO) Alma Ata Declaration introduced the concept of citizens having both the duty and right to participate in the implementation and planning of their healthcare [1]. It was in 1998 that the global worldwide disability movement took on the slogan 'nothing about us without us'. This slogan embodies the principle that no health policy, programme or other initiative that has a potential impact on patients should be undertaken without the participation of those patients [2, 3]. Principles behind involvement and engagement with patients include justice, equity and inclusion, diversity, and to counter any systemic discrimination [4].

We live in a world with ever-increasing patient-clinician expectations, a strong biopharmaceutical industry and growing inequalities in healthcare. Digital technologies, machine learning and artificial intelligence (AI) are seen as essential tools to help with maintaining healthcare. We need patients as equal stakeholders. Health services have over recent years shifted from paternalistic approaches to healthcare that dictate treatment regimens to placing patients at the centre of their care [5, 6]. Patients have a right to a voice in their own healthcare, and the policies and decisions that govern that care, but only some have the knowledge and resources, or capacity, to contribute in an active and productive manner. Empowerment is a multidimensional process that helps people gain control over their lives and increases their capacity to act on issues that are important to them [7]. Patient advocates can speak on behalf of other patients and, by working together in groups or organisations patients can provide mutual support and a stronger patient voice. Collective empowerment is a process through which individuals and communities can express their needs, present their concerns, devise strategies for involvement in decision making, and take political, social, and cultural action to meet those needs [8]. Patient advocacy covers the full span of healthcare including individual care, services and how healthcare is delivered, interventions and treatments that are available, and the policies that direct health services and the health system. The connections between the different parts of a healthcare system, and patient involvement across them, can be limited even though the system as a whole is looking to improve healthcare and outcomes for patients [9]. Engagement in care at a service level, the organisation and the health system are treated in separate streams with little attention paid to the interaction of patient engagement efforts at the different levels [10]. At service level, hospitals are challenged to address 'what matters to patients' and provide kind and considerate, value-based patient-centred care [11, 12]. Within health services, public and patient and carer engagement is expected to contribute to health system transformation but has had limited influence on overall healthcare delivery and design [13]. Over the years the focus has moved from people's management of chronic diseases to quality and safety improvements [14, 15] to determination of value, co-design and co-production, but with underutilization of patient experience and patient-reported outcome measures [9]. Patient engagement is generally provider-led in its initiation, by invitation, and within specified areas of service delivery [16, 17]. The negative impact of the COVID-19 pandemic on patient engagement in healthcare highlighted that patient participation was not well established in the work routines of providers, institutions and governments [18–21].

People's initial expectations and the health system's response to those expectations can determine the responsiveness of a health system [22]. Both past and current care encounters influence expectations, framed by social structures and relations. Individually, socioeconomic status, age, health status and past experiences shape our expectations, influenced by wider social, cultural, historical, and political contexts. Expectations are formed within a social construct, with social accountability and a collective nature that can be contested and negotiated through broad, equitable participation [23]. Collective judgements are reinforced by the authorisation of higher authorities. Perceptions of 'legitimacy' can change in line with individual and collective-level social norms and values [23]. Deliberation and decision-making about health financing are shaped by the political environment, and power asymmetries in society that can increase or decrease equity of access to healthcare. The potential of medical innovation is limitless, as evidenced by the websites of the European Federation on Pharmaceutical Industries and Associations (EFPIA) and the Pharmaceutical Research and Manufacturers of America (PhRMA) in their missions of patient-centred innovation and access to life-saving medicines [24, 25].

In this chapter we address the role of meaningful patient advocacy to strive for equitable, fair and just access to innovative medical products. We start with the AIDS activists in the 1980s and 1990s, evidence-based medicine and the regulatory pathway, through to how patient advocates and leaders are changing the spheres of action for collaborative efforts with the biopharmaceutical industry, using the European Union as a case study. Our approach is that of storylines in a meta-narrative pragmatic review of the literature [26], as adapted by Ulster and Denis [13]. A storyline is the unfolding 'plot' as set out in key publications. Our storylines follow the literature from a patient advocacy perspective in three interrelated but distinct pathways.

2. Storyline one. Access to innovative medical products: from AIDS activists to key players in this space today

2.1 AIDS/HIV activists and the US food and drug agency (FDA)

Access to new and innovative medical products was key for acquired immunodeficiency syndrome (AIDS) activists with the onset of the AIDS epidemic in the 1980s. At this time the affected community was being devastated with many dying as a result of contracting the mysterious illness. Many activist leaders were young to middle aged, relatively affluent, and well educated white gay men. The first cases in the United States of America (US) became evident in 1981. The term AIDS was established in 1982 and human immunodeficiency virus (HIV) was identified as the cause of AIDS only in 1984. The AIDS movement called for heightened commitment to studying this new condition and the provision of resources including research funding. People with AIDS became knowledgeable and involved in the clinical trials for the development of antiviral medications. The HIV/AIDS epidemic extended from the 1980s to the early 1990s in the US and during this time the activists changed the medical research paradigm. The focus of discontent was the slow regulatory process and the randomised controlled trial (RCT). Initial eligibility criteria meant that although AIDS was a life-threatening disease, the comparator was standard available treatment or placebo. Furthermore, trial participants were not permitted to take other medications during the trials (even though they also needed to use treatments to deal with opportunistic infections that were also killing people). And so, many refused to enter the trials. Through their activism the inclusion criteria were expanded and they were able to keep people in trials to fulfil the government regulator the US Food and Drug Agency (FDA) requirements so that the drugs could be marketed [27, 28].

The first antiretroviral drug for HIV/AIDS was approved by the FDA in 1987, and the Investigational New Drug (IND) Program was initiated based on surrogate outcomes rather than clinical outcomes, and compassionate use of treatments became available. The AIDS Coalition to Unleash Power (ACT UP) was established in the same year. This group brought a very sophisticated understanding of the situation and specific problems concerning the scientific and regulatory issues associated with making medications available. They educated themselves, found mentors to help them, opened the door to the regulator and introduced a new model of advocacy that included the patient expert. As patient advocates, they learned the concepts and language and overall gained scientific and research knowledge. In this way they were able to give alternative suggestions, ask reasonable questions, push for specific changes, and became positive contributors to the process. In the process they were able to build a community to focus people's fear and anger. People did not feel alone and developed fellowship. The movement had an inside and outside strategy. Over time, AIDS/HIV went from a death sentence to a chronic manageable illness [27].

2.2 Women with breast cancer claim their seats at the table

Breast cancer activists in the US quickly stepped in during the early 1990s. They wanted to actively contribute to the research process and for more women to be included in clinical trials [29]. The women adopted a 'seat at the table' approach to their advocacy with the development and implementation of an intensive science training course for breast cancer activists by the National Breast Cancer Coalition (NBCC) [30]. It was clear to these advocates that if they wanted a seat at the table where research decisions were being made—and to participate fully in making those decisions—they had to adapt to the dominant culture and understand the science. The programme termed Project LEAD (leadership, education and advocacy development) was developed offering in-depth immersion in epidemiology, molecular biology, clinical trials, and evidence-based healthcare, and building a base for ongoing learning [31]. To have a seat is a status within a group that gives one sufficient authority to be taken seriously, give a group perspective, to listen and be heard, share, define and influence, and make a difference. Through this approach, the NBCC was successful in gaining specific funding for breast cancer research through the US Department of Defence [29].

One breast cancer advocate who held a formal role with the FDA shared her experiences. She was able to work with industry and research groups to offer feedback on clinical trial design, serve on data monitoring committees and on steering committees for registry studies. Her questions included: should we wait for larger studies to provide conclusive evidence or take a chance that data will eventually confirm what we all hope to be true? Do the studies measure outcomes that actually help patients? Should we heed the speakers in the Open Public Hearings (a part of every FDA advisory committee) and get the proposed drug to market at the earliest possible moment or are there imperatives to wait for longer-term safety and efficacy data; and what about extenuating circumstances where alternative treatments do not exist? [32].

2.3 FDA committed to patient-focused drug development (PFDD)

The FDA as a government agency and under its congressional funding arrangement of accepting fees from medical product sponsors (Prescription Drug User Fee Act or PDUFA) launched the Patient-Focused Drug Development initiative (PFDD) in 2012 [33]. Public meetings have an important role and are designed to engage patients to elicit their perspectives on the most significant symptoms of a health condition, its impact on their daily life, and their views on current approaches to treatment [34, 35]. As a result, patient preferences, patient-reported outcome measures, patient experience data, and tolerability are patient-relevant clinical outcomes systematically included in clinical trials as part of drug development and evaluation. The FDA states that "as experts in what it is like to live with their condition, patients are uniquely positioned to inform the understanding of the therapeutic context for drug development and evaluation". This patient-centred approach has been developed to facilitate enrolment in clinical trials, reduce the burden of participation, and provide an understanding of trade-offs between treatment benefits and harms. A series of methodological guidance and core outcome sets have been developed, and the FDA continues to set up health condition-based meetings to gather patient experiences [33]. The Patient Engagement Collaborative (PEC) is a legislated joint project between the FDA and the Clinical Trials Transformation Initiative (CTTI) that was initiated in 2017. Its purpose is to provide an ongoing, shared setting in which the patient community (PEC members), FDA, and CTTI can discuss topics for improving communication, education, and patient engagement related to medical product regulation [36]. The PEC was modelled on the European Union regulator the European Medicines Agency's (EMA) Patient and Consumer Working Party, formed in 2014. The FDA and EMA have collaborated on patient engagement since 2016 [37]. They were both aware of the importance of public education resources and knowledge about the role of regulators and the safe use of medical products.

The EMA considers patient engagement along the regulatory lifecycle of medical products to be an integral part of its work, where patients and caregivers bring a unique perspective and offer real life insights including quality of life issues, unmet needs and the current therapeutic environment [38]. Representative patients first became scientific committee members in 2000; and the EMA has had a patients and consumers working party of patient organisations since 2006. As a community, patient advocates are on the Management Board, involved in consultations and workshops, and act as patient experts in various activities (scientific advice procedures; expert meetings; committee consultations; review of documents). EMA recognises the importance of patients working with clinicians and now better informs patient advocates with improved access to some of the data in the clinical reports submitted to the agency [39]. A biennial report summarises interactions with patients, consumers, healthcare professionals, academic researchers and their organisations, incorporating both quantitative and qualitative data [40].

2.4 Perceived and real competing interests

As is common practice, including for regulatory and payer or health technology assessment bodies, EMA takes care to ensure that its staff, scientific experts and board do not have any financial or other interests that could affect their impartiality. EMA's policy on handling competing interests allows it to restrict or exclude the potential involvement of an expert or scientific committee member with interests in the pharmaceutical industry or in the medical-device industry [41]. The relevance of competing interests was noted by the breast cancer advocate referenced earlier: "it is impossible not to be acutely aware of the ways in which financial incentives shape both the conduct and outcomes of research. In an age when clever marketing and clinical trials are sometimes so intertwined as to be indistinguishable, trained advocates would do well to question the source of data and the design and conduct of trials. But it's hard to maintain a critical perspective, to be the sceptic when others are so hopeful about this or that promising new agent..." [32]. These remarks apply not only to patients but the desire of patients to find relief and to participate in research and clinical trials can be inaccurately interpreted as competing interests.

Patient organisations face many challenges including a lack of formal recognition. The associated lack of resources and funding is an ongoing problem [42]. Many patient groups receive some funding from the pharmaceutical industry, either on a project basis or for operational activities. Others receive government funding aligned with current health policy and political interests. To maintain transparency and mitigate any perceived competing interests, patient organisations develop clear rules for ethical conduct and terms of engagement. Some groups choose not to accept such funding. Government, public health, and health research funding is limited, and donations and philanthropic funding are not enough [8]. Questions about the independence of groups that accept industry funding are raised. Patient organisations that are aligned with companies' approved drug portfolios and research and development pipelines, including rare diseases, appear more likely to receive funding [43]. Industry funding can decrease public trust in the independence and the representativeness of those organisations yet patient organisations are expected to make themselves available and to act in a professional manner in health policy debate [8, 42]. A balance is needed because as groups acquire the highest levels of integrity and competence, and become more 'professional', they can become distanced from their patient members and so lose their representativeness and familiarity with the everyday needs of patient, carers and families [8, 42].

In the past, biopharmaceutical codes of practice and regulations covering engagement with patients and patient groups were in the marketing domain and were bureaucratic and restrictive. This has led to a lack of information on new and innovative medical products for patients and patient advocates wishing to give input to HTA bodies on the potential value of those products [44]. The restrictions also interfered with patient involvement in clinical trials and drug development research [45], as highlighted in a survey of patient groups, industry and academia in the US identified through the CTTI and Drug Information Association (DIA) [46]. Growing numbers of clinical trial sponsors recognised the benefits of continuous and meaningful patient group engagement in clinical trials. There was some resistance [47], as well as mismatched expectations [48]. Engagement activities have the potential to avoid protocol amendments, improve clinical trial enrolment, adherence, and retention could add considerable financial value [49, 50]. Overall, a culture change was needed [51].

2.5 The biopharmaceutical industry - what is the price?

The biopharmaceutical industry develops new and innovative medical products to counter disease and life-threatening conditions. Severe acute respiratory syndrome (SARS) is a viral respiratory disease caused by the SARS-CoV-2 coronavirus. During the COVID-19 pandemic, the biopharmaceutical industry was able to provide rapid access to innovative vaccines [52]. These received emergency use approval by regulators and funding from payers and so could be used to decrease the severity of infections and the number of deaths. The pandemic raised public awareness of the role of regulators in ensuring the safety of new vaccines and treatments, and the role of innovation. Innovation is often derived from publicly funded scientific research, including from patient groups, and numerous research and development-intensive start-up companies come out of academic institutions [53, 54]. It is possible that some end-products may therefore be largely due to decades of research funded by public investment, billions in grants for development and production, and tens of billions in Advanced Purchase Agreements (APAs) with governments [55]. Legal issues are a part of its business. The industry is looking to 'game-changing science', new breakthrough therapies and, eventually, large company profits [54]. One company can control the market. An example is the situation with innovative medications for the treatment of cystic fibrosis (CF), an hereditary condition present at birth that markedly reduces lifespan. New medications are very effective and significantly extend life expectancy. The CF transmembrane conductance regulator (CFTR) modulator drug combination is only available in high income countries [56].

3. Storyline two. Adapting evidence-based practice to be more relevant to patients with timely access to innovation

3.1 Evidence-based practice in healthcare

The term 'evidence-based medicine' (EBM) was introduced in the 1990s to formalise the scientific basis of medicine. The intent was to move away from expert opinion, actions led by individual senior physicians, and ingrained behaviours, which were causing waste and unwarranted variations in care [57, 58]. EBM was envisaged to reduce uncertainties in medical decision-making and to improve the quality of care [59, 60]. It was defined initially by Sackett as "the conscientious, explicit, and judicious use of current best evidence in making decisions about the care of individual patients" [61] and subsequently modified to include clinical expertise and the patient's views and preferences, or values. The best available evidence comes from randomised controlled trials (RCTs). These are carefully controlled studies in which participants are randomly allocated to 'intervention' and 'control' groups, where the control group receives an inactive placebo or 'standard treatment'. The participants are systematically followed, and predefined quantitative outcomes measured over a set time period generally up to 1 year. Bias, or factors that can influence the findings and result in systematic deviation from the true findings are in this way minimised. EBM operates at the population level but is applied to individuals, and healthcare is delivered within relationships, meaning that values, including patient values, are an inherent part of EBM [62]. Healthcare interventions can be multifactorial and complex, making it difficult or impractical to carry out definitive RCTs [63]. Long-term effects of interventions are also difficult to follow, as are any potential adverse effects. Greenhalgh et al. highlighted 'biases' against patients and carers in EBM including limited patient input into published materials, low value put on patient or carer experience, power imbalances that may suppress the patient's voice, hard-to-reach populations may be missed, and the humanistic, person-centred aspects of clinical consultations (empathy, compassion, the therapeutic alliance) may be overlooked [64].

3.2 Need for measurable, standardised patient-relevant outcomes that give patients a voice

It is the patient who best understands the life experience of living with a disease or health condition. Quality of life measures and other patient-reported outcome measures (PROMs), patient-reported experience measures (PREMs), patient experience data and patient preference studies [65–68] provide ways in which a person-centred approach to regulatory assessment can be incorporated [69]. Such measures can help clinicians to understand patient experiences and needs, and so enhance consultations and the delivery of individualised care [8, 70]. They also provide a person-centred approach with standardised tools for clinical trials [71, 72]. Patient-relevant outcomes capture patient data on the burden of disease and its treatment by following symptoms, ability to function, experiences and health-related quality of life over time and with interventions. New and innovative medical products, such as immuno-oncology treatments for cancer and weight reduction medications, can have high toxicities for some patients. Development of tolerability patient-reported outcomes (PROs) are therefore also important [73].

These measures are now collected electronically (as ePROs), which improves adherence to their collection, increases reliability, and reduces data entry errors [74]. Information can at the same time be gathered about the data collection process itself and device setups can be altered, training and resources provided, and better PROs developed as a result [74]. Overall, remote data gathering reduces the participant burden of collecting the data and in interpreting outcomes [75] to inform research and clinical services. Industry has the adaptability and resources to involve patients to provide specific validated tools that capture patient experience data and new methodologies in clinical trial design, particularly involving digital technologies. The in-depth descriptions of how companies invest into going deep into experiences of the health conditions and their treatment to develop PROMs [71] and patient preference studies [67, 72] are good examples. It is important that patients can relate to the measures, that they are relevant to them and capture what matters to them so including their voice [76].

3.3 Access to innovative medicines: what makes one need this?

The biopharmaceutical industry needs rapid access to market to maximise sales during the patent protected period [77]. From the patient perspective, accelerated or early access schemes have value when targeted toward innovative technologies with the potential for significant clinical benefit. This is particularly so for people with serious disease burden and high unmet needs where the stakes are high, if the medical product goes on to deliver significant clinical value [78]. Patients, medical professionals and their clinical communities, policymakers and the manufacturers of innovative technologies are all seeking rapid access to new medical products, and regulators, reimbursement or HTA bodies and payers are working to meet these demands [79]. Early access requires investment from payers and is associated with significant risk, since not all technologies will go on to be routinely reimbursed or show benefits over existing treatments [80, 81] and only be slowly withdrawn from the market worldwide [78]. Furthermore, complex technologies may present a significant step-change in care that poses challenges for implementation with alterations to health services, diagnostic requirements or treatment pathways. With early access schemes, payers need to determine the period of reimbursement, ensure fair competition for comparators, and consider both the possibility of new competitive technologies and future innovation in the area. The corporate relative balance of risks and benefits of early access schemes may vary according to the strategic importance of the healthcare system for industry, and patients may find their access to the medical product stopped at the end of contractually agreed early access scheme [82]. It is also relevant that shorter time to medical product regulation can mean that less clinical evidence is available on regulation and for funding approval considerations. This makes it difficult for HTA bodies and payers, patients and medical practitioners to understand the full profile of the product compared to existing treatment approaches.

The WHO's health systems framework emphasises the importance of a well-functioning system that provides equitable access to essential medical products, vaccines, and technologies with assured quality, safety, efficacy, and cost-effectiveness, while promoting their scientifically sound and cost-effective use [83]. Healthcare systems are often passive, unplanned recipients of innovation. The activities of regulators and HTA bodies are very much set by companies, as they determine the medical products they seek market approval for, and for which indications [62]. Health Technology Assessment (HTA) provides a method to determine the clinical utility and value of a product within a health system to inform payment or reimbursement. It can also determine cost-effectiveness. A multi-stakeholder committee that often includes patient or public members appraises the evidence [84]. HTA has the potential to create a balance between population health and individual patient needs, so that limited resources are equitably distributed and people with, for example, rare diseases are considered [75]. Medical product lifecycle activities can, however, map poorly to need in terms of the burden of disease and so represent an opportunity cost for patients and health services. If biopharmaceutical science is defined in terms of commercially viable innovations, there will be less available funding or political will to address other areas of healthcare and the greatest societal good. The ways in which evidence is generated and interventions are developed and implemented for common chronic diseases including heart disease, cancer, Alzheimer's disease, diabetes, and chronic lung, liver, and kidney diseases leave room for improvement [85] as does how they are prioritised for value assessment [86].

Governments want to be able to provide innovative medical products and make them available to their people. Australia, for example, has a National Medicines Policy that provides a highly supportive medicines policy environment to support better healthcare and reduce regulatory costs [87]. The European Commission in its proposed revised pharmaceutical strategy for aims to make sure all patients across the EU have timely and equitable access to safe, effective, and affordable medicines with secure supply; and continue to offer an attractive and innovation-friendly environment for research, development, and production of medicines [88]. To reduce medical product development time, both regulatory and HTA bodies need to adapt their processes. This was evident when the FDA approved a drug for Alzheimer's disease before good clinical evidence was publicly available, effectively supporting 'compassionate use and hope' [11, 79, 89, 90]. Regulators are harmonising their work across comparable jurisdictions, through agreements such as with Project Orbis for promising new cancer treatments [91]. The initial stages of HTA in Europe are being brought together through EU Joint Clinical Assessments working closely with EMA and Regulation (EU) 2021/2282 on health technology assessment (HTAR) [92]. Regulators and HTA bodies use horizon scanning and offer early scientific advice to help with evidence generation challenges and new types of evidence [75, 82, 93–95]. Patient input adds value as it can offer a different perspective to other experts; bring experience of living with the condition and its treatment into the discussion, and leads to concrete additions to the final scientific advice given [96].

Real-world data sources include electronic medical records, billing and registries. Gathering real-world data to develop real-world evidence is a key priority area for investment [82, 97] but which requires protection of patients [75]. While RCTs are good for studying causal effects, real-world studies offer the ability to follow larger populations of patients for longer periods of time to capture the lived experience of patients. Registries and large databases can be used for less common and rare diseases [98] as well as capture less-common events such as side effects and exacerbations of disease. Making PROM data available beyond clinical trials can capture how people feel and function, reported by the patients themselves [66]. Not doing so is a missed opportunity for learning about the therapeutic use of interventions. Patient experience data reflect patients' lived experience, their symptoms, interactions with the healthcare system, information-seeking behaviours, any misdiagnoses, lifestyle changes, treatments, side effects, and comorbidities adding to the completeness of the data to enhance person-centred care [99]. Patient groups themselves can collect data, as with Duchenne disease [100].

4. Storyline three. Empowering patient advocates in medical product research and development: the European Union as a case study

The European Patients Forum (EPF) was formed with the backing of EU institutions, including with commercial interests, as a pan-European umbrella body for patients, with national bodies as its members and not individuals. Early in its existence concerns about the independence of patient organisations from the drug industry and the power of more established interests within the healthcare system were seen by academic researchers as serious challenges [101]. Patient organisations focus on representing, mobilising and empowering patients and advocate for their rights. They are able to 'speak with one voice', with visibility and credibility, and ensure a coordinated presence of patient-related issues in health and non-health policies and programmes. While patient advocates and patient organisations are routinely challenged on their representativeness and ability to distinguish between personal and collective views, other stakeholders are not [8].

EPF has been a strong facilitator in placing an emphasis on collaboration and new ways of working, including working with EFPIA to build opportunities [51, 102]. They recognised that irrespective of the strong rationale for engagement, any relationship between patient organisations and pharmaceutical industry can be seen as commercially motivated. To encourage interactions and ensure ethical practice, EFPIA co-created with its Patient Think Tank a set of principles to govern relationships between patient organisations and the pharmaceutical industry (Working together with patient groups, September 2017) and principles for renumeration, with recognition of work of EUPATI, The Change Foundation, PFMD, and WECAN (Working together with patients. Principles for renumerating, June 2019). In 2019, the EFPIA board endorsed its patient engagement strategy (relationships). These documents are in addition to the EFPIA Code members for the Promotion of Medicinal Products to healthcare professionals (HCPs) and the interactions with HCPs, healthcare organisations and patients' organisations [103].

4.1 European Union: innovative medicines initiative and EUPATI

The Innovative Medicines Initiative (IMI) programme, now the Innovative Health Initiative, is a public-private partnership between the European Commission and EFPIA to improve the drug development process by supporting a more efficient discovery and development of better and safer medicines for patients. The programme was launched in 2008 to support collaborative research projects, develop networks of industrial and academic experts in Europe as a way of boosting innovation in healthcare and to build a more collaborative ecosystem for pharmaceutical research and development. In 2010, an applicant Consortium of umbrella patient advocacy groups operating at European level submitted a project entitled 'Fostering Patient Awareness on Pharmaceutical Innovation', in the third IMI call for projects [104]. The patient groups were involved with EMA, active in EU Pharmaceutical Policy (that dictates EMA activities), and with academic partners, DIA and the International Society for Pharmacoeconomics and Outcomes Research (ISPOR). The project, which set up the European Patients' Academy on Therapeutic Innovation (EUPATI), ran from 2012 to 2017, extended to 2020 and beyond. An infrastructure was built for educational materials and develop patient experts through education and training - provide resources to learn the technical skills to aid them in being full participants in a relationship where each side has knowledge that the other does not - and a common language to communicate effectively with each other. It was important that the project was accepted by the patient community and was seen to be objective, transparent, and independent. The project coordinator and executive committee were appointed through EPF. The project also had a Steering Committee and Advisory Board. Well-balanced working parties or task forces from a network of all stakeholders and chaired by the coordinator and other patient experts were tasked with developing the EUPATI course. The course objective was to promote knowledgeable patient advocates and patient support groups to work effectively with government authorities, healthcare professionals, and industry to meaningfully contribute to medicines research and development [105].

Parsons et al. [106], as part of the EUPATI work, provided an academic perspective and identified that the pharmaceutical industry was becoming increasingly interested in how medicines research and development could with patient involvement be patient-centred. Such involvement could also have other benefits such as identifying new areas of research, promoting innovation, providing new insights, identifying solutions to problems in running trials, and improving acceptability of new medicines to patients. Companies previously had little contact with patients in their day-to-day working. The authors also identified a need to work with media to build understanding and communication about medicines research and development, to build public trust.

A large number of EUPATI graduates now hold leadership positions in patient organisations [75]. They ensure patients' needs are at the heart of drug development, by joining science, ethical and regulatory committees and getting involved in clinical trial design. The EUPATI programme currently includes an in-depth training course, an e-learning platform (Open Classroom), an online toolbox, national platforms and more. It has been a game-changer for patient empowerment in Europe and beyond. Japan now has its own national platform. EUPATI became an independent, non-profit foundation toward the end of 2020. A subsequent project, IMI PARADIGM, Patients Active in Research and Dialogues for an Improved generation of Medicines (2018 to 2020) was co-led by EPF and EFPIA to further patient engagement and involvement in research priority setting, design of clinical trials and early dialogue for regulatory and HTA purposes by developing processes and tools. A set of metrics to measure the impact of patient engagement was also produced [107]. In 2019, IMI PARADIGM, EUPATI, and EPF joined forces with Patient Focused Medicines Development (PFMD) to initiate the Patient Engagement Open Forum (PEOF) to hold regular events [108]. These provide opportunities to share patient engagement tools, discuss challenges and facilitate collaboration.

Patient Focused Medicines Development (PFMD) was established in 2015 under the umbrella of The Synergist, an incubator that brings key players together in 'people-public-private' partnerships to solve societal problems through collective action [109]. It is working collaboratively with stakeholders to develop patient engagement tools, frameworks, training and events [110, 111]. Their work includes a Patient Engagement Quality Guidance (PEQG) tool [112], 'how-to guides' for patient engagement in medicines development [113] and a Global Patient Experience Data Navigator tool [114] as well as Patient Engagement Country Guidelines to help navigate country codes of conduct and other regulations. A co-created Fair Patient Engagement (PE) Planner applies activity and expertise frameworks to support patient engagement partners in defining the level of expertise required for activities, an important step. This will enable dialogue among patient involvement partners to agree on fair renumeration [110].

At an international level, patient involvement in HTA processes is well established [115–117] but is largely concentrated on the appraisal stage of an assessment. This leaves room for broader involvement at all stages of an HTA [69, 118]. Public knowledge about HTA is still limited. Following the successful negotiation for the new EU Regulation on HTA, EUPATI [119] and EUCAPA, a collaboration between EPF, EURORDIS and Tyrolean Private University (UMIT) [120], have been funded under the EU4Health programme to provide training.

4.2 We have moved a long way from patients as subjects in clinical trials

It can be asked why the biopharmaceutical industry has taken so long to consult and partner with its end users. EUPATI provided opportunities for biopharmaceutical company representatives to work closely with patient advocates and leaders. At the same time, public knowledge is being increased about medical product development in the EU and beyond. Patient-centred healthcare recognises individual patient preferences, needs, and values in the context of their own social worlds. Inclusion of patient voices helps develop treatments that improve people's lives and in ways that matter most to them, how they feel, function, and set their personal goals. It also makes good economic sense [75, 82]. Industry is making patient-centredness its' goal and now biopharmaceutical companies can empower patients by including them throughout product development [51]. While advances made in recent years are promising, there is still a long way to go to secure the systematic involvement of patients across companies and as true partners at many levels of internal decision making.

Patients can use their insights to identify target areas/questions that have meaning for them, and inform clinical trial design [51, 95]. Relevant outcome measures must relate to patients' experiences, perspectives, needs, and priorities – and be seen as meaningful to patients - core outcome assessments for clinical trials that form part of the regulatory submission [51]. Patients can help identify biases in large datasets, so that they can be corrected, anticipate barriers to applying results that others could miss, and assist in safety surveillance during trials. On study completion, patients can take part in interpreting results and then go on to communicate with their communities and increase health literacy and knowledge [75]. Patient input is required for economic models to reflect true value based on lived experience and produce more realistic models [75]. Social media provides a way of gathering perspectives from informal conversations, and the use of language. Adverse events can be detected in postings on public sites. This is particularly useful for pharmacovigilance because historically patients do not routinely report side effects [75]. Interests, perspectives or insights relevant to more than one person are mobilised and acted upon, with validation through interactions with other patients and gathering community knowledge [111].

5. Conclusions: vision for the future, possible steps

Patient advocates deserve recognition as equal stakeholders and partners in promoting fair and affordable access to quality innovative products across diverse populations. If the impact of their involvement is to be measured then so should that of all stakeholders. The issue of competing interests needs to be re-assessed and declarations co-designed by regulatory and HTA bodies, academia, patients and patient groups, and industry for all stakeholders. Patient advocates and their patient groups need funding considerations with development of models that allow for best practice management that allow them to be equal stakeholders.

Are we trying to solve the right problems, and is it time for process improvement? We need accountable care – where providers, both healthcare and medical product providers, are enabled with advanced technologies that help them communicate with, engage, and inform patients so that they become empowered with information. Their behaviours can then better align with actions that improve healthcare. Healthcare currently falls well short of having truly informed patients and patient advocates. We need multidisciplinary ownership of the care experience over time, greater information sharing across all dimensions of care, a focus on patient, family and support systems, a true measure of outcomes, and a strong focus on improvement and affordability. We would benefit from strengthened relationships with healthcare professionals themselves.

- Many tools and resources have been developed to help different stakeholders work with patient advocates. How can these be collated into a searchable library that enables easy access? We would benefit from improving the links between advances being made in industry with patient involvement within health services, to better meet the needs of patients, for example PROMs and related materials, patient education and training, funding opportunities, recognition as partners and opportunities to become patient experts and leaders including in less-well serviced communities.

- Greater transparency and availability of information on new medical products (e.g., less commercial in confidence materials/redacted information in EMA reports) to enable patients and their organisations to assess the value of the products from their own perspective and for their voices to be heard more meaningfully on access within health systems.

- Reassessment of competing interests in relation to participating in the research undertaken by bio-pharmaceutical and related companies comparable to healthcare professionals. And recognition of patient advocates as able to make their own carefully considered decisions on competing interests, as with clinicians. At the same time identify the power base from which people come, to give greater accountability. Work collaboratively to identify other funding models of patient groups as recognition of their evolving place within health systems; allocating budgets to build their skills and capacity.

- Provide clear information on medical product mechanism of action, possible interactions with other medical products and the level of overall scientific development. When medical products have the same mechanism of action as existing medical products highlight any real and potential differences e.g. route and frequency of administration, possible side effects. Make public the marketing strategies for new medical products, in which countries and where, to inform access and enable action to promote diversity. Enable patients and patient organisations to be co-decision makers and arbiters on access to medical products. Work on a disease basis in lifecycle negotiations, aligned to clinical services.

Acknowledgements

We would like to thank the people in the global HTA patient advocacy community who helped construct this chapter through many hours of discussion and learning experiences. We particularly thank Neil Bertelsen, Heidi Livingstone, Catherine Voutier, and Stella O'Brien. We are also grateful to Trisha Greenhalph for her fresh thinking in approaching methodological issues in evidence-informed healthcare.

Conflict of interest

No funding was received for the development of this manuscript. Janet Wale is a previous chair of the HTAi Patient and Citizen Involvement in HTA Interest Group and a current active member of the Cochrane Collaboration and declares no conflicts of interest.

Dominique Hamerlijnck (DH) is a member of the patient advisory boards for European Lung Foundation (ELF), European Federation of Allergy and Airways Diseases Patients' Associations (EFA), Dutch Lung Foundation, EU Innovative Health Initiative, Global Initiative on Asthma (GINA). She is an independent patient advisor to Novartis, Chiesi, Pfizer, and Roche; and a member of the patient advisory board for the following projects: EU SafePolyMed, ERS Severe Heterogeneous Asthma Research Collaboration, Patient-centered, IMI/IHI 3 TR, IMI/IHI Mobilise-D, IMI/IHI Digital and data DAG+. DH is also a member of scientific advisory committees for ZonMW (Dutch organisation for funding of research). She is a member of HTAi and ISPOR.

Nomenclature

The term 'patients' is used to refer to patients, caregivers, consumers, potential patients, and any organisation that represents people who use health services.

Author details

Janet L. Wale[1*] and Dominique Hamerlijnck[2]

1 Independent Patient Advocate, Melbourne, Australia

2 Independent Patient Leader, Amsterdam, The Netherlands

*Address all correspondence to: janneylw@gmail.com

References

[1] World Health Organization Declaration of Alma Ata [Internet]. 1978. Available from: https://www.who.int/docs/default-source/documents/almaata-declaration-en.pdf [Accessed: March 2, 2024]

[2] Charlton JI. Nothing about us without us. In: Disability Oppression and Empowerment. Berkeley: University of California Press; 1998. ISBN: 9780520224810

[3] United Nations. International Day of Disabled Persons [Internet]. New York: Department of Economic and Social Affairs; 2004. Available from: https://www.un.org/development/desa/disabilities/international-day-of-persons-with-disabilities-3-december/international-day-of-disabled-persons-2004-nothing-about-us-without-us.html [Accessed: March 2, 2024]

[4] Phillips KA, Marshall DA, Adler L, Figueroa J, Haeder SF, Hamad R, et al. Ten health policy challenges for the next 10 years. Health Affairs Scholar. 2023;**1**(1):qxad010. DOI: 10.1093/haschl/qxad010

[5] WHO Framework on integrated people-centred health services [Internet]. 2016. Available from: https://apps.who.int/gb/ebwha/pdf_files/WHA69/A69_39-en.pdf?ua=1&ua=1 [Accessed: April 22, 2024]

[6] North J. In: Nolte E, Merkur S, Anell A, editors. Achieving Person-Centred Health Systems: Evidence, Strategies and Challenges [Internet]. Cambridge: Cambridge University Press; 2020. DOI: 10.1017/9781108855464 [Accessed: March 17, 2024]

[7] Bravo P, Edwards A, Barr PJ, Scholl I, Elwyn G, McAllister M. Cochrane healthcare quality research group, Cardiff University. Conceptualising patient empowerment: A mixed methods study. BMC Health Services Research. 2015;**15**:252. DOI: 10.1186/s12913-015-0907-z

[8] Sienkiewicz D, van Lingen C. The Added Value of Patient Organisations [Internet]. In: Bedlington N, Bullot C, Immonen K, editors. European Patients Forum (EPF). Brussels; 2017. Available from: https://www.eu-patient.eu/globalassets/library/publications/epf_added_value_report_final.pdf [Accessed: February 14, 2024]

[9] Stamm T, Bott N, Thwaites R, Mosor E, Andrews MR, Borgdorff J, et al. Building a value-based care infrastructure in Europe: The health outcomes observatory. NEJM Catalyst. 2021;**2**(3):1-14. DOI: 10.1056/CAT.21.0146. Available from: https://catalyst.nejm.org/doi/abs/10.1056/CAT.21.0146

[10] Miller T, Reihlen M. Assessing the impact of patient-involvement healthcare strategies on patients, providers, and the healthcare system: A systematic review. Patient Education and Counseling. 2023;**110**:107652. DOI: 10.1016/j.pec.2023.107652

[11] Montori VM. The Good Doctor. Care to Hope. Virtues & Vocations. Notre Dame, Indiana: University of Notre Dame. [Internet]. Jan 2024. Available from: https://socialconcerns.nd.edu/virtues/magazine/care-to-hope/ [Accessed: March 2, 2024]

[12] Heath I, Montori VM. Responding to the crisis of care. BMJ. 2023;**380**:464. DOI: 10.1136/bmj.p464

[13] Usher S, Denis J-L. Exploring expectations and assumptions in

the public and patient engagement literature: A meta-narrative review. Patient Education and Counseling. 2022;**105**(22):2683-2692. DOI: 10.1016/j.pec.2022.04.001

[14] Institute of Medicine (US). In: Kohn LT, Corrigan JM, Donaldson MS, editors. Committee on Quality of Health Care in America. To Err Is Human: Building a Safer Health System. Washington (DC): National Academies Press (US); 2000. DOI: 10.17226/9728

[15] Bombard Y, Baker GR, Orlando E, Fancott C, Bhatia P, Casalino S, et al. Engaging patients to improve quality of care: A systematic review. Implementation Science. 2018;**13**(1):98. DOI: 10.1186/s13012-018-0784-z

[16] Crawford MJ, Rutter D, Manley C, Weaver T, Bhui K, Fulop N, et al. Systematic review of involving patients in the planning and development of health care. BMJ. 2002;**325**(7375):1263. DOI: 10.1136/bmj.325.7375.1263

[17] Rowland P, Fancott C, Abelson J. Metaphors of organizations in patient involvement programs: Connections and contradictions. Journal of Health Organization and Management. 2021;**35**(2):177-194. DOI: 10.1108/JHOM-07-2020-0292

[18] Shih P, Hallam L, Clay-Williams R, Carter SM, Brown A. Reimagining consumer involvement: Resilient system indicators in the COVID-19 pandemic response in New South Wales, Australia. Health Expectations. 2022;**25**(4):1988-2001. DOI: 10.1111/hex.13556

[19] van de Bovenkamp H, de Graaff B, Kalthoff K, Bal R. The patient representation struggle during the COVID-19 pandemic: Missed opportunities for resilient healthcare systems. Health Expectations. 2023;**27**(1):e13877. DOI: 10.1111/hex.13877

[20] Marcinow M, Sandercock J, Cadel L, et al. A qualitative study exploring how patient engagement activities were sustained or adapted in Canadian healthcare organizations during the COVID-19 pandemic. PLoS One. 2023;**18**(3):e0282890. DOI: 10.1371/journal.pone.0282890

[21] Tripp L, Vanstone M, Canfield C, Leslie M, Levasseur MA, Panday J, et al. The impact of COVID-19 on patient engagement in the health system: Results from a pan-Canadian survey of patient, family and caregiver partners. Health Expectations. 2022;**25**(2):744-753. DOI: 10.1111/hex.13421

[22] Lakin K, Kane S. Peoples' expectations of healthcare: A conceptual review and proposed analytical framework. Social Science & Medicine. 2022;**292**:114636. DOI: 10.1016/j.socscimed.2021.11463

[23] Lakin K, Kane S. What can one legitimately expect from a health system? A conceptual analysis and a proposal for research and action. BMJ Global Health. 2023;**8**:e012453. DOI: 10.1136/bmjgh-2023-012453

[24] European Federation on Pharmaceutical Industries and Associations (EFPIA). IMAGINE. The Potential of Medical Innovation Is Limitless. If Europe Fully Seizes this Opportunity, Just Imagine What we Could Achieve [Internet]. Brussels; 2024. Available from: https://www.efpia.eu/ [Accessed: February 16, 2024]

[25] Pharmaceutical Research and Manufacturers of America (PhRMA). We're Working to Drive Patient-Centered Progress in Innovation, Affordability and Access to Life Saving Prescription

Medicines. We Believe there's a Better Way to Approach Health Care in the United States [Internet]. Washington, DC; 2024. Available from: https://phrma.org/en [Accessed: February 16, 2024]

[26] Greenhalgh T, Robert G, Macfarlane F, Bate P, Kyriakidou O, Peacock R. Storylines of research in diffusion of innovation: A meta-narrative approach to systematic review. Social Science & Medicine. 2005;**61**(2):417-430. DOI: 10.1016/j.socscimed.2004.12.001, Available from: https://www.sciencedirect.com/science/article/pii/S0277953604006471

[27] Faster Cures, HCM Strategists. Back to Basics. HIV/AIDS Advocacy as a Model for Catalysing Change [Internet]. Washington, DC; 2011. Available from: www.fastercures.org/documents/file/Back2BasicsFinal(1).pdf [Accessed: February 16, 2024]

[28] FDA's role in preventing the spread of HIV/AIDS [Internet]. 2019. Available from: https://www.fda.gov/about-fda/fda-history-exhibits/history-fdas-role-preventing-spread-hivaids [Accessed: February 16, 2024]

[29] Dresser R. Advocates on the research team -- shaping and assessing science. Chapter 2. In: When Science Offers Salvation: Patient Advocacy & Research Ethics. New York: Oxford University Press; 2001

[30] National Breast Cancer Coalition (NBCC), a collaboration of activists, survivors, researchers, policy-makers, grassroots groups and national organizations founded in 1991 [Internet]. 2024. Available from: https://www.stopbreastcancer.org/who-we-are/about-us/ [Accessed: April 2, 2024]

[31] Dickersin K, Braun L, Mead M, Millikan R, Wu AM, Pietenpol J, et al. Development and implementation of a science training course for breast cancer activists: Project LEAD (leadership, education and advocacy development). Health Expectations. 2001;**4**(4):213-220. DOI: 10.1046/j.1369-6513.2001.00153.x

[32] Mayer M. A seat at the table: A research advocate's journey [Internet]. Journal of Participatory Medicine. 2009;**1**(1):e14. Available from: https://participatorymedicine.org/journal/evidence/case studics/2009/10/21/a-seat-at-the-table-a-research-advocates-journey/ [Accessed: January 23, 2024]

[33] United States Food & Drug Administration (FDA). FDA Patient-Focused Drug Development Guidance Series for Enhancing the Incorporation of the Patient's Voice in Medical Product Development and Regulatory Decision Making [Internet]. Silver Spring; 2024. Available from: https://www.fda.gov/drugs/development-approval-process-drugs/cder-patient-focused-drug-development [Accessed: February 24, 2024]

[34] US Food and Drug Administration. Evolution of Patient Engagement at the FDA [Internet]. Silver Spring; 2019-2023. Available from: https://www.fda.gov/patients/learn-about-fda-patient-engagement/evolution-patient-engagement-fda-text-description [Accessed: February 16, 2024]

[35] Chalasani M, Vaidya P, Mullin T. Enhancing the incorporation of the patient's voice in drug development and evaluation. Research Involvement and Engagement. 2018;**2**(4):10. DOI: 10.1186/s40900-018-0093-3

[36] Patient Engagement Collaborative (PEC). 2024. Available from: https://www.fda.gov/patients/learn-about-fda-patient-engagement/patient-engagement-collaborative [Accessed: February 16, 2024]

[37] Food and Drug Administration (FDA) and European Medicines Agency (EMA) collaboration on patient engagement [Internet]. 2016. Available from: https://www.ema.europa.eu/en/news/ema-fda-reinforce-collaboration-patient-engagement [Accessed: February 16, 2024]

[38] EMA patients and consumers [Internet]. 1995-2024. Available from: https://www.ema.europa.eu/en/partners-networks/patients-and-consumers [Accessed: February 16, 2024]

[39] EMA now better informs patient advocates with improved access to some of the data in the clinical reports submitted to the agency [Internet]. 2023. Available from: https://clinicaldata.ema.europa.eu/web/cdp/background [Accessed: April 2, 2024]

[40] Engagement framework: European Medicines Agency and patients, consumers and their organisations (europa.eu) [Internet]. First published: 14/02/2006, last updated: 07/02/2022. Available from: https://www.ema.europa.eu/en/documents/other/engagement-framework-european-medicines-agency-and-patients-consumers-and-their-organisations_en.pdf [Accessed: February 16, 2024]

[41] Handling competing interests. 2023. Available from: https://www.ema.europa.eu/en/about-us/how-we-work/handling-competing-interests [Accessed: February 16, 2024]

[42] O'Mara-Eves A, Brunton G, McDaid D, Oliver S, Kavanagh J, Jamal F, et al. Community Engagement to Reduce Inequalities in Health: A Systematic Review, Meta-Analysis and Economic Analysis. Southampton (UK): NIHR Journals Library; 2013

[43] Gentilini A, Parvanova I. Industry funding of patient organisations in the UK: A retrospective study of commercial determinants, funding concentration and disease prevalence. BMJ Open. 2023;**13**:e071138. DOI: 10.1136/bmjopen-2022-071138

[44] Cook N, Livingstone H, Dickson J, Taylor L, Morgan K, Coombes M, et al. Development of an international template to support patient submissions in health technology assessments. International Journal of Technology Assessment in Health Care. 2021;**37**(1):e50. DOI: 10.1017/S0266462321000167

[45] Lowe MM, Blaser DA, Cone L, Arcona S, Ko J, Sasane R, et al. Increasing patient involvement in drug development. Value in Health. 2016;**19**(6):869-878. DOI: 10.1016/j.jval.2016.04.009

[46] Smith SK, Selig W, Harker M, Roberts JN, Hesterlee S, Leventhal D, et al. Patient engagement practices in clinical research among patient groups, industry, and academia in the United States: A survey. PLoS One. 2015;**10**(10):e0140232. DOI: 10.1371/journal.pone.0140232

[47] Bloom D, Beetsch J, Harker M, Hesterlee S, Moreira P, Patrick-Lake B, et al. The rules of engagement: CTTI recommendations for successful collaborations between sponsors and patient groups around clinical trials. Therapeutic Innovation & Regulatory Science. 2018;**52**(2):206-213. DOI: 10.1177/2168479017720247

[48] Boudes M, Robinson P, Bertelsen N, Brooke N, Hoos A, Boutin M, et al. What do stakeholders expect from patient engagement: Are these expectations being met? Health Expectations. 2018;**21**(6):1035-1045. DOI: 10.1111/hex.12797

[49] Levitan B, Getz K, Eisenstein EL, Goldberg M, Harker M, Hesterlee S,

et al. Assessing the financial value of patient engagement: A quantitative approach from CTTI's patient groups and clinical trials project. Therapeutic Innovation & Regulatory Science. 2018;**52**(2):220-229. DOI: 10.1177/2168479017716715

[50] Vat LE, Finlay T, Jan Schuitmaker-Warnaar T, Fahy N, Robinson P, Boudes M, et al. Evaluating the "return on patient engagement initiatives" in medicines research and development: A literature review. Health Expectations. 2020;**23**(1):5-18. DOI: 10.1111/hex.12951

[51] Boutin M, Dewulf L, Hoos A, Geissler J, Todaro V, Schneider RF, et al. Culture and process change as a priority for patient engagement in medicines development. Therapeutic Innovation & Regulatory Science. 2017;**51**(1):29-38. DOI: 10.1177/2168479016659104

[52] Lurie N, Saville M, Hatchett R, Halton J. Developing covid-19 vaccines at pandemic speed. The New England Journal of Medicine. 2020;**382**(21):1969-1973. DOI: 10.1056/NEJMp2005630

[53] Eisenstein M, Garber K, Landhuis E, et al. Nature biotechnology's academic spinouts 2021. Nature Biotechnology. 2022;**40**:1551-1562. DOI: 10.1038/s41587-022-01530-9

[54] Eisenstein M, Schmidt C, DeFrancesco L. Nature biotechnology's academic spinouts 2022. Nature Biotechnology. 2023;**41**:1669-1678. DOI: 10.1038/s41587-023-02023-z

[55] de Haan E, ten Kate A. Pharma's pandemic profits pharma profits from COVID-19 vaccines [Internet]. SOMO. 2023. Available from: https://www.somo.nl/wp-content/uploads/2023/02/SOMO-Pharmas-Pandemic-Profits.pdf [Accessed: February 14, 2024]

[56] Hoen 'tE. Wrapping up 2023 with some Noteworthy Medicines, Law and Policy Developments: See November International Campaign to Increase Access to Cystic Fibrosis (CF) Treatments. Medicines Law and Policy; 2023. Available from: https://medicineslawandpolicy.org/2023/12/wrapping-up-2023-with-some-noteworthy-medicines-law-and-policy-developments/ [Accessed: December 27, 2023]

[57] Forest PG. A new synthesis. International Journal of Health Policy and Management. 2014;**2**(2):55-57. DOI: 10.15171/ijhpm.2014.13

[58] Guyatt G, Cairns J, Churchill D, et al. Evidence-based medicine. A new approach to teaching the practice of medicine. Journal of the American Medical Association. 1992;**268**:2420-2425. DOI: 10.1001/jama.1992.03490170092032

[59] Grol R. Improving the quality of medical care: Building bridges among professional pride, payer profit, and patient satisfaction. Journal of the American Medical Association. 2001;**286**(20):2578-2585. DOI: 10.1001/jama.286.20.2578

[60] Sackett DL, Straus SE, Richardson WS, Rosenberg W, Haynes RB. Evidence-Based Medicine: How to Practice and Teach EBM. Edinburgh: Churchill Livingstone; 2000

[61] Sackett DL, Rosenberg WM. The need for evidence-based medicine. Journal of the Royal Society of Medicine. 1995;**88**(11):620-624. DOI: 10.1177/014107689508801105

[62] Kelly MP, Heath I, Howick J, Greenhalgh T. The importance of values in evidence-based medicine. BMC Medical Ethics. 2015;**16**:69. DOI: 10.1186/s12910-015-0063-3

[63] Greenhalgh T, Papoutsi C. Studying complexity in health services research: Desperately seeking an overdue paradigm shift. BMC Medicine. 2018;**16**(1):95. DOI: 10.1186/s12916-018-1089-4

[64] Greenhalgh T, Snow R, Ryan S, Rees S, Salisbury H. Six 'biases' against patients and carers in evidence-based medicine. BMC Medicine. 2015;**13**:200. DOI: 10.1186/s12916-015-0437-x

[65] Pushparajah DS. Making patient engagement a reality. Patient. 2018;**11**(1):1-8. DOI: 10.1007/s40271-017-0264-6

[66] Calvert MJ, O'Connor DJ, Basch EM. Harnessing the patient voice in real-world evidence: The essential role of patient-reported outcomes. Nature Reviews. Drug Discovery. 2019;**18**:731-732. DOI: 10.1038/d41573-019-00088-7

[67] Cook NS, Cave J, Holtorf A-P. Patient preference studies during early drug development: Aligning stakeholders to ensure development plans meet patient needs. Frontiers in Medicine. 2019;**6**:82. DOI: 10.3389/med.2019.00082

[68] The PREFER framework [Internet]. 2021. Available from: https://www.imi-prefer.eu/public-consultation/the-prefer-framework/ [Accessed: February 16, 2024]

[69] Wale JL, Chandler D, Collyar D, Hamerlijnck D, Saldana R, Pemberton-Whitely Z. Can we afford to exclude patients throughout health technology assessment? Frontiers in Medical Technology. 2022;**3**:796344. DOI: 10.3389/fmedt.2021.796344

[70] The Health Outcomes Observatory: The power of patient-reported outcomes. 2023. Available from: https://health-outcomes-observatory.eu/wp-content/uploads/2023/10/The-Health-Outcomes-Observatory-The-Power-of-Patient-Reported-Outcomes.pdf [Accessed: February 14, 2024]

[71] Morel T, Schroeder K, Cleanthous S, Andrejack J, Blavat G, Brooks W, et al. The value of co-creating a clinical outcome assessment strategy for clinical trial research: Process and lessons learnt. Research Involvement and Engagement. 2023;**9**(1):98. DOI: 10.1186/s40900-023-00505-7. Erratum in: Res Involv Engagem. 2024;10(1):5

[72] Holtorf A-P, Cook NS. The role of patients in market access. In: Koçkaya G, Wertheimer A, editors. Pharmaceutical Market Access in Developed Markets. Seed Medical Publishers; 2018. pp. 267-288. DOI: 10.7175/747.ch18. Available from: https://books.seedstm.com/index.php/seed/catalog/view/Pharmaceutical_MA_developed/PDF/747.ch18

[73] Regulatory Science. Understanding and Measuring Treatment Tolerability of Immune-Oncology (IO) Treatment in Selected Cancers [Internet]. Regulatory Science; 2024. Available from: https://www.diaglobal.org/en/resources/research/regulatory-science?utm_source=db&utm_medium=email&utm_campaign=publication&utm_content=PUB_GSU_2023_12_29&mkt_tok=NjI3LVZKWS03ODUAAAGQVT29vn54KDy743yKx1cFiGlRMn5r9xI3HjSLtY4YVvVWTSz3_hamo-leN2whOWM2_f0L1nZccsS8jjA3GTT9C-SUS4bnKHdolQcPMEw [Accessed: April 16, 2024]

[74] Nowojewski A, Bark E, Shih VH, O'Quinn S, Dearden R. Leveraging ePRO paradata for patient-centered trial designs [Internet]. Value & Outcomes Spotlight. 2023, 2023;(9, 6). Available from: https://www.ispor.org/publications/journals/value-outcomes-spotlight/vos-archives/issue/view/

patient-centricity-in-heor/leveraging-epro-paradata-for-patient-centered-trial-designs?utm_medium=email&utm_source=database&utm_campaign=value_and_outcomes_spotlight&utm_content=leveraging_epro_paradata_for_patient_centered_trial_designs&utm_term=heor_articles&_zs=3hXOX&_zl=XuOr3 [Accessed: December 16, 2023]

[75] Watkins J. Including patients as partners in clinical and outcomes research. Value & Outcomes Spotlight [Internet]. 2023;**9**(6). Available from: https://www.ispor.org/publications/journals/value-outcomes-spotlight/vos-archives/issue/view/patient-centricity-in-heor/including-patients-as-partners-in-clinical-and-outcomes-research?utm_medium=email&utm_source=database&utm_campaign=value_and_outcomes_spotlight&utm_content=including_patients_as_partners_in_clinical_and_outcomes_research&utm_term=featured&_zs=3hXOX&_zl=SuOr3 [Accessed: December 16, 2023]

[76] Addario B, Geissler J, Horn MK, Krebs LU, Maskens D, Oliver K, et al. Including the patient voice in the development and implementation of patient-reported outcomes in cancer clinical trials. Health Expectations. 2020;**23**(1):41-51. DOI: 10.1111/hex.12997

[77] Brown DG, Wobst HJ, Kapoor A, et al. Clinical development times for innovative drugs. Nature Reviews. Drug Discovery. 2021;**21**:793-794. DOI: 10.1038/d41573-021-00190-9

[78] Akhade A, Sirohi B, Gyawali B. Global consequences of the US FDA's accelerated approval of cancer drugs. The Lancet Oncology. 2022;**23**(2):201-203. DOI: 10.1016/S1470-2045(21)00709-9

[79] Bellberry Ltd. International Scientific Congress 'Towards a Coordinated Approach for Managing Accelerated Patient Access to Potentially Beneficial Medicines' Balancing Patient, Regulator, HTA, Payer, and Other Stakeholder Needs 20-23 June 2023 Adelaide, Australia [Internet]. Bellberry Ltd; 2023. Available from: https://bellberry.com.au/wp-content/uploads/BbL-SYMPOSIUM-REPORT.pdf [Accessed: February 14, 2024]

[80] Brinkhuis F, Goettsch WG, Mantel-Teeuwisse AK, Bloem LT. Added benefit and revenues of oncology drugs approved by the European medicines agency between 1995 and 2020: Retrospective cohort study. BMJ. 2024;**384**:e077391. DOI: 10.1136/bmj-2023-077391

[81] Lichtenberg FR. The relationship between pharmaceutical innovation and cancer mortality in Spain, from 1999 to 2016. Value in Health. 2023;**26**(12):1711-1720. DOI: 10.1016/j.jval.2023.08.011

[82] Farmer C, O'Toole B, Barnish MS, Trigg LA, Hayward S, Crathorne L, et al. Early access schemes for innovative health technologies: The views of international stakeholders. International Journal of Technology Assessment in Health Care. 2023;**39**(1):e45. DOI: 10.1017/S0266462323000429

[83] Chow CK, Ramasundarahettige C, Hu W, AlHabib KF, Avezum A, Cheng X, et al. Availability and affordability of essential medicines for diabetes across high-income, middle-income, and low-income countries: A prospective epidemiological study. The Lancet Diabetes and Endocrinology 2018;**6**(10):798-808. DOI: 10.1016/S2213-8587(18)30233-X

[84] Wale J, Scott AM, Hofmann B, Garner S, Low E, Sansom L. Why patients should be involved in health technology assessment. International

Journal of Technology Assessment in Health Care. 2017;**33**(1):1-4. DOI: 10.1017/S0266462317000241

[85] Warraich HJ, Marston HD, Califf RM. Addressing the challenge of common chronic diseases - a view from the FDA. The New England Journal of Medicine. 2024;**390**(6):490-492. DOI: 10.1056/NEJMp2313217

[86] Richardson M, Sander B, Daneman N, Mighton C, Miller FA. Moving from intervention management to disease management: A qualitative study exploring a systems approach to health technology assessment in Canada. International Journal of Technology Assessment in Health Care. 2023;**39**(1):e67. DOI: 10.1017/S0266462323002696

[87] Australian Government Department of Health and Aged Care National Medicines Policy [Internet]. 2022. Available from: https://www.health.gov.au/sites/default/files/2022-12/national-medicines-policy.pdf [Accessed: March 15, 2024]

[88] The European Commission proposed revised pharmaceutical strategy for Europe [Internet]. 2023. Available from: https://health.ec.europa.eu/medicinal-products/pharmaceutical-strategy-europe/reform-eu-pharmaceutical-legislation_en [Accessed: March 2, 2024]

[89] Venkataramani AS. Affirmative action, population health, and the importance of opportunity and hope. The New England Journal of Medicine. 2023;**389**(13):1157-1159. DOI: 10.1056/NEJMp2307766

[90] Fernandez Lynch H, Kearns L, Moch KI, Caplan AL. What's the worst that could happen? A toothless FDA. Health Affairs Forefront. 2023;**2023**. DOI: 10.1377/forefront.20231109.520330. Available from: https://www.healthaffairs.org/content/forefront/s-worst-could-happen-toothless-fda [Accessed: November 26, 2023]

[91] FDA Oncology Center of Excellence Project Orbis. A Framework for Concurrent Submission and Review of Oncology Products. Silver Spring; 2024. Available from: https://www.fda.gov/about-fda/oncology-center-excellence/project-orbis [Accessed: April 26, 2024]

[92] European Commission Regulation on Health Technology Assessment. Regulation (EU) 2021/2282 [Internet]. Brussels; 2024. Available from: https://health.ec.europa.eu/health-technology-assessment/regulation-health-technology-assessment_en [Accessed: February 16, 2024]

[93] EMA Scientific advice and protocol assistance. 2024. Available from: https://www.ema.europa.eu/en/human-regulatory-overview/research-and-development/scientific-advice-and-protocol-assistance [Accessed: February 16, 2024]

[94] Fameli A, Paulsson T, Altimari S, Gutierrez B, Cimen A, Nelsen L, et al. Looking beyond survival data: How should we assess innovation in oncology reimbursement decision making. Value Outcomes Spotlight [Internet]. 2023;**9**(5):S1. Available from: https://www.ispor.org/publications/journals/value-outcomes-spotlight/vos-archives/issue/view/looking-beyond-survival-data-in-oncology-reimbursement-decisions/looking-beyond-survival-data-how-should-we-assess-innovation-in-oncology-reimbursement-decision-making?utm_medium=email&utm_source=vos&utm_campaign=value_and_outcomes_spotlight&utm_content=vos_gsk_suppl_article&utm_term=vos_gsk_

suppl_article&_zs=3hXOX&_zl=avEf3 [Accessed: April 26, 2024]

[95] Perfetto EM, Oehrlein EM, Love TR, Schoch S, Kennedy A, Bright J. Patient-centered core impact sets: What they are and why we need them. Patient. 2022;**15**(6):619-627. DOI: 10.1007/s40271-022-00583-x

[96] Murphy A, Bere N, Vamvakas S, Mavris M. The added value of patient engagement in early dialogue at EMA: Scientific advice as a case study. Frontiers in Medicine. 2022;**8**:811855. DOI: 10.3389/fmed.2021.811855

[97] HMA-EMA Catalogues of real-world data sources and studies [Internet]. 2024. Available from: https://catalogues.ema.europa.eu/ [Accessed: February 26, 2024]

[98] Geissler J, Makaroff LE, Söhlke B, Bokemeyer C. Precision oncology medicines and the need for real world evidence acceptance in health technology assessment. European Journal of Cancer. 2023;**193**:113323. DOI: 10.1016/j.ejc.2023.113323

[99] Oehrlein EM, Schoch S, Burcu M, JF MB, Bright J, Pashos CL, et al. Developing patient-centered real world evidence: Emerging methods recommendations from a consensus process. Value in Health. 2023;**26**(1):28-38. DOI: 10.1016/j.jval.2022.04.1738

[100] van Lin N, Paliouras G, Vroom E, et al. How patient organizations can drive FAIR data efforts to facilitate research and health care: A report of the virtual second international meeting on Duchenne data sharing, March 3, 2021. Journal of Neuromuscular Diseases. 2021;**8**:1097-1108. DOI: 10.3233/JND-210721

[101] Baggott R, Forster R. Health consumer and patients' organizations in Europe: Towards a comparative analysis. Health Expectations. 2008;**11**(1):85-94. DOI: 10.1111/j.1369-7625.2007.00472.x

[102] Geissler J, Ryll B, di Priolo SL, Uhlenhopp M. Improving patient involvement in medicines Research and Development: A practical roadmap. Therapeutic Innovation & Regulatory Science. 2017;**51**(5):612-619. DOI: 10.1177/2168479017706405

[103] EFPIA Relationships & Code. 2024. Available from: https://www.efpia.eu/relationships-code/ [Accessed: February 14, 2024]

[104] EUPATI [Internet]. Available from: https://www.imi.europa.eu/projects-results/project-factsheets/eupati [Accessed: February 14, 2024]

[105] The European Patients' Academy on Therapeutic Innovation (EUPATI) [Internet]. Available from: https://eupati.eu/about-us/history/ [Accessed: February 14, 2024]

[106] Parsons S, Starling B, Mullan-Jensen C, Tham SG, Warner K, Wever K. What do pharmaceutical industry professionals in Europe believe about involving patients and the public in research and development of medicines? A qualitative interview study. BMJ Open. 2016;**6**(1):e008928. DOI: 10.1136/bmjopen-2015-008928

[107] IMI PARADIGM Patient Engagement Toolbox [Internet]. 2021. Available from: https://imi-paradigm.eu/ [Accessed: February 14, 2024]

[108] Patient Engagement Open Forum (PEOF) [Internet]. 2024. Available from: https://patientengagementopenforum.org/ [Accessed: February 14, 2024]

[109] The Synergist. We Build Partnerships [Internet]. The Synergist;

2024. Available from: https://www.thesynergist.org/ [Accessed: February 24, 2024]

[110] Patient Focused Medicines Development (PFMD) Mission and Strategy, Our work [Internet]. 2024. Available from: https://patientfocusedmedicine.org/mission-and-strategy/# [Accessed: February 24, 2024]

[111] Egher C, Zvonareva O. Knowledge-based representation: Patient engagement in drug development. Health Expectations. 2023;**27**:e13912. DOI: 10.1111/hex.13912

[112] Deane K, Delbecque L, Gorbenko O, Hamoir AM, Hoos A, Nafria B, et al. Co-creation of patient engagement quality guidance for medicines development: An international multistakeholder initiative. BMJ Innovations. 2019;**5**(1):43-55. DOI: 10.1136/bmjinnov-2018-000317

[113] Feldman D, Kruger P, Delbecque L, Duenas A, Bernard-Poenaru O, Wollenschneider S, et al. Patient focused medicines development working groups 1; patient focused medicines development working groups 2A; patient focused medicines development working groups 2B. Co-creation of practical "how-to guides" for patient engagement in key phases of medicines development-from theory to implementation. Research Involvement and Engagement. 2021;**7**(1):57. DOI: 10.1186/s40900-021-00294-x

[114] Willgoss T, Escontrias OA, Scrafton C, Oehrlein E, Livingstone V, Chaplin FC, et al. Co-creation of the global patient experience data navigator: A multi-stakeholder initiative to ensure the patient voice is represented in health decision-making. Research Involvement and Engagement. 2023;**9**(1):92. DOI: 10.1186/s40900-023-00503-9

[115] Weeks L, Polisena J, Scott AM, Holtorf AP, Staniszewska S, Facey K. Evaluation of patient and public involvement initiatives in health technology assessment: A survey of international agencies. International Journal of Technology Assessment in Health Care. 2017;**33**(6):715-723. DOI: 10.1017/S0266462317000976

[116] Gagnon MP, Tantchou Dipankui M, Poder TG, Payne-Gagnon J, Mbemba G, Beretta V. Patient and public involvement in health technology assessment: Update of a systematic review of international experiences. International Journal of Technology Assessment in Health Care. 2021;**37**:e36. DOI: 10.1017/S0266462321000064

[117] Campbell B, Sedrakyan A. Patient involvement in regulation: An unvalued imperative. Lancet. 2021;**397**(10290):2147-2148. DOI: 10.1016/S0140-6736(21)00977-6

[118] Bertelsen N, Dewulf L, Ferrè S, et al. Patient engagement and patient experience data in regulatory review and health technology assessment: A global landscape review. Therapeutic Innovation & Regulatory Science. 2024;**58**:63-78. DOI: 10.1007/s43441-023-00573-7

[119] EUPATI HTA4patients [Internet]. 2024. Available from: https://eupati.eu/hta4patients/ [Accessed: April 4, 2024]

[120] EUCAPA particularly targets patients impacted by cancer and rare diseases to support capacity building for Patient Involvement in HTA [Internet]. 2023. Available from: https://www.eucapa.eu/ [Accessed: April 4, 2024]

Chapter 11

Perspective Chapter: Sedentary Behaviors – Implications for the Future of Health

Brett Baker

Abstract

Sedentary behaviors have become ubiquitous in modern societies. Once considered synonymous with physical inactivity, it is now known that sedentary behavior is its own distinct form of activity on the 24-hour activity continuum separate from both physical inactivity and physical activity. While the positive health ramifications of physical activity on health disease risk and mortality have been known for decades, the negative health risks associated with prolonged and extensive sedentary behaviors are just starting to be recognized. With increased reliance on technology for work (e.g. computers and smart tablets) and leisure (e.g. televisions, video games, social media), screen time and thus time spent in a sedentary posture is increasing around the world. This chapter will address how sedentary behavior influences chronic disease risk, the economic costs associated with sedentary behavior, and future directions pertaining to the interaction between physical activity and sedentary behavior.

Keywords: sedentary behavior, physical activity, chronic disease, economic costs, public health

1. Introduction

Physical activity—a behavior requiring energy expenditure and use of large skeletal muscles [1]—is one of the most modifiable behaviors to decrease chronic disease risk. Accumulating evidence has increasingly demonstrated the health benefits of living a physically active lifestyle [2–5]. In contrast, physical inactivity has been recognized as a global health problem and is one of the leading contributors to the worldwide epidemic on non-communicable diseases [6]. Ever since the Industrial Revolution, new technologies have allowed individuals to perform more tasks with less energy expenditure [7]. While the goal of many new technological advancements is increased efficiency and decreased physical labor at work, they have also led to an increase in physical inactivity.

To counteract physical inactivity, in 2008 the Centers for Disease Control and Prevention (CDC) created the Physical Activity Guidelines for Americans [8]. These guidelines stipulate what amount, type, and intensity of physical activity is recommended for health benefits and are commonly used to classify individuals as "physically active." For optimal disease reducing benefits, the CDC recommends that adults 18 years and older engage in at least 150 minutes of moderate-intensity aerobic activity a week and muscle strengthening activities twice a week; or 75 minutes of vigorous-intensity aerobic activity a week and two days of muscle strengthening activities; or an equivalent combination of moderate and vigorous aerobic activity mixed with two days of muscle strengthening. Differentiating between someone who is physically active and someone who is physically inactive is determined on if they meet the physical activity guidelines (e.g., someone who performs 85 minutes of vigorous aerobic activity and muscle strengthening activities twice per week is physically active). Yet, only 23% of Americans meet these guidelines, and 25% of Americans perform no aerobic or strength training activity [8].

Technological advances have not only influenced participation in physical activities, but also sedentary behaviors. Once thought to be synonymous and interchangeable with physical inactivity, sedentary behavior—defined as any activity of less than 1.5 MET's while in a seated or reclining posture [9]—is now recognized as its own activity state independent of both physical activity and physical inactivity. Based on this definition, there is an activity continuum in which someone can be highly active and highly sedentary at the same time (e.g., someone who meets the physical activity guidelines by running 30 minutes, 5 times per week, but then sits for 10 hours every day at work). To be clear, physically active = meeting CDC guidelines, physically inactive = not meeting CDC guidelines, sedentary = someone may meet or not meet guidelines, but still experiences long bouts of sitting throughout the day.

Emerging technologies have made sedentary behaviors ubiquitous in modern societies [10]. Increased sedentary behavior, or prolonged bouts of sitting, come primarily from increases in digital screen time. In 2005, just 5% of U.S. adults used social media, but currently, more than 80% of U.S. adults report habitual social media use [11]. Further, streaming video sites such as Netflix saw an 842% increase in viewership between 2011 and 2020 [12]. Lastly, Twitch, the global leader in video game streaming, has more than 140 million monthly users, compared to only 55 million in 2015 [13]. In total, it is estimated that U.S. adults spend 18 hours a day in sedentary behaviors [14, 15]. These increases in sitting are alarming given the negative health ramifications of such behavior.

Prolonged sitting (e.g., uninterrupted sitting with no breaks) and total sitting time are both negatively associated with chronic disease risk [16], metabolic health [17] and premature mortality [18]. A recent systematic review and meta-analysis demonstrated a dose-dependent relationship between sitting time with cancer, cardiovascular disease, and all-cause mortality, with each 1-hour increment of total daily sitting time accounting for hazard ratios of 1.01 (95% Cis 1.00–1.02), 1.04 (1.02–1.07) and 1.03 (1.02–1.03), respectively [19]. Furthermore, compared to more physically active counterparts, all-cause mortality is increased by 15% for individuals who sit for more than 8 hours per day and increased by 40% for those who sit for more than 11 hours per day [20]. With sedentary behaviors having increased following the coronavirus pandemic [21–24], and with the expectation that they will continue to do so, it is important we understand how sedentary behavior influences health risk.

2. Sedentary behavior influences on chronic disease physiology

While we now have objective measures of physical activity, physical inactivity, and sedentary behavior, parsing out *how each* or *if each* activity independently influences chronic disease risk has been more difficult. To some degree, debates between physical activity and sedentary behavior are artificial, as these behaviors are clearly interdependent [10]. It is not possible to change time spent in sedentary behaviors without also altering time spent in some form of physical activity (other than sleep). While the physiological mechanisms of how sedentary behavior and physical inactivity might differentially affect health are not well understood, it is clear time spent sedentary affects chronic disease pathophysiology. Sedentary behaviors are associated with increased risks of developing type 2 diabetes mellitus [25], hypertension [26], dyslipidemia [27] and cancer risk [28]. Although chronic diseases can manifest independently of one another, there are comorbidities within cardiovascular diseases and its risk factors. Although the manifestation of chronic diseases does not always happen in a linear progression as described below, many diseases are characterized by metabolic disturbances that are exacerbated by other diseases. As such, many diseases are associated with or develop from obesity, which is highly influenced by sedentary behavior and physical activity.

2.1 Obesity

Obesity—a disease characterized by excessive body fatness—is caused by an imbalance of energy expenditure and energy intake [29]. Measured using height and weight, obesity is defined as a body mass index greater than 30. The worldwide obesity rate has tripled since 1975, and in 2016, 650 million individuals were obese [30].

To be clear, obesity is a complex and multifaceted disorder with multiple causes (e.g., endocrine disorders such as hypothyroidism). Additionally, many people around the world live in communities in which there is little, if any, access to healthy food options. Known as a "food desert," these areas have little to no fruits, vegetables, healthy grains, or unprocessed meats. These individuals do not have access to healthy foods and must rely on sodium rich, sugar-sweetened, ultra-processed food and beverages to obtain nutrients. Even if the proper number of calories are ingested, the poor quality of the food results in obesity. Therefore, obesity may be a result of illness, metabolic disorders, or unfavorable living conditions, independent of the individuals choice of foods.

The topic of this section is not to negatively stereotype obesity, but to explain the physiological processes underlying obesity. When an individual ingests more energy than they expend, a positive energy balance develops and the excess energy is stored as fat [31]. Rather than serving as a passive deposit for excess fat, adipose tissue is considered an endocrine organ which secretes adipokines (e.g. hormones) that negatively influence metabolism [32, 33]. The majority of these adipokines are harmful as they lead to a chronic pro-inflammatory state. Leptin, resistin, and tumor necrosis factor-alpha, are pro-inflammatory adipokines that are secreted in proportion to the amount of fat in adipose tissue [34]. In contrast, adiponectin—an adipokine with anti-inflammatory properties—is secreted in indirect proportion to the amount of fat in adipose tissue. Taken together, these secretory molecules released by excessive adipose tissue promote a chronic inflammatory state, characterized by a pro-atherogenic environment, endothelial dysfunction and dyslipidemia [35].

The association between sedentary behavior and obesity is clear. Yet, the link distinguishing the effects of sedentary behavior versus the effects of physical inactivity on obesity is unknown. More time spent in sedentary behavior means less energy expenditure. Without an equivalent reduction in caloric intake, excessive weight gain will ensue, leading to obesity and an obesity-driven inflammatory state.

2.2 Type 2 diabetes mellitus

Perhaps the most well-known disease associated with obesity is type 2 diabetes mellitus (T2DM). T2DM is a complex disease characterized by hyperglycemia due to defects in insulin action. Currently, 10.5% of the global adult population has diabetes, with 1 in 8 adults projected to be living with diabetes by the year 2045 [36]. Further, an estimated 80% of individuals with T2DM are overweight or obese [30], demonstrating a link between excessive adiposity and defects in insulin.

When individuals ingest food, blood sugar levels elevate stimulating the release of insulin from the pancreas. Insulin binds to a receptor on target tissues (most notably the liver and skeletal muscle), leading to an intracellular signaling cascade of enzymatic reactions. Following, glucose transporter type 4 (GLUT4) is released and moves to the cell membrane, stimulating the cellular uptake and storage of glucose and the subsequent reduction in blood sugar levels. Yet, in T2DM individuals, target tissues responsible for storing glucose do not respond to insulin as they should, resulting in hyperglycemia. It is presumed that the primary cause of T2DM is obesity-driven insulin resistance [37].

The obesity-stimulated release of adipokines increases insulin resistance—the decreased physiological effects of circulating insulin [38]. Resistin and leptin, pro-inflammatory adipokines, negatively interfere with the intracellular signaling cascade of insulin-responsive cells [39]. These adipokines inhibit enzymatic reactions from happening once insulin binds to its target receptor, ultimately inhibiting GLUT4 movement to the cellular membrane, which inhibits the uptake and storage of circulating glucose. Resistin and leptin are insulin antagonists, increasing insulin resistance. Adiponectin, an anti-inflammatory adipokine, is an insulin agonist which can decrease insulin resistance. However, obesity leads to reductions in adiponectin and elevations of resistin and leptin, increasing insulin resistance.

As insulin-responsive cells do not respond to insulin as they should due to obesity-driven insulin resistance, glucose is not properly cleared from the blood, resulting in chronic hyperglycemia. To try and overcome hyperglycemia, the pancreas responds by secreting increased amounts of insulin. As insulin resistance worsens, the individual is left with a metabolic state characterized by insulin resistance, hyperglycemia and hyperinsulinemia. Increased amounts of time spent sedentary exacerbates the effects of obesity and the subsequent obesity-driven metabolic disturbances that characterize T2DM.

2.3 Dyslipidemia and atherosclerosis

Dyslipidemia is a disorder characterized by an imbalance of lipids. Dyslipidemia normally manifests as an increased concentration of low-density lipoprotein (LDL-C) and very low-density lipoprotein (VLDL) and a decreased reduction of high-density lipoprotein (HDL). Normally known as "bad" and "good" cholesterol respectively, LDL and HDL have opposing effects on metabolic health. Excessive levels of LDL and VLDL float in the bloodstream and increase the risk for plaque formation and blood vessel blockages while HDL promotes the excretion of LDL.

In contrast to what some may believe, VLDL and LDL are a normal byproduct of metabolism and healthy within certain amounts. Only when the concentrations of these molecules become excessive do they pose a risk to human health. As humans eat, the ingested dietary fat is broken down into free fatty acids. Free fatty acids can be stored as triglycerides (the storage form of fat) in adipose tissue and muscle. The free fatty acids that are not stored are diverted to the liver and converted into LDL and VLDL where they aid in transporting cholesterol.

Obesity-driven insulin resistance is a precursor to dyslipidemia. Insulin resistance leads to increased lipolysis—the breakdown of stored triglycerides into free fatty acids. These free fatty acids are moved into the bloodstream, diverted to the liver and converted to LDL and VLDL. Over time the chronic elevations and accumulations of lipids leads to atherosclerosis, a disease marked by plaque buildup in arteries. Arterial walls typically have tight cell-to-cell junctions which are impermeable to cholesterol and blood cells. However, in the presence of chronic elevations of LDL and VLDL, the arterial walls become "leaky" and permeable to these molecules.

LDL molecules enter the arterial walls, followed by immune cells to overcome this disrupted barrier. While located within the arterial wall, these LDL molecules and immune cells undergo oxidation and are transformed into foam cells which further exacerbate the inflammatory process [40]. Over time, the accumulation of molecules within the arterial wall causes the wall to increase in size and directly decreases the diameter of the vessel, reducing blood flow. These plaques can remain stationary and disrupt blood flow or they can rupture, leading to a blood clot and a further reduction in vessel diameter and blood flow.

2.4 Hypertension

Hypertension is a complex disorder marked by chronic elevations in blood pressure and is prevalent in 1.28 billion people worldwide [41]. Hypertension is a multifaceted disease due to either a narrowing of the vessel diameter or to increased stiffness of the vessel, both leading to increases in pressure.

As blood flows through the arteries, it places pressure on the arterial walls as it is constantly pushed back and forth on the artery. Similar to a water hose increasing in pressure when squeezed, when the artery diameter decreases, blood pressure increases. As the diameter of the vessel becomes narrower, the blood is in contact with the artery walls more forcefully, as it pulses back and forth against the vessel more often. There is a clear link between the previously discussed diseases and hypertension.

Increased release of adipokines from excessive adipose tissue stimulates the sympathetic nervous system, leading to increases in vasoconstriction and decreases in vessel diameter. Insulin resistance from T2DM promotes vasoconstriction due to inhibition of vasodilatory molecules [42]. As lipids accumulate in vessel walls, plaques form, vessel diameter is decreased, and blood pressure increases.

Independent of disease, sedentary behavior directly influences hypertension. It is known that physical activity promotes endothelial function, namely by increasing the concentration of nitric oxide, a vasodilatory molecule. As humans move, the amount of blood pumped from the heart increases, increasing the stress placed on the vessel walls. To compensate, the vessels release nitric oxide, causing the vessel walls to relax, allowing the vessel diameter to increase, and decreasing blood pressure. In contrast, sedentary behavior leads to blood pooling in the lower extremities, decreases venous return to the heart, decreasing blood flow from the heart, decreasing stress placed on the vessel walls. Because of this, nitric oxide release is decreased, inhibiting vessel relaxation and leading to vessel constriction, increasing blood pressure.

2.5 Chronic disease summary

While the precise link underscoring how sedentary behavior influences metabolic health and chronic disease risk remains to be determined, it is clear there is an association between sedentary behaviors and total sitting time on chronic disease development and progression. Reductions in energy expenditure due to sedentary behavior increases obesity risk, which increases risk of T2DM, dyslipidemia, atherosclerosis, and hypertension. Again, these diseases do not necessarily progress in a linear fashion in each individual, as one disease can develop without the other. Yet, there is a clear association between these diseases as 1 in 3 Americans has Metabolic Syndrome—defined as having 3 or more of the following conditions: obesity, hypertension, hyperglycemia, hypertriglyceridemia, dyslipidemia [43]. Although, these diseases can manifest independent of activity level, due to environmental factors, diet, genetics, etc., with sedentary behaviors and chronic disease prevalence increasing, the associations between the two must continue to be investigated.

3. Associated economic costs with sedentary behavior

The economic costs associated with chronic diseases continues to be staggering. Yet, only a handful of studies have investigated the economic costs related specifically to sedentary behavior. Each study retrospectively determined the economic impact of sedentary behaviors, ranging in time from the year 2009–2019. As each study used slightly different methodologies, each will be briefly summarized [44–48].

In 2014, Peeters and colleagues determined the health care costs associated with prolonged sitting in a population of middle-aged Australian women [44]. This was a longitudinal study with four follow up periods spaced every three years (2001, 2004, 2007, and 2010). At each follow-up period, the participants answered surveys regarding their time spent sitting and in leisure related activities. Sitting time was categorized as low (0–4 hours/day), moderate (5–7 hours/day) and high (>8 hours/day). To determine healthcare costs, Medicare-subsidized health services were calculated per participant for the entire study duration (years 2001–2010) and health insurance claims data were averaged over the survey year ±1 year to calculate average annual costs. Unsurprisingly, healthcare costs were highest in the high sitting group AU$709 (IQR = 283–1575) and lowest in the low sitting group AU$671 (IQR = 273, 1551). However, there were no differences in costs between high and low levels of daily sitting time.

The methodology used to determine associations between sedentary behavior and health care expenditures in Chinese older adults by Yu & Schwingel was similar [45]. The Physical Activity Scale for the Elderly questionnaire and self-reported health care expenditures were used to determine sedentary behavior and health care costs, respectively. Regression analyses revealed that for each additional hour spent sedentary, health care costs increased by $37 ($p$ < 0.001).

Heron et al. [46], Kolu et al. [47] and Chaput et al. [48] all utilized population attributable fractions to determine the direct or indirect costs of sedentary behavior in the United Kingdom, Finland, and Canada, respectively [46–48]. To determine the population attributable fractions, three items were needed: the relative risks of selected diseases, the prevalence of sedentary behavior, and the direct or indirect economic costs.

First, each study extracted the relative risks (RR) of selected non-communicable diseases consistently associated with sedentary behavior from suitable meta-analyses. The RR's were adjusted for age, physical activity, body mass index, smoking and education. The RR's were defined as the probability of having a disease for individuals with excessive sedentary behavior divided by the probability of having a disease for individuals without excessive sedentary behavior.

Second, each study determined the prevalence of sedentary behavior. Using the Health Survey for England, which reports the percentage of adults spending at least 6 hours/day sedentary on weekdays and on weekends, Heron et al. estimated the percentage of United Kingdom adults who are sedentary on any given day [46]. Kolu et al. utilized self-reports and accelerometer data from Finnish population studies to classify excessive sedentary behavior as at least 8 hours of sitting/reclining/lying during 16 waking hours [47]. Chaput et al. used accelerometer data from the Canadian Health Measures Survey to define excessive sedentary behavior as greater than 8 hours per day sedentary [48].

Third, each study determined the direct or indirect economic costs of their chosen non-communicable diseases. Heron et al. [46] used the National Health Service to obtain healthcare budgets, Kolu et al. [47] used Finnish registries to determine direct economic costs (outpatient visits, days of inpatient care, medication) and indirect economic costs (sickness-related absences, disability pensions, all-cause mortality), and Chaput et al. [48] used the Economic Burden of Illness in Canada to determine direct costs (physician, hospital care and prescription drug expenditures) and indirect costs (lost productivity due to premature mortality) [46–48].

Following, population attributable fraction percent's were calculated for each selected disease by combining the RR with the prevalence of sedentary behavior. The population attributable fraction for each disease was then multiplied by the direct and indirect costs of each disease to determine the economic costs of sedentary behavior. These population attributable fractions estimate the contribution of sedentary behavior to the total burden of disease [46].

Total costs of sedentary behavior in the United Kingdom were 761 million pounds, with the largest economic costs attributable to cardiovascular disease and type 2 diabetes (**Tables 1** and **2**). These results suggested that 11.6% of all-cause mortality in the year 2017 was associated with sedentary behavior. In Finland, excessive sedentary behavior was associated with 469 million euros of direct costs and 1034 million euros of indirect costs (**Table 1**), with type 2 diabetes representing 91% and 63% of direct and indirect costs, respectively (**Table 2**). Lastly, direct and indirect costs associated with sedentary behavior in Canada were $2.1 billion and $50.4 million, respectively (**Table 1**), with the two most expensive diseases being cardiovascular disease and diabetes (**Table 2**).

Taken collectively, these studies demonstrate the negative ramifications of sedentary behavior on economic costs. However, as these studies varied in their determination of sedentary behavior, diseases measured, different time points, what constitutes direct and indirect costs, fluctuations in inflation, etc., it is difficult to compare cost estimates across countries. Even so, the total economic costs associated with sedentary

	Heron et al. [46]*	**Kolu et al. [47]****	**Chaput et al. [48]*****
Direct Costs	761.80	469.2	2144
Indirect Costs	______	1034.3	50.4
Total Costs	761.80	1503.5	2194.4

Note: Adapted from Heron et al. [46], Kolu et al. [47], and Chaput et al. [48]. *Measured in millions of Pounds.*
**Measured in millions of Euros.*
***Measured in millions of Canadian dollars.*

Table 1.
Mean direct and indirect costs associated with sedentary behavior.

	Heron et al. [46]*			Kolu et al. [47]**			Chaput et al. [48]***		
	Direct costs	Indirect costs	Total costs	Direct costs	Indirect costs	Total costs	Direct costs	Indirect costs	Total costs
Cardiovascular Disease	424.38		424.38				725.4	22.5	747.9
Coronary Heart Disease				14.6	4.3	18.9			
Type 2 Diabetes	281.34		281.34	426.5	661.2	1087.7	607.4	2.0	609.4
Breast Cancer				11.6	3.3	14.9	48.1	3.3	51.4
Colon Cancer	29.64		29.64	8.0	2.1	10.1	141.2	6.3	147.5
Lung Cancer	19.16		19.16				115.5	14.9	130.4
Endometrial Cancer	7.29		7.29				22.6	1.3	23.9
Dementia							161.6	0.2	161.8
Depression				8.6	65.4	74.0	322.3	0.02	322.3
All-cause mortality					298.1	298.1			

*Note: Adapted from Heron et al. [46], Kolu et al. [47], and Chaput et al. [48].*Measured in millions of Pounds.*
***Measured in millions of Euros.*
****Measured in millions of Canadian dollars.*

Table 2.
Mean direct and indirect costs of chronic diseases associated with sedentary behavior.

behavior are likely a conservative estimate of the true burden of sedentariness. The prevalence of sedentary behavior used in these studies' cost estimates were based on data collected before the coronavirus (COVID-19) pandemic. Time spent in sedentary behaviors substantially increased during and immediately following the COVID-19 outbreak [24, 49, 50]. Thus, a higher prevalence of sedentary behavior would result in higher economic cost estimates, meaning the overall burden of sedentary behavior is likely larger than these studies suggest.

4. More physical activity or less sedentary behavior?

Much evidence demonstrates the associations between sedentary behavior and chronic disease risk. Recent evidence also demonstrates the association between sedentary behavior and economic costs. In contrast, the positive metabolic health ramifications of acute and chronic physical activity participation are known and dose-responsive. Even more, physical activity and sedentary behavior may influence health through overlapping pathways, one such example being energy balance [51]. The absence of muscle contractions characterized by sedentary behaviors suppresses lipoprotein lipase (LPL), a key enzyme for triglyceride metabolism [16]. Thus, reductions in LPL activity will increase fat accumulation. In contrast, physical activity increases LPL activity, increasing triglyceride metabolism and reducing fat accumulation.

A meta-analysis examining associations between sedentary behaviors, physical activity, and all-cause mortality seems to support the notion of an interaction between sedentary behaviors and physical activity on health risk [52]. Using data from more than 1 million individuals, participants were stratified into one of four quartiles of physical activity, and then further stratified by time in sedentary behavior within each physical activity quartile. Individuals in the highest quartile of physical activity (60–75 min/day) who sat for more than 8 hours per day had a significantly lower risk of mortality than individuals who sat for less than 4 hours per day in the least active quartile (5 min/day). Further, across sitting time categories, all-cause mortality was diminished with higher levels of physical activity. These results suggest that high levels of physical activity (60–75 min/day—which is above recommended guidelines) is necessary to attenuate the harmful effects of prolonged sedentary behavior. Those in the middle quartiles of activity—which encompasses current recommended physical activity guidelines—had marked reductions in all-cause mortality, but the increased risk of sitting was not completely eliminated when compared to the least active quartile. When compared with other health risk factors, the increased all-cause mortality risk for individuals who sat for more than 8 hours per day and were least active is similar to that of smoking and obesity [53, 54].

The question these interactions pose for health researchers is: What's more important for health, increasing physical activity or reducing sedentary behavior? In 2008, when much less was known regarding sedentary behavior, the CDC guidelines focused on improving physical activity: "all adults should avoid inactivity. Some physical activity is better than none, and adults who participate in any amount of physical activity gain some health benefits" [8]. In 2018, with the second edition of the CDC Physical Activity guidelines, it was acknowledged that not only would individuals benefit from increased physical activity, but also with decreasing sedentary behavior: "Adults should move more and sit less throughout the day. Some physical activity is better than none. Adults who sit less and do any amount of moderate-to-vigorous physical activity gain some health benefits" [55].

Although the CDC and the Global Action Plan on Physical Activity have both adopted strategies to increase physical activity and reduce sedentary behavior [56] to prevent chronic disease, the optimal time, frequency and dosage of sedentary behavior remains elusive. As found in the work published by Ekelund et al. [52], some health risks associated with sedentary behavior are related to time spent in physical activity [52]. The independence of sedentary behavior and physical activity remains arbitrary, as one cannot be edited without altering the other.

While the call is to increase time in physical activity and reduce time spent sedentary, an individual's budget and time are crucial barriers to these behavior changes. Some of the most common reasons given for not being physically active are a lack of money (e.g., gyms/fitness centers and exercise classes are too expensive) and a lack of time. More money or time might make participation in a physically active lifestyle more appealing. At the same time, having more time or money means a decision on how to spend those increased resources. Studies investigating time spent in physical activity and sedentary behavior during the COVID-19 pandemic—a time period in which individuals had increased free time at home—resulted in significant reductions in physical activity minutes and significant increases in sedentariness [21–24]. The issue is not always the time, but how we spend time. The importance of having the money and time needed to live a physically active lifestyle cannot be overstated. Yet there are things we can do to be more active and less sedentary without changes in finances and time. To optimize our behavior towards more activity, consider alternating time spent sitting with time spent standing at work, take the stairs instead of elevators, and park further away at businesses to spend more time walking.

5. Conclusions

Sedentary behavior—activity of less than 1.5 MET's while in a seated or reclining posture—has become a global health issue associated with increased health disease and all-cause mortality risk. Rather than the opposite physical inactivity, sedentary behavior is its own activity state independent of both physical inactivity and physical activity. Because of this definition, all people are susceptible to long bouts of sedentariness, regardless of time spent in moderate-to-vigorous physical activity.

Many questions remain as researchers aim to determine how exactly sedentary behavior influences health dependently *and or* independently from physical activity. Are continuous bouts of sedentary behavior without breaks or intermittent sedentary behavior stints more hazardous for health [57]? Are the specific pathophysiological mechanisms in which sedentary behavior influences health different from the pathophysiological mechanisms in which physical activity promotes health, or do they overlap (e.g. triglyceride metabolism) [10]? Is the relationship between sedentary behavior and health disease risk dose-responsive as is the relationship between physical activity and health promotion? Given the limited knowledge to these questions, there are no "optimal" amounts or patterns of sedentary behavior and as such, only general recommendations can be given: Sit less, move more [10].

Unfortunately, the human race has evolved into a sedentary phenotype [58, 59] and time spent in sedentary behavior should only increase as social media and technological innovations continue to manifest. With much emphasis in the past on increasing physical activity levels, more emphasis is needed on lowering time spent in sedentary behavior. It is unarguable that sedentary behavior has negative health ramifications—from associations with obesity, diabetes and atherosclerosis to increased economic costs—and it is imperative that we reduce time spent in sedentary behavior as much as feasible [60].

Conflict of interest

The author declares no conflict of interest.

Author details

Brett Baker
Huston-Tillotson University, Austin, TX, USA

*Address all correspondence to: brettdbaker77@gmail.com

References

[1] Physical Activity. Available from: https://www.who.int/europe/news-room/fact-sheets/item/physical-activity#

[2] Morris JN, Heady JA, Raffle PAB, Roberts CG, Parks JW. Coronary heart-disease and physical activity of work. The Lancet. 1953;**262**:1111-1120

[3] Paffenbarger RS, Robert H, Wing AL, Chung-cheng H. Physical activity, all-cause mortality, and longevity of college alumni. New England Journal of Medicine. 1986;**314**:605-613

[4] Wen CP et al. Minimum amount of physical activity for reduced mortality and extended life expectancy: A prospective cohort study. The Lancet. 2011;**378**:1244-1253

[5] Lee I-M et al. Effect of physical inactivity on major non-communicable diseases worldwide: An analysis of burden of disease and life expectancy. The Lancet. 2012;**380**:219-229

[6] Alwan A. Global status report on noncommunicable diseases 2010. World Health Organization; 2011

[7] Hallal PC et al. Global physical activity levels: Surveillance progress, pitfalls, and prospects. The Lancet. 2012;**380**:247-257

[8] U.S. Department of Health and Human Services. Physical Activity Guidelines for Americans 2008-2018. Washington, DC: U.S. Department of Health and Human Services; 2008

[9] Tremblay MS et al. Sedentary behavior research network (SBRN)—Terminology consensus project process and outcome. International Journal of Behavioral Nutrition and Physical Activity. 2017;**14**:75

[10] Dempsey PC et al. Sedentary behavior and chronic disease: Mechanisms and future directions. Journal of Physical Activity and Health. 2020;**17**:52-61

[11] NW, 1615 L. St, Washington, S. 800 & Inquiries, D. 20036 U.-419-4300 | M.-857-8562 | F.-419-4372 | M. Social Media Fact Sheet. Pew Research Center: Internet, Science & Tech. Available from: https://www.pewresearch.org/internet/fact-sheet/social-media/

[12] Netflix Revenue and Usage Statistics. Business of Apps. 2023. Available from: https://www.businessofapps.com/data/netflix-statistics/

[13] Durrani A. Top Streaming Statistics in 2024. Forbes Home. Available from: https://www.forbes.com/home-improvement/internet/streaming-stats/ (2024)

[14] Aittasalo M et al. Moving to business–changes in physical activity and sedentary behavior after multilevel intervention in small and medium-size workplaces. BMC Public Health. 2017;**17**:1-14

[15] Hadgraft NT et al. Office workers' objectively assessed total and prolonged sitting time: Individual-level correlates and worksite variations. Preventive Medicine Reports. 2016;**4**:184-191

[16] Hamilton MT, Hamilton DG, Zderic TW. Role of low energy expenditure and sitting in obesity, metabolic syndrome, type 2 diabetes, and cardiovascular disease. Diabetes. 2007;**56**:2655-2667

[17] Healy GN, Matthews CE, Dunstan DW, Winkler EAH, Owen N. Sedentary time and cardio-metabolic biomarkers in US adults: NHANES 2003-06. European Heart Journal. 2011;**32**:590-597

[18] Dunstan DW et al. Breaking up prolonged sitting reduces postprandial glucose and insulin responses. Diabetes Care. 2012;**35**:976-983

[19] Zhao R, Bu W, Chen Y, Chen X. The dose-response associations of sedentary time with chronic diseases and the risk for all-cause mortality affected by different health status: A systematic review and meta-analysis. The Journal of Nutrition, Health and Aging. 2020;**24**:63-70

[20] van der Ploeg HP, Chey T, Korda RJ, Banks E, Bauman A. Sitting time and all-cause mortality risk in 222 497 Australian adults. Archives of Internal Medicine. 2012;**172**:494-500

[21] Castañeda-Babarro A, Arbillaga-Etxarri A, Gutiérrez-Santamaría B, Coca A. Physical activity change during COVID-19 confinement. International Journal of Environmental Research and Public Health. 2020;**17**:6878

[22] Bertrand L et al. The impact of the coronavirus disease 2019 (COVID-19) pandemic on university students' dietary intake, physical activity, and sedentary behaviour. Applied Physiology, Nutrition, and Metabolism. 2021;**46**:265-272

[23] Czenczek-Lewandowska E et al. Health behaviours of young adults during the outbreak of the Covid-19 pandemic—A longitudinal study. BMC Public Health. 2021;**21**:1038

[24] Baker BD, Castelli DM. Impact of a global pandemic on young adult sedentary behavior and physical activity. AJPM Focus. 2024;**3**(3):100202

[25] Biswas A et al. Sedentary time and its association with risk for disease incidence, mortality, and hospitalization in adults. Annals of Internal Medicine. 2015;**162**:123-132

[26] Beunza JJ et al. Sedentary behaviors and the risk of incident hypertension*: The SUN cohort. American Journal of Hypertension. 2007;**20**:1156-1162

[27] Zhou J et al. Associations of sedentary behavior and physical activity with dyslipidemia. Beijing Da Xue Xue Bao Yi Xue Ban. 2017;**49**:418-423

[28] Schmid D, Leitzmann MF. Television viewing and time spent sedentary in relation to cancer risk: A meta-analysis. JNCI: Journal of the National Cancer Institute. 2014;**106**:dju098

[29] Gadde KM, Martin CK, Berthoud H-R, Heymsfield SB. Obesity. Journal of the American College of Cardiology. 2018;**71**:69-84

[30] Jin X et al. Pathophysiology of obesity and its associated diseases. Acta Pharmaceutica Sinica B. 2023;**13**:2403-2424

[31] Haas B, Schlinkert P, Mayer P, Eckstein N. Targeting adipose tissue. Diabetology and Metabolic Syndrome. 2012;**4**:43

[32] Gaspar RC, Pauli JR, Shulman GI, Muñoz VR. An update on brown adipose tissue biology: A discussion of recent findings. American Journal of Physiology-Endocrinology and Metabolism. 2021;**320**:E488-E495

[33] Hermano E et al. Heparanase accelerates obesity-associated breast

cancer progression. Cancer Research. 2019;**79**:5342-5354

[34] Gjermeni E et al. Obesity–an update on the basic pathophysiology and review of recent therapeutic advances. Biomolecules. 2021;**11**:1426

[35] Redinger RN. The pathophysiology of obesity and its clinical manifestations. Gastroenterología y Hepatología. 2007;**3**:856-863

[36] Galicia-Garcia U et al. Pathophysiology of type 2 diabetes mellitus. International Journal of Molecular Sciences. 2020;**21**:6275

[37] Rohm TV, Meier DT, Olefsky JM, Donath MY. Inflammation in obesity, diabetes, and related disorders. Immunity. 2022;**55**:31-55

[38] Lebovitz HE. Insulin resistance: Definition and consequences. Experimental and Clinical Endocrinology & Diabetes. 2001;**109**:S135-S148

[39] Czech MP. Insulin action and resistance in obesity and type 2 diabetes. Nature Medicine. 2017;**23**:804-814

[40] Jebari-Benslaiman S et al. Pathophysiology of atherosclerosis. International Journal of Molecular Sciences. 2022;**23**:3346

[41] Hypertension. Available from: https://www.who.int/news-room/fact-sheets/detail/hypertension

[42] Tabit CE, Chung WB, Hamburg NM, Vita JA. Endothelial dysfunction in diabetes mellitus: Molecular mechanisms and clinical implications. Reviews in Endocrine & Metabolic Disorders. 2010;**11**:61-74

[43] Metabolic Syndrome—What is Metabolic Syndrome? | NHLBI, NIH. 2022. Available from: https://www.nhlbi.nih.gov/health/metabolic-syndrome

[44] Peeters GMEE(G), Mishra GD, Dobson AJ, Brown WJ. Health care costs associated with prolonged sitting and inactivity. American Journal of Preventive Medicine. 2014; **46**:265-272

[45] Yu H, Schwingel A. Associations between sedentary behavior, physical activity, and out-of-pocket health care expenditure: Evidence from Chinese older adults. Journal of Aging and Physical Activity. 2019;**27**:108-115

[46] Heron L, O'Neill C, McAneney H, Kee F, Tully MA. Direct healthcare costs of sedentary behaviour in the UK. Journal of Epidemiology and Community Health. 2019;**73**:625-629

[47] Kolu P et al. Economic burden of low physical activity and high sedentary behaviour in Finland. Journal of Epidemiology and Community Health. 2022;**76**:677-684

[48] Chaput J-P, Janssen I, Lang JJ, Sampasa-Kanyinga H. Economic burden of excessive sedentary behaviour in Canada. Canadian Journal of Public Health. 2023;**114**:165-174

[49] Schuch FB et al. Moderate to vigorous physical activity and sedentary behavior changes in self-isolating adults during the COVID-19 pandemic in Brazil: A cross-sectional survey exploring correlates. Sport Sciences for Health. 2022;**18**:155-163

[50] Stockwell S et al. Changes in physical activity and sedentary behaviours from before to during the COVID-19 pandemic lockdown: A systematic review. BMJ Open Sport & Exercise Medicine. 2021;7:e000960

[51] Stranahan AM, Mattson MP. Bidirectional metabolic regulation of neurocognitive function. Neurobiology of Learning and Memory. 2011;**96**:507-516

[52] Ekelund U et al. Does physical activity attenuate, or even eliminate, the detrimental association of sitting time with mortality? A harmonised meta-analysis of data from more than 1 million men and women. Lancet. 2016;**388**:1302-1310

[53] Martin S, Gerta R, Guido S. Meta-analysis and the surgeon General's report on smoking and health. New England Journal of Medicine. 2014;**370**:186-188

[54] Collaboration, P. S. Body-mass index and cause-specific mortality in 900 000 adults: Collaborative analyses of 57 prospective studies. The Lancet. 2009;**373**:1083-1096

[55] U.S. Department of Health and Human Services. Physical Activity Guidelines for Americans, 2nd edition. Washington, DC: U.S. Department of Health and Human Services; 2018

[56] Global action plan on physical activity 2018-2030: More active people for a healthier world. Geneva: World Health Organization; 2018. License: CC BY-NC-SA 3.0 IGO

[57] Diaz KM et al. Potential effects on mortality of replacing sedentary time with short sedentary bouts or physical activity: A National Cohort Study. American Journal of Epidemiology. 2019;**188**:537-544

[58] Dumith SC, Hallal PC, Reis RS, Kohl HW. Worldwide prevalence of physical inactivity and its association with human development index in 76 countries. Preventive Medicine. 2011;**53**:24-28

[59] Kohl HW et al. The pandemic of physical inactivity: Global action for public health. The Lancet. 2012;**380**:294-305

[60] Park JH, Moon JH, Kim HJ, Kong MH, Oh YH. Sedentary lifestyle: Overview of updated evidence of potential health risks. Korean Journal of Family Medicine. 2020;**41**:365-373

Chapter 12

Healthcare Accessibility: Metrics, Assessment, Policies, and Barriers

Kawtar Zahidi, Majdouline Obtel and Saida Naji

Abstract

This chapter delves into the multifaceted concept of healthcare accessibility, examining how it can be measured, evaluated, and improved through various policies. While terms such as "measures," "interventions," and "strategies" are used throughout this text, each plays a unique role in the broader context of health policies designed to enhance access to healthcare. This chapter begins by exploring different metrics and indicators used to assess accessibility, highlighting the strengths and limitations of these tools. It transitions into an analysis of national and international policies aimed at enhancing healthcare access, alongside discussions on local and community-level policies. A critical evaluation of the effectiveness of these policies provides insights into best practices and areas for improvement. Furthermore, the chapter addresses the diverse barriers that impede access to healthcare services, including financial, cultural, linguistic, geographical, and stigma-related challenges. Through this comprehensive examination, the chapter aims to shed light on the complex interplay of factors influencing healthcare access and to suggest pathways toward more equitable healthcare systems.

Keywords: healthcare accessibility, healthcare disparities, barriers to healthcare access, metrics and indicators, health policy

1. Introduction

Health is a fundamental and universal right, yet accessibility to healthcare remains a major global concern. The effectiveness of health systems is often judged by their ability to provide equitable and universal health coverage. However, the barriers that limit access to essential health services vary widely from region to region and from population to population, influenced by a complex spectrum of socio-economic, cultural, geographic, and policy factors.

This chapter offers an exhaustive examination of the measures and indicators of accessibility to care, while questioning the relevance and limits of these evaluation tools. It explores the multiple determinants that influence access to care, highlighting not only physical and financial barriers but also less visible, yet equally significant, barriers, such as cultural norms or institutional policies.

We also examine the deep disparities that exist in accessibility to healthcare, highlighting differences by region, socio-economic class, gender, age, and ethnicity, and assessing the impact of these inequalities on public health. Finally, we discuss policies and interventions implemented nationally and internationally, as well as local and community initiatives intended to improve access to care, and we question their effectiveness.

Through this chapter, our aim is to provide in-depth reflection on accessibility to healthcare and to contribute to the development of strategies to overcome barriers to equitable access to health services for all.

2. Measures and indicators of accessibility to care

In the field of health, accessibility to care is a key indicator of the efficiency and equity of health systems. It reflects the ability of individuals to obtain necessary and timely health services, based on their needs. Understanding and improving accessibility requires accurate assessment through a series of measures and indicators, which serve to map barriers, identify gaps in services, and guide policies and interventions for better health coverage.

2.1 Accessibility measurement methods

In this subsection, we will explore the diverse and complex approaches used to assess accessibility to healthcare services. These methods, ranging from quantitative analyses to qualitative surveys, are essential for understanding the multiple dimensions of accessibility and for guiding public health interventions and policies.

2.1.1 Conceptual approaches

Accessibility to healthcare is a multidimensional concept that goes beyond simple physical proximity to health services. It encompasses the ease with which individuals can obtain adequate care when they need it, without undue constraints or barriers. Penchansky and Thomas [1] helped to clarify this concept by breaking it down into five distinct dimensions: availability, accessibility, acceptability, affordability, and adequacy. Each of these dimensions highlights a crucial aspect of access to care:

- *Availability* refers to the sufficient presence of health services and professionals to meet the needs of the population.
- *Accessibility* focuses on geographic distance and time required to access health services.
- *Acceptability* concerns the match between the attitudes and characteristics of patients and providers (including cultural and social norms).
- *Affordability* refers to the financial ability of individuals to pay for health services without suffering economic harm.
- *Adequacy* assesses the extent to which health services respond effectively and appropriately to patients' needs.

These dimensions highlight the fact that accessibility is not limited to geography but also includes economic, social, and cultural considerations that can affect individuals' ability to receive quality care.

Several theoretical frameworks have been developed to understand and measure accessibility to health care. The Penchansky and Thomas model is fundamental in this area, providing a framework for understanding different aspects of accessibility and for assessing the fit between health services and user needs.

Furthermore, Levesque et al. [2] proposed an enriched framework that describes accessibility through five dimensions corresponding to the capacities of health services and the needs of populations. This framework highlights the importance of the capacity of health systems to be accessible, available, and acceptable to all individuals, while recognizing the need for populations to have the capacity to seek, reach, pay, and engage in health care. This model highlights the dynamic interaction between health services and users, considering accessibility as a meeting between the supply and demand of care.

These theoretical frameworks are essential to guide research and policies regarding access to care. They provide a basis for developing measurement methods and for evaluating the effectiveness of interventions aimed at improving access to health services. By taking a holistic and multidimensional approach, these models help recognize and respond to various barriers to accessibility, ensuring that healthcare is equitable and responsive to the needs of all populations.

2.1.2 Quantitative methods

Quantitative methods play a crucial role in measuring healthcare accessibility, providing objective, measurable data that can be statistically analyzed. These methods assess various aspects of accessibility, ranging from the availability of services to the geographic distribution of healthcare resources.

2.1.2.1 Geospatial analytics

One of the most popular quantitative methods for measuring geographic accessibility to healthcare services is geospatial analysis, often implemented through Geographic Information Systems (GIS). These tools allow the mapping of healthcare facilities and populations, helping to identify underserved areas and calculate distances or travel times. Shah et al. [3] demonstrated the effectiveness of GIS analyses in identifying underserved neighbourhoods in Canadian urban settings, highlighting the importance of these tools for planning and improving access to primary healthcare services at a local level.

2.1.2.2 Statistical indicators

Statistical indicators provide another dimension to quantitative methods, providing clear and comparable measures of accessibility. These indicators may include the ratio of health professionals per capita, the percentage of the population living within a certain distance of a health facility, or vaccination coverage rates. These quantitative data are essential for assessing the availability and distribution of health services. Gulliford et al. [4] discussed the importance of these indicators in understanding what it means to "have access" to health care, highlighting the need for quantitative measures to evaluate public health policies.

2.1.2.3 Optimization models

Optimization models are another important quantitative method, using mathematical techniques to improve the allocation and efficiency of healthcare resources.

These models can help determine optimal locations for new healthcare facilities or optimize the distribution of healthcare professionals across different regions. The objective is to maximize accessibility for the population while minimizing costs and necessary resources.

2.1.2.4 Use of telemedicine

In response to geographic limitations and barriers to physical access to care, telemedicine has emerged as an area of growing interest. Bauer and Weber [5] highlighted how telemedicine can improve healthcare accessibility, particularly in rural or isolated communities, by allowing patients to access healthcare services remotely. This approach may be particularly relevant to overcoming geographic challenges and improving access to specialists.

In conclusion, quantitative methods provide essential tools for measuring and analyzing healthcare accessibility. Whether through geospatial analyses, statistical indicators, optimization models, or the use of telemedicine, these approaches provide a precise and detailed understanding of accessibility challenges and guide decisions, policies, and interventions to improve access to healthcare for all.

2.1.3 Qualitative methods

Qualitative methods bring essential depth and nuance to understanding healthcare accessibility, focusing on the experiences, perceptions, and lived experiences of individuals. These approaches help explore aspects of accessibility that are not always quantifiable, such as cultural barriers, personal preferences, and the subjective experiences of patients and providers.

2.1.3.1 Surveys and interviews

Surveys and interviews with patients and healthcare professionals constitute a pillar of qualitative methods. These tools make it possible to collect direct testimonies on obstacles to access to care, experiences of care, and perceptions of the quality of services. Gulliford et al. [4] highlighted the importance of these methods for understanding the multiple dimensions of accessibility, recognizing that qualitative data offer irreplaceable insights into the factors that influence the use of health services.

2.1.3.2 Discussion groups

Focus groups are another valuable qualitative method, facilitating the exchange of ideas and perspectives between different participants. This approach helps capture a range of views and experiences regarding accessibility to care, providing a richer understanding of the social, cultural, and community dynamics that can influence access to health services.

2.1.3.3 Participatory observations

Participatory observation, where researchers immerse themselves in healthcare settings, allows for a first-hand understanding of interactions between patients and healthcare providers, as well as operational processes within healthcare settings. This qualitative method can reveal aspects of accessibility that are not evident through surveys or data analysis, such as non-verbal barriers to communication or informal practices that facilitate or hinder access to care.

2.1.3.4 Content analysis and case studies

Content analysis of health policy documents, medical records, and media can provide valuable insights into public discourses and priorities regarding healthcare accessibility. Similarly, in-depth case studies of specific situations or contexts allow for detailed examination of how policies and practices affect access to care for various population groups.

2.1.3.5 Integrating qualitative data into mixed analyses

Integrating qualitative data into mixed-methods analyses enriches the understanding of quantitative measures of accessibility, providing context and interpretation to trends and statistical patterns. This combination helps create a comprehensive picture of healthcare accessibility, recognizing the complexities and nuances that characterize the health experiences of individuals and communities.

In conclusion, qualitative methods play an indispensable role in assessing healthcare accessibility. By focusing on individuals' lived experiences and perceptions, these approaches provide a deep and nuanced understanding of the challenges and opportunities associated with accessing care. Integrating qualitative perspectives into accessibility analyses is essential for developing policies and interventions sensitive to the specific needs and contexts of the populations served.

2.1.4 Mixed approaches

Adopting mixed approaches, combining quantitative and qualitative methods, is crucial for a comprehensive assessment of healthcare accessibility. This hybrid approach leverages the strengths of each method, providing a richer, more nuanced overview of accessibility.

2.1.4.1 Integration of quantitative and qualitative data

The integration of quantitative data, such as statistical indicators and geospatial analyses, with qualitative data from interviews, focus groups, and satisfaction surveys, enriches the understanding of accessibility to care. This combination captures not only measurable aspects of accessibility, such as distance to health services or the ratio of health professionals per capita, but also the personal experiences, perceptions, and barriers experienced by patients and providers. of care. By recognizing the importance of qualitative data to complement quantitative data, researchers and policymakers can obtain a more complete picture of the multiple dimensions of accessibility.

2.1.4.2 Case studies and longitudinal analyses

Mixed approaches benefit greatly from the use of case studies and longitudinal analyses to examine changes in access to care over time and in specific contexts. Case studies can provide detailed insights into the unique challenges faced by different populations or regions, while longitudinal analyses can track changes in accessibility resulting from new policies, demographic shifts, or the introduction of innovative technologies such as telemedicine. These approaches help understand how interventions affect accessibility and identify emerging trends or persistent problems in healthcare access.

2.1.4.3 Ethical considerations and fairness

Mixed approaches must also take into account ethical considerations and health equity issues. Incorporating patient perspectives, particularly those from marginalized or vulnerable groups, is essential to ensure that accessibility measures reflect the needs and experiences of all populations. The blended approach helps identify and address disparities in access to care, ensuring that interventions are equitable and inclusive.

In summary, mixed approaches offer a robust methodology for assessing healthcare accessibility, combining the benefits of quantitative and qualitative analyses. This hybrid approach allows for a deeper understanding of the multiple facets of accessibility, integrating objective data with personal and contextual perspectives. By adopting such an approach, researchers and policymakers can develop more effective and equitable strategies to improve access to healthcare for all.

2.1.5 New technologies and innovations

The advent of new technologies and digital innovations is radically transforming healthcare accessibility, providing new avenues to overcome traditional barriers and improve health service delivery.

2.1.5.1 Telemedicine and remote care

Telemedicine, which enables the delivery of healthcare remotely via digital platforms, is at the forefront of this transformation. Bauer and Weber [5] highlighted how telemedicine has improved access to care during the COVID-19 pandemic, allowing patients to consult healthcare professionals without the risks associated with in-person visits. This technology is particularly beneficial for rural and isolated communities, where access to health services may be limited by geographic factors.

2.1.5.2 Mobile applications and digital health

Mobile health apps and digital platforms provide patients with tools to manage their health, access medical information, and communicate with healthcare providers. These technologies increase patient autonomy and facilitate continued access to health advice and support, potentially improving treatment adherence and disease prevention.

2.1.5.3 Big data and artificial intelligence

The use of Big Data and Artificial Intelligence (AI) in the healthcare sector opens new possibilities for analyzing health trends, predicting epidemics, and optimizing the distribution of healthcare resources. These technologies can help identify unmet healthcare needs and target interventions to improve accessibility. AI, in particular, can improve the accuracy of diagnoses and personalize treatments, making healthcare more efficient and accessible.

2.1.5.4 Electronic health records

Electronic Health Records (EHR) facilitate the secure management and sharing of health information between patients and the various healthcare professionals involved in their care. By improving communication and coordination between providers, EHRs can reduce wait times and improve the efficiency of care, thereby contributing to greater accessibility.

2.1.5.5 Impact on accessibility and inequalities

Although new technologies offer significant opportunities to improve accessibility to care, they also raise questions regarding digital inequalities. Unequal access to the internet and digital technologies can exacerbate existing health disparities, highlighting the need to address these inequities as part of efforts to improve accessibility to care.

In conclusion, new technologies and innovations play a crucial role in transforming healthcare accessibility, providing solutions to overcome traditional barriers, and improving the quality and efficiency of care. However, to fully realize their potential, it is essential to address the challenges of digital inequality and ensure that these technologies benefit all segments of the population.

2.1.6 Ethical issues and equity

Questions of ethics and equity are at the heart of debates about accessibility to healthcare, emphasizing the need to ensure that all individuals, regardless of their socio-economic, geographic, or cultural circumstances, have equitable access to necessary care.

2.1.6.1 Ethical considerations in access to care

Ethical issues related to accessibility to care include the right to health, confidentiality of patient data, and informed consent, particularly in the context of the growing use of digital technologies in health. Respecting the dignity of patients and protecting their personal information are essential to maintaining trust in health systems and to promoting ethical use of health data. The need to ensure informed consent in the use of telemedicine technologies and electronic health records is crucial to respecting patient autonomy and health rights.

2.1.6.2 Equity in access to care

Equity in access to healthcare is a major concern, with persistent disparities based on factors such as ethnicity, income, gender, and geography. Braveman and Gruskin [6] emphasize the importance of defining and measuring health equity to identify and combat these inequalities. Ensuring equitable access to care requires special attention to the needs of vulnerable and marginalized populations, ensuring that health policies and interventions are designed to be inclusive and meet the needs of all segments of the population.

2.1.6.3 Impact of new technologies on equity

Although new health technologies offer considerable potential to improve access to care, they also pose challenges in terms of equity. Unequal access to digital technologies and the internet can exacerbate existing health inequalities, creating new divides between those with access to these technologies and those who are excluded. Recognizing and addressing these digital inequities is essential as part of efforts to improve accessibility to care, ensuring that the benefits of health innovations are accessible to all.

2.1.6.4 Strategies to promote equity

Promoting equity in access to care involves developing targeted strategies to reach underserved and marginalized populations. This may include allocating additional resources to underserved areas, developing health services tailored to the cultural and linguistic needs of diverse populations, and implementing policies to reduce financial barriers to accessing care.

In summary, ethical issues and equity are central in the discussion on accessibility to health care. It is imperative to address health inequities and ensure that technological advances benefit all people equitably. This requires a continued commitment to assess and address the ethical and equitable dimensions of accessibility to care, ensuring that health systems are inclusive, fair, and respectful of the rights and dignity of all patients.

2.2 Commonly used indicators

The use and calculation of geographical accessibility indicators has become widespread thanks to the automated functions of software such as MapInfo or ArcView [7]. The approach adopted is to measure this dimension using criteria that can be calculated by the software in a given territory for a category of service and target population [7]. Then, the identification of areas of low or high accessibility will pose the problem of planning policy [7].

The notion of service refers to the spatial distribution of medical personnel (supply) in relation to potential demand in a given area. This indicator takes into account accessibility by combining supply and demand in a specific area, for example, one doctor per 500 inhabitants. Service maps make it possible to visualize the balances (and therefore inequalities) between the health resources that are available for a given population in a delimited region. Coverage, for its part, measures the proportion of the population which benefits from the existence of a service (% of the population served by a health resource, % of municipalities equipped with a service) [8].

In other words, service and coverage are two complementary indicators that make it possible to assess access to care in a given region. Access allows us to analyze the spatial distribution of medical resources in relation to potential demand, while coverage measures the proportion of the population served by these resources. These two indicators are essential for understanding inequalities in access to care and for developing public policies aimed at improving accessibility to health services.

We must differentiate it from medical density (rate of doctors in a certain specialty compared to the population likely to use it), which is expressed rather on the population at risk and in relation to the medical expertise of which we measure the density (and not in relation to the total population), for example, pediatricians in relation to the young age group of the population [9].

The spatial concentration of health resources (N doctors per km^2 = resources per surface unit) is also of little interest in addressing accessibility if this indicator is not linked to a demand indicator. (large areas can be population deserts) [9].

There is the geographic equity indicator E [9]. The geographic equity indicator E makes it possible to assess equity in the geographic distribution of health services by measuring the distance or cost of transportation to the nearest service. This is an important indicator because it allows us to determine whether the distribution of this variable is homogeneous or heterogeneous in a given territory, thus signaling important differences.

When all people live the same distance or below a threshold distance from a service location, equity is considered achieved. Thus, the mapping of this indicator, after discretization of the variable, makes it possible to visualize the spatial hierarchies and to highlight the areas where geographic equity is respected or not.

In summary, the geographic equity indicator E makes it possible to assess the spatial distribution of health services in terms of equity and to highlight areas where actions must be taken to guarantee equitable access to health services.

The concepts of social, economic, and physical distance between the demand for healthcare and the supply of medical resources are closely linked, allowing the determination of a level of accessibility that results in the use of services and an improvement in the state of health of populations [10].

Indeed, a demand for health, which can be influenced by factors such as population density, age, prevalence of diseases, poverty, etc., can be satisfied by a supply of care, which is generally provided by healthcare professionals, hospitals, and clinics. The physical distance between the demand and supply of care is often considered a key indicator of accessibility.

However, physical distance alone is not enough to determine accessibility. It is also important to consider social and economic distances, which are often linked to factors such as culture, language, ethnicity, social class, etc. These factors can influence people's ability to access healthcare services because they can affect their ability to navigate the healthcare system, their trust in healthcare professionals, and their ability to pay costs associated with care.

Ultimately, the level of accessibility is measured by the effective use of health services and the improvement in the health status of populations. This means that health services must be accessible enough for people to use them regularly, depending on their health needs. Additionally, accessibility should be assessed on an ongoing basis to ensure that inequalities and potential barriers to accessing health services are identified and addressed.

The dimensions of accessibility, namely social, economic, and physical distances, are closely linked and result in the definition of a level of accessibility which translates into the use of health services and the improvement of health status of populations. These dimensions, as well as the factors that describe them, in particular their components and their statistical variables, make it possible to identify inequalities in terms of accessibility and to determine overall or specific accessibility to care. As a result, we can attempt to modify these inequalities, especially regarding spatial aspects [11].

2.3 Limitations and criticisms of indicators

Healthcare accessibility indicators are essential for evaluating and improving health systems. However, they have several limitations and are subject to important criticisms that must be considered for appropriate use and interpretation.

2.3.1 *Validity and reliability*

The validity and reliability of indicators are often questioned. Validity concerns the ability of an indicator to measure what it is intended to measure. For example, the number of doctors per capita, although frequently used, may not reflect actual accessibility if doctors are unevenly distributed or if their specialty does not match the needs of the population [12]. Reliability, in turn, refers to the consistency of indicators over time and across different contexts. Variations in data collection methods or definitions of indicators can compromise their reliability and, therefore, their usefulness for monitoring progress or comparing different health systems.

2.3.2 *Data coverage and granularity*

Indicators may suffer from a lack of disaggregated data, thus masking disparities within populations [13]. For example, national averages may hide significant inequalities between urban and rural regions or between different socio-economic groups. Additionally, reliance on often self-reported data can introduce bias, affecting the accuracy of indicators.

2.3.3 *Contextualization and interpretation*

Indicators may lack context, limiting their ability to provide a comprehensive understanding of access to care. They may not consider factors such as quality of care, language or cultural barriers, and patients' personal experience [14]. Additionally, the interpretation of indicators can be complicated by the diversity of health systems and populations, requiring nuanced analysis that considers local specificities and social determinants of health.

2.3.4 *Power dynamics and politicization*

Healthcare accessibility indicators are also subject to political and economic influences, which can bias the selection, interpretation, and use of indicators [15]. Decision-makers may favor certain indicators that favorably reflect their policies or their performance, to the detriment of a more objective assessment of accessibility to care.

2.3.5 *Toward more inclusive measures*

In the face of these criticisms, there are calls for the development of more inclusive and holistic indicators, which incorporate qualitative measures, and which reflect a wider range of dimensions of accessibility, including patient satisfaction and aspects of health equity [16]. It is also crucial to take a participatory approach in developing indicators, including patient and community perspectives to ensure that measures are relevant and meaningful to those directly affected by access issues in care.

In summary, although healthcare accessibility indicators are valuable tools for evaluating health systems, they have significant limitations that must be considered. A critical and thoughtful approach is necessary to interpret the indicators, considering their limitations and seeking to develop more comprehensive and equitable measures that accurately capture the complexity of healthcare accessibility.

DOI: http://dx.doi.org/10.5772/intechopen.1006821

3. Determinants of access to care

Access to healthcare concerns helping people obtain appropriate health resources to maintain or improve their health [4]. This access involves several aspects: the availability of services, which must be adequate; the absence of financial, organizational, and socio-cultural barriers that would limit use; the relevance and effectiveness of services to achieve satisfactory health outcomes; and assessing the availability of services and barriers to their use in the context of the varied perspectives, health needs, and material and cultural environments of different social groups.

3.1 Geographic and demographic factors

Accessibility to healthcare services is profoundly influenced by geographic and demographic factors, which often determine where and how services are provided and used. According to McLafferty [17], the use of geographic information systems (GIS) in public health can reveal significant disparities in the accessibility of care between urban and rural regions. These tools make it possible to visualize trends in access to care and define targeted improvement strategies.

Frenk [18] addresses health systems reform by emphasizing the importance of considering demographic distribution and geographic infrastructure when planning and implementing health services. This perspective is crucial to ensure that health services adequately respond to the distribution and specific needs of populations.

Furthermore, Hart's Law of Inverse Care [19] illustrates how healthcare resources are often distributed unequally, with fewer services available to those who need them most. This law highlights the need for an equitable approach in the distribution of health services to counter geographic and demographic inequalities.

Dixon and Le Grand [20] examined whether greater choice for patients is compatible with equity in the English National Health Service (NHS). They suggest that without adequate consideration of geographic and demographic factors, increasing patient choice may actually exacerbate inequalities in access to care.

These sources indicate that policymakers must understand and address geographic and demographic complexities to improve access to care. Effective health policy must therefore incorporate strategies that recognize and address regional disparities and demographic distribution to promote equitable access to health care.

Studies specializing in rural health highlight unique challenges related to access to care for populations far from urban centers. Research published in the *Journal of Rural Health* suggests that difficulties accessing care in these regions are compounded by several factors. First, the significant distances that rural residents must travel to access healthcare represent a significant barrier, especially in emergency situations or for specialized care that is not available locally.

Additionally, the lack of health professionals in rural areas, especially specialists, is a major concern. Low population densities in these areas make it difficult to maintain full-time specialists, leading to gaps in available services. This phenomenon is illustrated by studies such as that of Casey et al. [21], who examined the characteristics of surgical practice in rural areas.

These problems are exacerbated by the fact that rural populations are often made up of demographically vulnerable groups, such as the elderly or low-income, who are already prone to experiencing health inequalities. Hartley [22] discussed how these demographic factors can influence the health of rural communities and their access to care.

In sum, the differences between health services available in rural versus urban areas require careful attention from policymakers and healthcare providers to develop tailored solutions that meet the unique needs of rural populations. To address these accessibility issues, initiatives such as increasing telemedicine services, incentivizing rural practice for new health professionals, and grant programs for rural health centers have been suggested and need to be explored further.

3.2 Economic factors

If there is no specific pathology of the poor, poverty is accompanied by a great vulnerability to a wide range of ordinary pathologies [23]. The frequency of depression and various psychological disorders related to anxiety generated by living conditions are often noted [24]. In addition, removing the most vulnerable people from care systems requires the implementation of specific support methods [25].

To reduce health inequalities, it is essential to not only focus on narrow health goals, but also to consider the material and social aspects of health. Indeed, health inequalities are often linked to broader social and economic factors, such as access to quality jobs, safe and affordable housing, healthy diets, quality education, a clean and safe environment., and positive social relationships [26].

People living in poverty may be particularly vulnerable to illness because they often have limited access to preventive and curative health care, which can lead to self-medication or resignation to illness; in poor households where several people are sick, limited resources can lead to difficult choices about which sick people will receive priority care, which can lead to a delay in medical care and risk to the patient's life.

Additionally, people with chronic or disabling illnesses may be vulnerable to poverty due to high healthcare costs, loss of income, and employment difficulties. These economic factors can have significant consequences for these individuals and their families.

On the other hand, reports from the World Health Organization (WHO) offer statistics on access to care in different age groups and socio-economic categories, showing how factors such as age, gender, and economic status can influence access to care. For example, older or economically disadvantaged populations may not have the same level of access to health services due to financial barriers, mobility, or systemic discrimination.

To reduce these social health inequalities, it is essential to put in place policies and programs that improve access to healthcare for the most vulnerable populations, as well as social and economic protection measures to prevent poverty and social exclusion. This may include community healthcare programs, healthcare subsidies, training and employment programs, and other measures to promote the economic and social inclusion of vulnerable populations [27].

Indeed, human beings are not all equal in terms of access to the benefits of life and face different difficulties. To achieve fairer living conditions, it is necessary to guarantee each individual equal opportunities to flourish and escape situations of vulnerability.

This can be achieved by adopting policies and practices that promote equality of opportunity and the redistribution of resources, focusing on the provision of health, education, housing, and employment services, and by ensuring that every person has access to the resources necessary to meet their basic needs.

It is important to work toward creating a world where every person can live with dignity and security without having to suffer the consequences of economic or social vulnerability. This requires international solidarity and cooperation, as well as national policies that take into account social inequalities in health and aim to reduce them.

The influence of financial factors on healthcare access and utilization is complex and multifaceted. Fees directly associated with health services, such as drug prescriptions, have been shown to have a disincentive effect on their use [28]. Likewise, indirect costs can represent significant barriers, particularly for disadvantaged populations and those living in rural areas. Current data on the impact of pricing structures on healthcare availability and utilization, however, remains limited and does not allow for easy generalization, indicating a need for further research in this area.

3.3 Cultural and social factors

Cultural beliefs and practices play a significant role in how individuals perceive illness and seek care. According to Kleinman [29], each culture has a unique belief system that influences the understanding of what an illness is and how it should be treated. Therefore, individuals may turn to traditional remedies or local healers, rooted in their cultural heritage, rather than conventional medicine. This preference for traditional methods may be due to a distrust of modern medicine, a greater faith in ancestral practices, or simply a matter of accessibility and familiarity. Such inclinations may not only delay seeking appropriate medical care but also create barriers to the adoption of essential preventive practices such as vaccination, negatively influencing public health programs and disease prevention efforts.

Language barriers are another major barrier to healthcare accessibility, hampering effective communication between patients and healthcare providers. As Airhihenbuwa [30] points out, cultural competence in health services goes beyond simple translation of words and encompasses a deep understanding of the cultural contexts that influence health communication. The inability to communicate in the patient's native language can lead to misunderstandings, misinterpretation of diagnoses and treatments, and ultimately, a decline in the quality of care. Therefore, establishing interpretation services and training healthcare professionals in intercultural communication is crucial to overcoming these barriers and ensuring that all patients, regardless of language, receive understandable and respectful care.

Additionally, stigma and discrimination associated with certain health conditions or specific social groups may discourage individuals from seeking care for fear of judgment or ostracization. Smedley et al. [31] highlight how bias, whether conscious or unconscious, within health systems can negatively influence access to care and health outcomes, particularly for ethnic minorities and marginalized groups. Combating stigma and promoting equity in healthcare requires a systems approach that addresses not only individual attitudes but also the institutional structures that perpetuate inequality and exclusion.

Family structures and community support networks are fundamental pillars that strongly influence health behaviors and decisions. The family, as the primary unit of social support, plays a crucial role in recognizing health problems, making decisions about seeking care, and providing support throughout the treatment process. Andrulis [32] highlights the importance of these dynamics by emphasizing that, depending on the family and community context, access to care can be significantly facilitated or hindered. For example, in some cultures, health decisions are made collectively, meaning that family opinions and beliefs can strongly influence the individual in their decision whether or not to seek medical care. This can be particularly beneficial when the family actively encourages its members to use available prevention and treatment services.

However, family or community norms and expectations can also constitute barriers to accessing care. In some cases, stigmas associated with certain health conditions or traditional beliefs may deter individuals from seeking external medical help [33]. Additionally, traditional gender roles within the family may impose additional constraints, particularly on women, who may be assigned primary responsibility for caring for other family members, thereby limiting their ability to seek care for themselves [34]. Pressure to adhere to community norms and values may also prevent individuals from seeking care that is perceived to be at odds with these beliefs.

To overcome these challenges, it is essential to promote public health interventions that actively engage families and communities in the healthcare process. This can include health education that respects and integrates cultural and family values, while providing information on the importance of medical and preventive care. Establishing community awareness programs and accessible health services within communities can help build trust and reduce stigma associated with seeking care. By recognizing and addressing family and community dynamics in the planning and implementation of health services, it is possible to create a more inclusive and supportive environment that promotes equitable access to care for all individuals.

3.4 Institutional and political factors

Institutional and political factors play a dominant role in the accessibility to health care, shaping health systems through decisions that affect the distribution of resources, healthcare infrastructure, and the regulatory framework. As Navarro and Shi [35] pointed out, the political context profoundly influences the structure of health care, creating environments that can either facilitate or hinder access to necessary medical services. Health policies focused on equity and inclusion are crucial to reducing barriers to accessing care, while the absence of such policies can worsen existing disparities.

Primary care reform is often cited as a key lever for improving access to care. Saltman et al. [36] discuss the importance of placing primary care at the heart of the health system, arguing that this helps ensure an accessible, affordable, and high-quality base of care for all. This strategy strengthens the health system's capacity to provide early interventions and ongoing disease management, helping to prevent complications and reduce the need for more expensive specialized care.

Social determinants of health, such as economic and social factors, also have a major impact on health inequalities, as highlighted by Marmot and Wilkinson [37]. Health policies must therefore encompass a broader perspective, addressing the roots of disparities by improving living conditions, access to education, and employment opportunities. These measures can help alleviate health inequalities by directly addressing the factors that negatively influence individuals' well-being.

The equitable availability and distribution of health resources is also essential to ensure universal access to care. Gulliford and Morgan [38] highlight the need for fair allocation of health professionals, medical facilities, and equipment to effectively meet the needs of all communities, including the most marginalized. Strategic planning and resource allocation based on the real needs of populations can greatly improve the accessibility and quality of health care.

Equity issues are at the center of concerns for health systems [39]. Health justice involves responding equitably to the varied health needs of different populations, ensuring that health systems are inclusive and responsive to the diversity of needs. This requires recognition and consideration of the specific vulnerabilities of certain groups, such as low-income populations, ethnic minorities, and rural areas, to ensure that no one is left behind.

The World Health Organization report [40] on financing health systems highlights the crucial importance of universal coverage to achieve equitable access to care. Financing mechanisms should be designed to remove financial barriers, allowing every individual to access necessary health services without incurring financial hardship. This involves reforms in health financing systems to ensure adequate and accessible coverage for all.

In conclusion, institutional and policy factors largely determine accessibility to health care. Establishing equitable and well-designed health policies, promoting primary care, paying attention to social determinants of health, equitable distribution of health resources, and a commitment to health justice are essential to building accessible and inclusive health systems. By acting on these levers, it is possible to move toward universal accessibility to care, thus guaranteeing that each individual has the opportunity to enjoy the best possible state of health.

4. Inequalities in access to care

Equitable access to healthcare is a cornerstone of modern health systems and a key indicator of social justice. However, despite progress, inequalities persist, impacting individuals' ability to obtain timely, quality care. The following section focuses on the multiple dimensions of inequalities in access to care and their impact on public health.

4.1 Regional and rural disparities

Regional and rural disparities in access to healthcare represent a major challenge for healthcare systems across the world [41]. These inequalities arise from various structural, geographic, and economic factors that hamper the availability, accessibility, and quality of health services for populations living in rural areas. The lack of primary and specialized health infrastructure in these areas is a central problem. As Ricketts pointed out [41], there is often a disproportionate concentration of medical facilities in urban areas, leaving rural communities underserved. This polarization is partly explained by economic considerations, such as the high costs associated with providing health services in sparsely populated areas, which can reduce the return on investment for healthcare providers.

Another critical aspect of regional disparities is the shortage of health professionals in rural areas. Hartley [22], in 2004, highlighted that doctors and other health professionals are often reluctant to settle and practice in these regions due to constraints such as limited career opportunities, isolation geographic, and restricted access to resources. This shortage compromises access to primary care and specialized services, leading to prolonged wait times and increased workload for the few available providers.

Rural populations also face significant barriers in terms of continued access to health care. Physical distance from health centers, combined with a limited supply of transportation, can discourage individuals from seeking care, especially for services requiring regular monitoring or management of chronic diseases. Larson and Fleishman [42] addressed these barriers, highlighting how economic challenges specific to rural areas, such as higher poverty levels, can make the costs of care prohibitive for many families.

Faced with these challenges, it is imperative to put in place strategies aimed at improving access and quality of care in rural regions. Possible initiatives include financial incentives to encourage health professionals to practice in rural areas, the development of telemedicine to overcome geographic barriers, and the implementation of mobile health programs to reach isolated populations. MacDowell and colleagues have discussed these approaches, highlighting their potential to significantly improve access to care in rural communities [43].

These regional and rural disparities require continued attention and innovative strategies to ensure that all individuals, regardless of where they live, have equitable access to health care. This involves a substantial investment in health infrastructure, an increased valorization of medical practice in rural areas and the adoption of healthcare technologies adapted to the specific needs of these populations. By addressing these issues head on, it is possible to build more inclusive and equitable health systems that effectively serve all sections of the population.

To conclude, the presence of regional and rural disparities represents a serious obstacle to the establishment of health systems that are both just and universal. Solving these issues requires a comprehensive and varied approach that takes into consideration the multiple facets — geographic, economic, and social — that characterize the provision of healthcare in rural areas. By implementing specifically tailored policies and devoting appropriate resources, it is possible to substantially increase access to health services for rural communities. This, in turn, will play a crucial role in reducing health disparities and promoting greater health equity.

4.2 Socio-economic inequalities

Social inequalities in health refer to unjust and avoidable differences in health status between groups of people belonging to different socio-economic categories. These inequalities often reflect broader inequalities in society, such as access to education, work, housing, food and the environment.

Social inequalities in health can have serious consequences for individuals and communities. People from disadvantaged groups often have shorter life expectancy, poorer mental health, and a higher prevalence of chronic diseases. These inequalities can also affect people's quality of life, their ability to work and participate fully in society, and are avoidable because they are socially constructed determinants [26]. Social inequalities can manifest themselves in the form of health inequalities, which are often linked to living and working conditions. In other words, some people may be socio-economically disadvantaged, which may result in avoidable and unjust health differences.

Each social position comes with a specific level of resources – whether material, behavioral or psychosocial resources – as well as exposure to different risk factors. In other words, an individual's social position can influence their level of access to resources and their exposure to conditions promoting or disfavoring health [26]. Indeed, social differences in health are the result of the combination of these resources and these risks. Depending on an individual's social position, this combination can have a significant impact on their health, contributing to the health inequalities observed between different population groups.

There are several models that seek to explain how social determinants can influence an individual's health status, and how these determinants can interact with each other. Indeed, it is important to understand how social factors can influence each other and have cumulative effects on health, to implement effective interventions to reduce social inequalities in health [26]. The most recent model is that developed by the WHO Commission on Health Determinants [44]. It distinguishes three fundamental components which are the socio-economic and political context, the structural determinants linked to the socio-economic position of individuals and the intermediate determinants (**Figure 1**).

Indeed, health inequalities and their determinants are closely linked to theories of social justice. Differences in access to health information, income level, and other social factors all impact health behaviors, which cannot be viewed solely as individual choices. In reality, health inequalities are often the result of broader social and economic factors that influence individual choices and behaviors, such as the environment in which a person lives, works and develops. Therefore, interventions to reduce health inequalities must consider these broader social and economic factors, and not simply focus on individual responsibility [45].

Following the previous clarifications, we will continue to clearly present the evaluation and measurement of accessibility to care, considering attendance and the potential for access to the service as a measurable reality.

4.3 Inequalities linked to gender, age, and ethnicity

Inequalities in access to healthcare related to gender, age, and ethnicity constitute significant barriers that reflect deep societal disparities and institutional biases. These inequalities can limit access to preventive care, treatment, and chronic disease management for certain groups, leading to long-term consequences on their well-being and overall health.

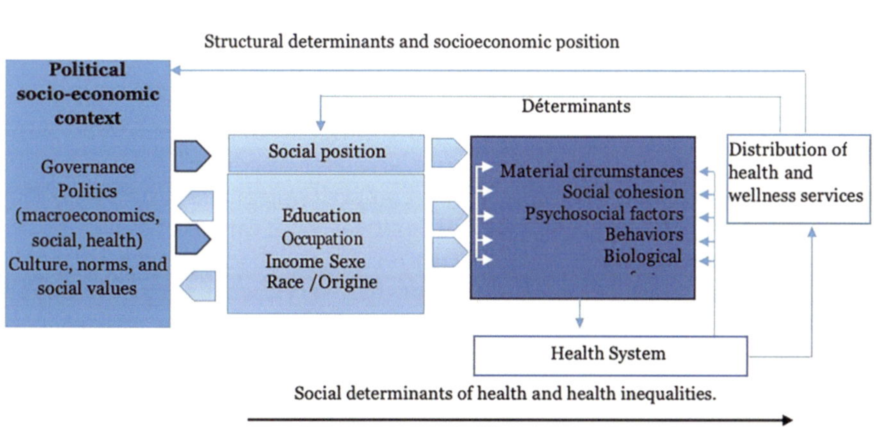

Figure 1.
WHO's model of social determinant of health. Source: Commission on Social Determinants of Health, WHO (2009).

4.3.1 Impact of gender on access to care

Women face distinct challenges in accessing health care, exacerbated by deeply ingrained cultural norms and gender roles that shape their experience with the healthcare system. The report by Sen et al. [46] for the WHO Commission on Social Determinants of Health highlights that gender inequalities in health are not simply the result of biological differences but are often rooted in unequal social structures that limit access for women to education, paid employment and autonomy in decision-making.

Reproductive healthcare represents a particularly critical area where gender inequalities are evident. Studies show that, in many regions, women are less likely than men to have adequate access to comprehensive reproductive health information and services such as contraception, maternal health and screenings for sexually transmitted diseases. Transmissible [47]. Financial barriers, lack of confidentiality, and social stigma are all obstacles that can prevent women from seeking and receiving quality reproductive health care.

Furthermore, women are often disadvantaged in terms of access to healthcare in general due to institutional biases and gender stereotypes within health systems themselves. Studies like that of Mead et al. [48] revealed that women's symptoms are more likely to be downplayed or misinterpreted by healthcare providers, which can delay diagnoses and treatments, and can negatively impact health outcomes.

Strategies to overcome these inequities require not only increasing access to health services but also changing attitudes and practices within the health system. Education and training of health professionals on gender bias, as well as the development of policies that specifically recognize and address the health needs of women, are crucial to reducing these inequalities [49].

To ensure more equal access to care, it is also essential to invest in public health programs that specifically target women, particularly in the areas of prevention and well-being, and to provide sufficient resources to fight against the social determinants of health that disproportionately affect women. Finally, increased representation of women in health decision-making bodies can contribute to better consideration of their specific perspectives and needs in the planning and implementation of health services.

4.3.2 Age-related vulnerabilities

Children and older adults, due to their specific life stages, face distinct barriers to accessing health care. Children, particularly those from disadvantaged backgrounds, may experience negative consequences for their development and future well-being due to insufficient access to preventive and curative health care. Services such as vaccinations, regular checkups and interventions for childhood illnesses are essential for this age group. The coverage and quality of these services can vary considerably depending on the region, the economic resources of families and the available public health infrastructure.

For older adults, access to care is often complicated by physical challenges, multiple chronic conditions, and a higher prevalence of frailty or dependency. Reduced mobility may limit the ability to travel to healthcare centers, and limited financial resources may restrict available care options. Older adults may also face gaps in insurance coverage plans that do not adequately address the long-term or specialized care needs that become more common with age. The work of Angel and Angel [50] shows that the need for care adapted to aging is crucial, and the absence of this can lead to deterioration of health and a reduction in quality of life for older people.

Public health programs and policies must recognize and adapt to the specific needs of children and older people to overcome these age-related vulnerabilities. This may include establishing home health services or specialized geriatric care, improving access to preventive care for children, and ensuring that insurance plans cover health needs throughout the lifespan. Throughout life. Initiatives such as home visits by healthcare professionals for the elderly and companion programs for children's medical appointments are examples of solutions that can improve accessibility.

Furthermore, it is essential to encourage research and investment in innovative health technologies that can facilitate access to care for these groups. For example, telemedicine can be particularly beneficial for older adults, allowing them to receive medical consultations without having to travel. For children, the development of mobile health applications that allow parents to track their children's health and receive reminders for vaccinations and checkups can contribute to better child health management.

It is therefore imperative to implement targeted strategies that address the unique needs of children and older adults, to ensure that these vulnerable age groups receive the care they need to lead healthy and productive lives.

4.3.3 Ethnic disparities

Ethnic disparities in access to healthcare are a serious public health problem that results from a complex set of social, economic, and systemic factors. Williams and Mohammed [49] highlight that individuals belonging to ethnic minorities often face systematic barriers that reduce their ability to obtain appropriate medical care. These obstacles include not only language and cultural barriers, but also prejudice and discrimination which can influence the quality of care provided.

People from ethnic minorities may have difficulty navigating a healthcare system that does not always recognize their language, cultural beliefs, or traditional practices. Communication is a critical aspect of quality care, and the lack of interpretation services or educational materials in their native language can lead to insufficient understanding of medical instructions and treatment options, as shown by content analysis by Read and Gorman [47].

Additionally, ethnic health disparities are often linked to broader socio-economic inequalities. Ethnic minorities are disproportionately represented among low-income populations, resulting in lower health insurance rates and less ability to pay for care not covered by basic plans [51]. Health insurance policies that do not take these disparities into account can worsen inequality of access to care.

The consequences of these ethnic disparities are wide-ranging and include higher prevalence of chronic diseases, higher infant mortality rates, and reduced life expectancy for minority groups. To effectively address these inequalities, it is imperative to put in place targeted and culturally adapted interventions. Healthcare providers must be trained to recognize and address implicit bias, and healthcare systems must commit to developing inclusive and welcoming environments for all ethnic groups.

Interventions must also go beyond medical care to address the social determinants of health that underlie ethnic disparities. This includes programs to improve education, housing, employment and living conditions, all of which have a profound impact on the health of individuals and communities. Furthermore, efforts to improve access to care must be accompanied by more accurate and disaggregated data collection that can inform policies and practices aimed at reducing ethnic health inequalities.

4.4 Impacts of inequalities on public health

Inequalities in access to healthcare have profound and widespread implications for public health, affecting not only the quality of life of individuals but also society as a whole. The impacts of these inequalities manifest across several dimensions, including health indicators, economic costs, and social cohesion.

4.4.1 Effects on health indicators

Inequalities in access to healthcare exacerbate health disparities across various social dimensions, including income, education, location, ethnicity, and gender. As Marmot [52] points out, socio-economic inequalities are intrinsically linked to negative health indicators. For example, people living in poverty or in disadvantaged neighborhoods tend to have higher rates of chronic diseases, premature mortality, and a higher incidence of mental health problems.

Differences in life expectancy between socio-economic groups clearly illustrate the impact of inequalities in access to care [52]. Individuals from disadvantaged backgrounds not only have a shorter life expectancy, but they also spend a greater part of their lives in poor health or with disability, reducing their quality of life and their ability to contribute to society.

Disparities related to gender, age, and ethnicity add an additional layer of complexity to health inequalities. Women, for example, may face specific barriers in accessing reproductive and sexual health care, which can impact their overall health and well-being. Children from low-income families or ethnic minorities may not receive necessary vaccinations on time, putting them at higher risks of preventable diseases.

Additionally, older adults and ethnic minorities often face systemic barriers that limit their access to quality care. These barriers can include prohibitive costs, a lack of culturally competent healthcare providers, and difficulty navigating a complex healthcare system. These barriers contribute to delayed disease detection, less effective treatments, and poor health outcomes for these populations.

To reverse these trends and improve health indicators for all, it is crucial to adopt a comprehensive approach that addresses not only the symptoms of health inequalities but also their root causes. This involves investing in social and economic interventions that target the social determinants of health, such as education, housing, and employment, in addition to strengthening universal access to high-quality health care. Such an approach requires close coordination between the public health, education, housing, and employment sectors to create environments that promote health and well-being for all members of society, regardless of their socio-economic status, age, gender, or ethnic origin.

4.4.2 Impact on social cohesion

The impact of inequalities in access to healthcare on social cohesion is a complex and multifaceted phenomenon. Perceived unfairness in access to healthcare can lead to feelings of exclusion and isolation among disadvantaged populations, which can, in turn, weaken the social fabric and decrease trust in public institutions. and health systems.

Sense of injustice and exclusion: The sense of injustice felt by individuals and communities who do not have equitable access to healthcare can have profound impacts on social cohesion. When people perceive that their right to health is not respected equally, this can lead to feelings of exclusion and marginalization. These perceptions of injustice may be exacerbated in communities where health disparities are visible, and stories of neglect or unequal treatment are common.

Erosion of trust: The erosion of trust in public institutions, particularly in the health system, is a direct consequence of inequalities in access to care. As Link and Phelan [53] point out, trust is an essential pillar of social cohesion and societal stability. When citizens believe that the healthcare system is inequitable or that institutions are not meeting their needs, trust can quickly erode, threatening the legitimacy of institutions and the willingness of individuals to participate in public health initiatives.

Social fragmentation: Health inequalities can also lead to social fragmentation, where divisions between different social groups widen due to differences in access to healthcare and health outcomes. This fragmentation is particularly concerning in diverse societies, where health inequalities may intersect and reinforce other social divides, such as those based on race, ethnicity, income, or geography.

Strategies for strengthening social cohesion: To mitigate the impact of inequalities in access to healthcare on social cohesion, it is essential to promote inclusive and equitable health policies that recognize and address the needs of all parts of the community. Population. This involves ensuring equitable representation of different social groups in the planning and implementation of health policies, as well as promoting community health initiatives that promote the engagement and participation of all citizens.

Additionally, efforts should be made to improve transparency and communication around public health decisions, to build trust and demonstrate commitment to health equity. Establishing accountability and feedback mechanisms that allow citizens to express themselves and contribute to decision-making can also help build trust in health systems and promote greater social cohesion.

5. Policies and interventions aimed at improving access to care

Continuing our exploration of healthcare accessibility, Section 5 of this chapter looks at policies and strategic interventions implemented nationally and internationally. These initiatives are crucial to reducing health disparities and ensuring that every individual can access quality care, regardless of their geographic or economic situation. This section examines the concerted efforts of governments, international organizations, and local actors to design and implement strategies that address the complex challenges of healthcare accessibility.

5.1 National and international strategies

To deepen the discussion on "National and International Strategies" regarding access to care, it is essential to consider the central role of public health policies and the regulatory frameworks that underpin these strategies. The World Health Organization (WHO) plays a leading role in setting international standards and promoting policies to ensure universal access to care. The Sustainable Development Goals (SDGs), notably SDG 3 which aims to ensure healthy lives and promote well-being for all at all ages, provide a framework for action for member countries.

At the national level, strategies vary considerably depending on the specific political, economic, and cultural contexts of each country. For example, health system reforms in Brazil with the "Estratégia Saúde da Família" (Family Health Strategy) initiative emphasized a family and community-centered primary healthcare approach, which contributed to notable improvements in access to care in rural regions and disadvantaged communities.

The family and community-centered approach to primary healthcare is recognized for its potential to improve accessibility and quality of care. This strategy involves close collaboration between health professionals and communities to identify and respond to specific health needs, promoting better acceptance and use of health services. A study by Macinko and Harris [54] showed how the Estrategia Saúde da Família in Brazil improved health indicators through this community-based approach.

Disease prevention and health promotion is another pillar of this method, emphasizing health education and healthy behaviors within communities. A systematic literature review by Berra et al. [55] highlighted the effectiveness of health promotion interventions in primary care to improve health behaviors and prevent chronic diseases.

Multidisciplinary care teams, made up of doctors, nurses, community health workers, and other professionals, play a crucial role in providing holistic and personalized care. According to a study by Starfield and Shi [56], the existence of well-structured primary care teams is strongly associated with better population health, greater equity, and reduced costs.

However, this approach faces challenges, including the need for sufficient resources, adequate training of health professionals, and political commitment. An analysis by Viana et al. [57] explored the challenges of implementing the Estrategia Saúde da Família in Brazil, highlighting the importance of investment in human resources and infrastructure.

The United Kingdom's healthcare model – like other countries in Europe – embodied by the National Health Service (NHS), represents an approach where services are mainly financed by the State, aiming to ensure equality of access to care for all citizens, regardless of their financial situation. This design is distinct from models where healthcare is largely dependent on private insurance and may be influenced by the ability of individuals to pay for health services.

One of the cornerstones of the NHS is its commitment to the provision of universal care, based on need rather than ability to pay. This means that every UK resident has access to a wide range of health services without direct costs at the point of care. This includes, but is not limited to, medical consultations, hospital treatment, emergency services, and certain types of dental and eye care.

However, the system is not without challenges. NHS health policy must constantly adapt to meet the changing needs of the population, which can be influenced by demographic factors, technological advances, changes in disease patterns, and increasing patient expectations. Dixon and Le Grand [20] notably discussed the tension between increasing patient choice in the NHS and maintaining equity of care. The central argument is how the NHS can enable patients to have more choices in healthcare without compromising equity, that is, without creating disparities in access and quality care between different social and economic groups.

Increasing patient choice can be seen as a way to improve patient satisfaction and personalize care. This could potentially lead to better treatment adherence and improved health outcomes. However, there is a risk that this could also lead to a "commodification" of care, where resources are unevenly distributed based on patients' ability to navigate the system, their level of information, or their geographic proximity to quality healthcare providers.

In response to these challenges, the NHS has undertaken various reforms and initiatives to improve the efficiency, accessibility, and quality of services. This includes efforts to further integrate health and social care services, improve value-based care delivery, and harness digital technologies to improve access to care and efficiency.

These examples illustrate the diversity of approaches adopted around the world to improve access to health care. Evaluating the effectiveness of these strategies is crucial for their continuous improvement. Data from research and policy evaluations provide valuable information for adjusting programs and guiding future public health initiatives.

5.2 Local and community interventions

Local and community interventions play a crucial role in improving access to healthcare, specifically targeting vulnerable and isolated populations. These initiatives take a grassroots approach, seeking to understand and respond to the specific needs of the communities they serve.

Community health initiatives: Community health initiatives, and particularly community health insurance programs in low- and middle-income countries, play an important role in improving access to healthcare and protecting against catastrophic healthcare costs. These programs are designed to mobilize resources within communities and provide collective health coverage, with a particular emphasis on including the most vulnerable individuals and families.

Community participation is a pillar of these programs, allowing community members to play an active role in health insurance management and decision-making regarding which health services to cover. This approach not only promotes a sense of belonging and responsibility among community members but also contributes to better matching of health services to local needs.

According to Ekman in his study [58], community health insurance initiatives can be particularly effective in reducing financial barriers to accessing healthcare and in promoting the use of necessary health services. Community participation and solidarity help spread health risks among members, thereby reducing the financial impact of healthcare on the most vulnerable individuals.

Additionally, a systematic review by Wiesmann and Jütting [59] highlights that these programs have the potential to improve health equity by providing financial protection and increasing access to health services for disadvantaged populations. The authors note that the effectiveness of these programs depends largely on their design, their implementation, and the socio-economic and cultural context in which they operate.

It is also important to recognize the challenges associated with these programs, particularly in terms of financial sustainability, quality of care, and capacity to cover a wide range of health services. Despite these challenges, community health insurance programs represent a promising strategy to improve access to healthcare and protect against catastrophic health expenditures in resource-limited settings.

Mobile health programs and ambulant clinics: Mobile health programs, such as those discussed in the article by Hill et al. [60], illustrate how providing health services directly in communities can overcome geographic barriers and improve access to care. These mobile clinics are particularly beneficial in remote or underserved areas, where health infrastructure is limited or absent. By bringing care directly to patients, these programs reduce the need for often costly and time-consuming travel for individuals living in these areas.

These clinics offer a diverse range of health services, including emergency care, preventive medicine, chronic disease management, and behavioral health services, helping to bridge the gaps between community health needs and traditional modes of care delivery [61].

Mobile clinics serve diverse populations, including those from ethnic and racial minorities, the homeless, displaced populations, recent immigrants, migrant workers, those without insurance, and children. These clinics have a significant impact onaccessibility to care for uninsured and low-income people, providing care often free or at reduced cost and eliminating logistical barriers such as transportation issues and administrative processes complex (102).

Additionally, mobile clinics have played a crucial role during the COVID-19 pandemic [62], filling gaps in healthcare delivery networks and reaching vulnerable people in both rural and urban areas. Their ability to quickly adapt to community needs and provide testing and triage services, as well as telehealth services, has been particularly valuable during this time.

Role of NGOs and local associations: Non-governmental organizations (NGOs) and local associations play a pivotal role in strengthening access to health care, particularly in regions where health systems are fragile or insufficiently developed. Their commitment to health service delivery, research, and health policy implementation contributes significantly to closing gaps in access to care for disadvantaged populations.

In post-conflict or low-resource contexts like Timor-Leste, international NGOs have played a crucial role in rebuilding devastated health infrastructure. Their ability to quickly mobilize resources and implement health programs effectively has accelerated the process of restoring essential health services to affected populations. These initiatives are not limited to the provision of medical care but also encompass the training of local health personnel, the provision of medical equipment and the construction of health facilities, thus demonstrating the versatility and impact of NGOs in the strengthening health systems [63].

Partnerships between NGOs, governments, and donors, as observed in Pakistan, illustrate the importance of strategic collaboration to improve access to health care. These partnerships leverage the strengths of each actor, combining the technical expertise and resources of NGOs with the institutional support and legitimacy of governments. By focusing on targeted interventions such as immunization, maternal and child health, or combating communicable diseases, these collaborations have the potential to significantly improve health outcomes for the communities served [64].

In Ghana, public-NGO partnerships have been recognized for their ability to innovate in health service delivery. By integrating health services within communities and ensuring that interventions are adapted to local contexts, these collaborations have succeeded in making healthcare more accessible and acceptable to local populations. This community-based service delivery model highlights the vital role that NGOs and local associations can play in designing and implementing health solutions that respect the cultural and social specificities of the communities they serve [65].

Finally, the involvement of NGOs in research for development in global health helps generate essential knowledge for the development of effective health policies. By participating in research and contributing to innovation in healthcare, NGOs help establish evidence-based practices that can be adopted more widely to improve the accessibility and quality of healthcare. This contribution to the global health knowledge base is fundamental to identifying the most effective strategies to respond to public health challenges [66].

These different facets of the role of NGOs and local associations in the field of health illustrate their essential contribution to achieving universal access to health care. By leveraging their flexibility, capacity for innovation, and proximity to communities, these organizations continue to play a central role in improving the health and well-being of populations around the world.

Awareness and health education projects: Awareness and health education projects are essential components in improving accessibility to health care, arming individuals with the knowledge and skills to make informed decisions about their health. These initiatives can have a significant impact on health behaviors and access to health services, especially in urban areas and socially disadvantaged communities.

A systematic review [67] on community-based health promotion interventions found that 75% of articles reviewed reported improvements in at least one health behavior, access to health services, health literacy, health, and/or a range of health outcomes. However, large-scale community health promotion programs have often resulted in limited or absent population-level changes, in part due to methodological limitations, competing contextual effects, and limitations of the interventions used. These findings highlight that community-based interventions hold promise for health promotion and disease prevention, but their potential is not yet fully realized. Going forward, these interventions should deliver proximal outcomes and invest in community capacity building.

Community engagement is central to public health, and this engagement should also be central to the work of schools and public health programs. Levin et al. [68] examined best practices and emerging innovations in community engagement for education, research, and practice, including critical service learning, community-based participatory research, and impact collective. Leadership, infrastructure, and culture are key institutional enablers of successful academic endeavors. The main challenges to overcome include distrust of community members, power imbalance, and unequal sharing of credit. Success in this work will advance equity and improve health in communities around the world.

A relevant example of the impact of health education and awareness programs is seen in the health education-based interventions that were implemented to increase awareness and prevention of dengue fever in Delhi, in India. The effectiveness of these health education programs has been demonstrated by a significant increase in knowledge and prevention practices within the community, highlighting the importance of education as a tool for behavioral change and disease prevention [69].

Additionally, health promotion interventions delivered in community settings such as barbers and hair salons in the United States illustrate an innovative approach to reaching specific populations. These programs were designed to reduce risk factors and improve health outcomes related to obesity and related chronic diseases, such as cardiovascular disease and type 2 diabetes, by leveraging trusted community venues to deliver relevant health messages [70].

In the field of oral health, school-based oral health promotion programs, extending from kindergarten to high school, have also demonstrated their effectiveness in improving knowledge, attitudes, and behaviors regarding oral health. Oral health in children and adolescents. These programs have contributed to significant improvements in various aspects of oral health, highlighting the potential of school-based educational interventions to positively influence the health and quality of life of young people [71].

Finally, the United States National Heart, Lung, and Blood Institute (NHLBI) implements health education and awareness programs that aim to effect positive change in public health. These initiatives focus on implementing national programs to help reduce the risk and consequences of heart, lung, blood, and sleep disorders by developing educational programs that address topics such as heart health and high blood pressure [72].

These examples illustrate the significant impact that NGOs, local associations, and health education programs can have on improving health knowledge, changing behaviors, and ultimately, reducing the risk of disease within communities.

5.3 Evaluating policy effectiveness

To further analyze the evaluation of health policy effectiveness, it is essential to understand the nuances of different evaluation methodologies and their application in the public health context.

The interrupted time series method, discussed by Shadish, Cook, and Campbell in "Experimental and Quasi-Experimental Designs for Generalized Causal Inference" [73], is particularly relevant for public health policies where it is difficult to set up trials randomized controlled trials. This approach allows us to observe the effects of a policy by examining trends before and after its implementation, while taking into account natural variations. This method is often used to evaluate public health interventions, such as vaccination campaigns or healthcare reforms, where effects can be observed on large populations over time.

The "Handbook on Impact Evaluation" by Khandker et al. [74] provides quantitative tools for rigorous evaluation of policy impacts. In the health sector, this may include the evaluation of access to care programs or disease prevention strategies. The use of quantitative methods makes it possible to accurately measure changes in health indicators, such as morbidity and mortality rates, access to health services, and the quality of care received.

Pawson and Tilley [75] propose a theory-based approach to understanding how and why a policy works in a given context. This perspective is crucial for evaluating health policies because it considers the complex mechanisms and contexts in which these policies are implemented. Understanding the contextual factors and the mechanisms by which policies produce effects makes it possible to better target interventions and improve their effectiveness.

The "Impact Evaluation in Practice" guide by Gertler et al. is aimed directly at public health practitioners and highlights the importance of carefully planning impact evaluations to ensure they provide reliable and relevant information. The book encourages the use of theoretical frameworks to understand the mechanisms by which policies produce effects, as well as the importance of collecting high-quality data and using appropriate analysis methodologies. Emphasis is placed on the need to communicate results in a transparent and accessible manner to inform decision-makers, practitioners, and the public.

The use of observational data to evaluate health policies is of paramount importance, especially when traditional experimental approaches prove inapplicable. In his book entitled "Observational Studies", Paul R. Rosenbaum [76] carefully addresses the structuring of these studies to draw solid conclusions despite the absence of randomization. It highlights the importance of using sophisticated statistical techniques such as propensity score matching and sensitivity analyses, which can adjust for differences between groups exposed and not exposed to a policy, thereby reducing the bias. These techniques offer researchers the opportunity to evaluate the effect of health policies more precisely by overcoming the constraints associated with non-experimental data.

Rosenbaum also emphasizes the need to employ sound methodological methods to extrapolate causal conclusions from observational studies, which are commonly used for health policy analysis. These studies are essential for evaluating policies in situations where it is neither ethical nor feasible to conduct controlled experiments. It examines strategies to adjust for bias and confounding factors, which is essential to correctly attribute observed results to the intervention being evaluated.

These documents together provide a solid basis for evaluating the performance of health policies, highlighting the need to overcome methodological obstacles and ensure scientific rigor. They also emphasize the importance of putting the results of evaluations into context in relation to health systems and targeted populations, so that health policies are not only effective but also fair and adapted to the needs of beneficiary communities.

These works provide an overview of methods for evaluating the effectiveness of health policies, emphasizing the importance of appropriate selection of methods based on the objectives of the evaluation, the context of the intervention, and the data available. Methodical evaluation is crucial to ensure that health policies achieve their goals and concretely improve access to healthcare for the populations concerned.

6. Conclusion

This chapter highlighted the complexity of accessibility to health care, a theme that is as essential as it is multidimensional. We explored the measures and indicators that make it possible to evaluate this accessibility, while recognizing their limitations and the criticisms they give rise to. In addition, we examined in detail the determinants of access to care, whether geographical, economic, cultural, or institutional, and highlighted the resulting inequalities in access to care, as well as their profound impact on public health.

The issue of regional and rural inequalities, socio-economic disparities, and differences in access related to gender, age, and ethnicity have been of particular concern, revealing how these intersecting factors can hinder health equity. Policies and interventions aimed at improving accessibility were discussed, and the evaluation of their effectiveness highlighted successes, as well as persistent challenges that require continued attention.

In conclusion, this chapter calls for collective and coordinated action to overcome accessibility barriers. The ultimate objective remains to ensure that everyone, regardless of their social status, geographic location, or individual characteristics, can access quality health care. To achieve this, it is imperative that we continue to innovate, evaluate, and reform our health systems with an unwavering commitment to inclusion and equity. This means addressing the social determinants of health, strengthening primary care, and ensuring equitable financing systems that provide universal protection.

The task is arduous, and the obstacles are numerous, but the stakes are high: the health and well-being of our societies. Sustained efforts and renewed commitments to the principles of social justice and solidarity are the only path to a future where accessibility to healthcare will be a reality for all.

Acknowledgements

The authors would like to thank their respective institutions for the support provided during the research and writing of this chapter. Special thanks to the Faculty of Legal, Economic, and Social Sciences Souissi, Mohammed V University in Rabat, and the Faculty of Medicine and Pharmacy, Mohammed V University in Rabat.

The author acknowledges the limited usage of ChatGPT for proofreading and grammar correction of this manuscript.

Author details

Kawtar Zahidi[1*], Majdouline Obtel[2] and Saida Naji[1]

1 Faculty of Legal Economic and Social Sciences Souissi, Mohammed V University in Rabat, Morocco

2 Faculty of Medicine and Pharmacy, Mohammed V University in Rabat, Rabat, Morocco

*Address all correspondence to: kawtar_zahidi@um5.ac.ma

References

[1] Penchansky R, Thomas JW. The concept of access: Definition and relationship to consumer satisfaction. Medical Care. 1981;**19**(2):127-140

[2] Levesque J-F, Harris MF, Russell G. Patient-centred access to health care: Conceptualising access at the interface of health systems and populations. International Journal for Equity in Health. 2013;**12**:18. DOI: 10.1186/1475-9276-12-18

[3] Shah TI, Bell S, Wilson K. Spatial accessibility to health care services: Identifying under-serviced neighbourhoods in Canadian urban areas. PLoS One. 2016;**11**(12):e0168208. DOI: 10.1371/journal.pone.0168208

[4] Gulliford M et al. What does 'access to health care' mean? Journal of Health Services Research & Policy. 2002;7(3):186-188

[5] Bauer S, Weber E. COVID-19: How the use of telemedicine helps rural communities manage the pandemic. Journal of Rural Health. 2020;**36**(4):648-650. DOI: 10.1111/jrh.12442

[6] Braveman P, Gruskin S. Defining equity in health. Journal of Epidemiology & Community Health. 2003;**57**(4):254-258. DOI: 10.1136/jech.57.4.254

[7] Ndonky A, Oliveau S, Lalou R, Dos Santos S. Mesure de l'accessibilité Géographique aux Structures de Santé Dans l'agglomération de Dakar. CyberGeo; 2015. DOI: 10.4000/cybergeo.27312

[8] Picheral H. Dictionnaire raisonné de géographie de la santé. Atelier Géographie de la santé. France: Université Montpellier 3 - Paul Valery; 2001. p. 307

[9] Peters J, Hall GB. Assessment of ambulance response performance using a geographic information system. Social Science and Medicine. 1999;**49**(11):1551-1566

[10] Rochaix L, Tubeuf S. Mesures de l'équité en santé: Fondements éthiques et implications. Revue économique. 2009;**60**(2):325-344

[11] Closing the Gap in a Generation: Health Equity through Action on the Social Determinants of Health - Final Report of the Commission on Social Determinants of Health. Geneva, Switzerland: Social Determinants of Health (SDH); 2008. p. 40

[12] Peter P, Evans T. Évaluation de l'accessibilité aux soins de santé: une revue critique des indicateurs et de leur utilisation dans les systèmes de santé. Bulletin de l'Organisation mondiale de la santé. 2003;**81**(10):762-770

[13] Goddard M, Smith P. Équité d'accès aux soins de santé: une revue des concepts, des principes et des pratiques. Social Science & Medicine. 2001;**53**(6):1149-1162

[14] Lynch J et al. Indicateurs de santé et inégalités: vers une réconciliation. Social Science & Medicine. 2004;**58**(4):587-597

[15] Kawachi I, Kennedy BP. Santé et inégalités sociales: une perspective des sciences sociales. The Lancet. 1997;**349**(9066):1498-1501

[16] Braveman P. Indicateurs de santé et inégalités: quelle est la question et pourquoi est-ce important? Health Policy. 2006;**78**(2-3):222-231. DOI: 10.1016/j.healthpol.2005.10.007

[17] McLafferty S. GIS and health care. Annual Review of Public Health.

2003;**24**:25-42. DOI: 10.1146/annurev.publhealth.24.012902.141012

[18] Frenk J. Dimensions of health system reform. Health Policy. 1992;**27**(1):19-34

[19] Hart JT. The inverse care law. The Lancet. 1971;**1**(7696):405-412

[20] Dixon A, Le Grand J. Is greater patient choice consistent with equity? The case of the English NHS. Journal of Health Services Research & Policy. 2006;**11**(3):162-166. DOI: 10.1258/135581906777641668

[21] Casey MM et al. Practice characteristics of rural and urban general surgeons. Journal of Rural Health. 2005;**21**(3):250-258. DOI: 10.1111/j.1748-0361.2005.tb00090.x

[22] Hartley D. Rural health disparities, population health, and rural culture. American Journal of Public Health. 2004;**94**(10):1675-1678

[23] De Saint PT. La santé des plus pauvres. Insee Première. 2007;**1161**:1-4

[24] La FD. pauvreté et la maladie mentale: est-ce que les pauvres sont plus malades et si oui pourquoi? Santé mentale au Québec. 1989;**14**(2):104-113

[25] Volovitch P. Égalité devant les soins, égalité devant la santé: quel rôle pour l'assurance-maladie? Revue de l'IRES. 1999;**30**(2):1-27

[26] Potvin L, Moquet M-J, Jones C. (sous la dir). Réduire les Inégalités Sociales en Santé. Saint-Denis: INPES, coll. Santé en action; 2010. p. 380

[27] Mupenda B et al. Pauvreté et santé comme indices de vulnérabilité dans les pays en développement: Pour une éthique de la libération. Ethica Clinica. 2011;**2011**:37-43

[28] Goldman DP, Joyce GF, Zheng Y. Prescription drug cost sharing: Associations with medication and medical utilization and spending and health. Journal of the American Medical Association. 2007;**298**(1):61-69. DOI: 10.1001/jama.298.1.61

[29] Kleinman A. Patients and Healers in the Context of Culture: An Exploration of the Borderland between Anthropology, Medicine, and Psychiatry. 1st ed. Vol. 5. University of California Press; 1980. DOI: 10.2307/jj.2711689

[30] Airhihenbuwa CO. Health and culture: Beyond the Western paradigm. Nursing Standard. 1995;**9**(42):54. DOI: 10.7748/ns.9.42.54.s53

[31] Smedley BD, Stith AY, Nelson AR, editors. Institute of Medicine (US) Committee on Understanding and Eliminating Racial and Ethnic Disparities in Health Care. Unequal Treatment: Confronting Racial and Ethnic Disparities in Health Care. Washington (DC): National Academies Press (US); 2003. PMID: 25032386

[32] Andrulis DP. Access to care is the centerpiece in the elimination of socioeconomic disparities in health. Annals of Internal Medicine. 1998;**129**(5):412-416. DOI: 10.7326/0003-4819-129-5-199809010-00012

[33] Alonzo AA, Reynolds NR. Stigma, HIV and AIDS: An exploration and elaboration of a stigma trajectory. Social Science & Medicine. 1995;**41**(3):303-315. DOI: 10.1016/0277-9536(94)00384-6

[34] Hankivsky O. Women's health, Men's health, and gender and health: Implications of intersectionality. Social Science & Medicine. 2012;**74**(11): 1712-1720. DOI: 10.1016/j.socscimed.2011.11.029. Epub 2012 Jan 25

[35] Navarro V, Shi L. The political context of social inequalities and health. Social Science & Medicine. 2001;**52**(3):481-491. DOI: 10.1016/s0277-9536(00)00197-0

[36] Saltman R, Rico A, Boerma W. Primary Care in the Driver's Seat? Organizational Reform in European Primary Care. 2006

[37] Marmot M, Wilkinson RG. Social determinants of health. 2nd edition. International Journal of Epidemiology. 2006;**35**(4):1111-1112. DOI: 10.1093/ije/dyl121c

[38] Morgan M, Gulliford M, Hudson M. Access to Health Care. Gulliford. London, New York: Routledge; 2003. pp. 189-202, 14 p

[39] Rid A. Just health: Meeting health needs fairly. Bulletin of the World Health Organization. 2008;**86**(8):653. DOI: 10.2471/BLT.08.054601

[40] World Health Organization. Health Systems Financing: The Path to Universal Coverage. World Health Report 2010. World Health Organization; 2010. p. 106. ISBN: 978 92 4 156402 1

[41] Ricketts TC. The changing nature of rural health care. Annual Review of Public Health. 2000;**21**:639-657

[42] Larson SL, Fleishman JA. Rural-urban differences in usual source of care and ambulatory service use: Analyses of national data using Urban Influence Codes. Medical Care. Jul 2003;**41**(7 Suppl):III65-III74. DOI: 10.1097/01.MLR.0000076053.28108.F2. PMID: 12865728

[43] MacDowell M, Glasser M, Fitts M, Nielsen K, Hunsaker M. A national view of rural health workforce issues in the USA. Rural Remote Health. Jul-Sep 2010;**10**(3):1531. Epub 2010 Jul 26. PMID: 20658893; PMCID: PMC3760483

[44] Organisation Mondiale de la Santé. Combler le fossé en une génération, Rapport de la Commission des Déterminants sociaux de la Santé, Organisation Mondiale de la Santé. 2017. Available from: http://apps.who.int/iris/bitstream/10665/69831/1 /WHO_IER_CSDH_08.1_fre.pdf [Accessed: April 14, 2024]

[45] Aïach P. Les inégalités sociales de santé. Médecine/Sciences. 2010;**26**(5):540. DOI: 10.1051/medsci/2010265540

[46] Sen G, Östlin P. Gender inequity in health: Why it exists and how we can change it. Global Public Health. 2008;**3**(sup1):1-12. DOI: 10.1080/17441690801900795

[47] Read JG, Gorman BK. Gender inequalities in US adult health: The interplay of race and ethnicity. Social Science & Medicine. 2006;**62**(5):1045-1065

[48] Mead H et al. The influence of income and race on Total knee arthroplasty in the United States. Journal of Bone and Joint Surgery. 2008;**88**(10):2159-2166

[49] Williams DR, Mohammed SA. Discrimination and racial disparities in health: Evidence and needed research. Journal of Behavioral Medicine. 2009;**32**(1):20-47. DOI: 10.1007/s10865-008-9185-0

[50] Angel JL, Angel RJ. Who Will Care for us? Aging and Long-Term Care in Multicultural America. New York University Press; 1997

[51] Lynch J, Smith GD, Harper S, Hillemeier M, Ross N, Kaplan GA,

et al. Is income inequality a determinant of population health? Part 1. A systematic review. The Milbank Quarterly. 2004;**82**(1):5-99. DOI: 10.1111/j.0887-378x.2004.00302.x

[52] Marmot M. Social determinants of health inequalities. The Lancet. 2005;**365**(9464):1099-1104

[53] Link BG, Phelan J. Social conditions as fundamental causes of disease. Journal of Health and Social Behavior. 1995;Spec No:80-94. PMID: 7560851

[54] Macinko J, Harris MJ. Brazil's family health strategy—Delivering community-based primary care in a universal health system. The New England Journal of Medicine. 2017;**374**(23):2273-2276

[55] Berra S et al. Interventions promoting health: Analysis of systematic reviews. Cadernos de Saúde Pública. 2015;**31**:1-15

[56] Starfield B, Shi L. Policy relevant determinants of health: An international perspective. Health Policy. 2002;**60**(3):201-218

[57] d'Ávila VAL et al. Access to healthcare for children and adolescents in Brazil. Health Policy and Planning. 2016;**31**(3):350-362

[58] Ekman B. Community-based health insurance in low-income countries: A systematic review of the evidence. Health Policy and Planning. 2004;**19**(5):249-270. DOI: 10.1093/heapol/czh031

[59] Wiesmann D, Jütting J. The emerging movement of community based health insurance in sub-Saharan Africa: Experiences and lessons learned. Africa Spectrum. 2010;**35**(2):193-210

[60] Hill CF, Powers BW, Jain SH, Bennet J, Vavasis A, Oriol NE. Mobile health clinics in the era of reform. The American Journal of Managed Care. 2014;**20**(3):261-264

[61] Yu SWY, Hill C, Ricks ML, Bennet J, Oriol NE. The scope and impact of Mobile health clinics in the United States: A literature review. International Journal for Equity in Health. 2017;**16**(1):178. DOI: 10.1186/s12939-017-0671-2

[62] Attipoe-Dorcoo S. Mobile Clinics: A Powerful Resource for Addressing Health Disparities. Boston, Massachusetts, USA: Harvard Medical School Center for Primary Care; 2020. Available from: https://info.primarycare.hms.harvard.edu/perspectives/articles/mobile-clinics-health-disparities [Accessed: April 14, 2024]

[63] Mercer MA, Thompson SM, de Araujo RM. The role of international NGOs in health systems strengthening: The case of Timor-Leste. International Journal of Health Services. 2014;**44**(2):323-335. DOI: 10.2190/HS.44.2.i

[64] Ejaz I, Shaikh BT, Rizvi N. NGOs and government partnership for health systems strengthening: A qualitative study presenting viewpoints of government, NGOs and donors in Pakistan. BMC Health Services Research. 2011;**11**:122. DOI: 10.1186/1472-6963-11-122

[65] Hushie M. Public-non-governmental organisation partnerships for health: An exploratory study with case studies from recent Ghanaian experience. BMC Public Health. 2016;**16**(1):963. DOI: 10.1186/s12889-016-3636-2

[66] Delisle H, Roberts JH, Munro M, Jones L, Gyorkos TW. The role of NGOs in global health research for development. Health Research

Policy and Systems. 2005;**3**(1):3. DOI: 10.1186/1478-4505-3-3

[67] Nickel S, von dem Knesebeck O. Effectiveness of community-based health promotion interventions in urban areas: A systematic review. Journal of Community Health. 2020;**45**(2):419-434. DOI: 10.1007/s10900-019-00733-7

[68] Levin MB, Bowie JV, Ragsdale SK, Gawad AL, Cooper LA, Sharfstein JM. Enhancing community engagement by schools and programs of public health in the United States. Annual Review of Public Health. 2021;**42**:405-421. DOI: 10.1146/annurev-publhealth-090419-102324. Epub 2020 Nov 11

[69] Lachyan A, Zaki RA, Banerjee B, Aghamohammadi N. The effect of community-based intervention on dengue awareness and prevention among poor urban communities in Delhi, India. Journal of Research in Health Sciences. 2023;**23**(4):e00596. DOI: 10.34172/jrhs.2023.131. Epub 2023 Dec 29

[70] Palmer KNB, Rivers PS, Melton FL, McClelland DJ, Hatcher J, Marrero DG, et al. Health promotion interventions for African Americans delivered in U.S. barbershops and hair salons- a systematic review. BMC Public Health. 2021;**21**(1):1553. DOI: 10.1186/s12889-021-11584-0

[71] Bramantoro T, Santoso CMA, Hariyani N, Setyowati D, Zulfiana AA, Nor NAM, et al. Effectiveness of the school-based oral health promotion programmes from preschool to high school: A systematic review. PLoS One. 2021;**16**(8):e0256007. DOI: 10.1371/journal.pone.0256007

[72] Education and Awareness. National Heart, Lung, and Blood Institute (NHLBI), National Institutes of Health (NIH). Available from: https://www.nhlbi.nih.gov/education [Accessed: April 14, 2024]

[73] Shadish WR, Cook TD, Campbell DT. Experimental and Quasi-Experimental Designs for Generalized Causal Inference. 2nd ed. Cengage Learning; 2002

[74] Khandker S, Koolwal G, Samad H. Handbook on Impact Evaluation: Quantitative Methods and Practices - Exercises 2009 [Data set]. World Bank, Development Data Group; 2011. DOI: 10.48529/YSS8-M484

[75] Pawson R, Tilley N. Realistic Evaluation. Available from: https://www.researchgate.net/publication/252160435_Realistic_Evaluation_An_Overview [Accessed: April 14, 2024]

[76] Rosenbaum PR. Observational Studies. Available from: https://obssr.od.nih.gov/sites/obssr/files/Observational-Studies.pdf [Accessed: April 14, 2024]